COMMUNICATIVE DISORDERS

COMMUNICATIVE DISORDERS
An Appraisal

Compiled and Edited by

ALAN J. WESTON, Ph.D.
Chairman, Department of Audiology and Speech Pathology
Director, Memphis Speech and Hearing Center
Memphis State University
Memphis, Tennessee

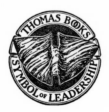

CHARLES C THOMAS • PUBLISHER
Springfield • Illinois • U.S.A.

Published and Distributed Throughout the World by
CHARLES C THOMAS • PUBLISHER
BANNERSTONE HOUSE
301-327 East Lawrence Avenue, Springfield, Illinois, U.S.A.
NATCHEZ PLANTATION HOUSE
735 North Atlantic Boulevard, Fort Lauderdale, Florida, U.S.A.

© *1972, by* CHARLES C THOMAS • PUBLISHER
ISBN 0-398-02437-5
Library of Congress Catalog Card Number 77-169891

With THOMAS BOOKS *careful attention is given to all details of
manufacturing and design. It is the Publisher's desire to present books
that are satisfactory as to their physical qualities and artistic possibilities and appropriate for their particular use.* THOMAS BOOKS *will
be true to those laws of quality that assure a good name and good will.*

Printed in the United States of America
N-1

CONTRIBUTORS

HARRY S. COOKER, PH.D.: *Associate Professor of Speech, University of Connecticut, Storrs, Connecticut.*

WILSON L. DIETRICH, ED.D.: *Chairman, Department of Special Education, University of Alabama, University, Alabama.*

ROBERT J. DUFFY, PH.D.: *Associate Professor of Speech, University of Connecticut, Storrs, Connecticut.*

THOMAS G. GIOLAS, PH.D.: *Professor of Speech, University of Connecticut, Storrs, Connecticut.*

ROBERT D. HUBBELL, PH.D.: *Assistant Professor of Speech Pathology and Director of Speech Clinic, California State College at Los Angeles.*

JOHN V. IRWIN, PH.D.: *Distinguished Pope M. Farrington Professor, Memphis State University, Memphis, Tennessee.*

JAY W. LERMAN, PH.D.: *Associate Professor of Speech, University of Connecticut, Storrs, Connecticut.*

HUGHLETT L. MORRIS, PH.D.: *Professor of Speech Pathology, University of Iowa, Iowa City, Iowa.*

ROBERT L. MULDER, PH.D.: *U. S. Office of Education, Bureau of Education for the Handicapped.*

DONALD L. RAMPP, PH.D.: *Associate Professor of Speech Pathology, Memphis State University, Memphis, Tennessee.*

CLYDE L. ROUSEY, PH.D.: *Director of Speech Pathology and Audiology, The Menninger Foundation.*

LOUISE M. WARD, M.A.: *Associate Professor of Speech Pathology, Memphis State University, Memphis, Tennessee.*

ELIZABETH J. WEBSTER, PH.D.: *Professor of Speech Pathology, Memphis State University, Memphis, Tennessee.*

ALAN J. WESTON, PH.D.: *Chairman, Department of Audiology and Speech Pathology; Director, Memphis Speech and Hearing Center, Memphis State University, Memphis, Tennessee.*

PREFACE

Some men see things as they are and say, why.
I dream things that never were and say, why not.

ROBERT F. KENNEDY

HUMAN COMMUNICATION has gained increasing attention in the scholarship of various disciplines. The professional specialists who are committed to alleviating disordered human communication are fortunate to have this increasingly broad base of scholarship from which they can draw and yet are presented a momentous task in identifying, evaluating, and selecting what is most useful for particular purposes. We are challenged in this age of accountability to continue to look at new ways to handle old problems, to become increasingly aware of the hypotheses upon which procedures are based, and to evaluate these hypotheses through pertinent research. We must select with great judiciousness what is good of the old and what is good of the new.

This text was conceived while the editor was completing a fellowship year in Washington, D.C. in the Bureau of Education for the Handicapped. This fellowship provided an opportunity to view the majority of speech and hearing programs granting master's level degrees and above, as well as a number of public school programs throughout the nation. This experience was impressive of the continuing need for literature which represents current thinking and practice related to disordered communication.

The authors have been selected to represent current movement in the fields of speech pathology and audiology. Therefore, they include some who would represent a more traditional point of view as well as some advocating newer ways of viewing and handling speech and hearing disorders. The text is intended to reflect some direction which these fields of speech pathology and audiology will begin to take, as well as to premote reevaluation of more traditional directions.

vii

I wish to acknowledge my indebtedness to those persons who authored the chapters, and especially to Mrs. Lorraine Cooper for her painstaking work in preparing the manuscript. A special thanks to Nancy Irwin for her editorial assistance.

Memphis, Tennessee   ALAN J. WESTON

CONTENTS

COMMUNICATIVE DISORDERS

CHAPTER ONE

COMMUNICATION

JOHN V. IRWIN

THE EMBRACING THEME of this book is disordered human communication. You are urged to read with two purposes: first, to seek understanding of the girl who does not talk, of the adolescent boy who stutters, of the housewife who is losing her hearing, and of the father whose thoughts have become silent, and, second, to play your part in helping these people to acquire, preserve, or regain the ability to communicate effectively with their fellows. To this end, starting point and final goal are one: Communication.

In the broadest sense, *communication* is the process by which one mechanism, animate or inanimate, interacts with other mechanisms, animate or inanimate. In a more conventional sense, *communication* includes all the ways, symbolic and nonsymbolic, with which one *human* interacts with other *humans*. In the narrowest sense, communication denotes the process by which humans stimulate and respond to other humans through oral and written language.

This chapter is your invitation to extend your study of mankind's most human characteristic, communication.

THE COMMUNICATION PROCESS

Communication has long been of concern to traditional academic fields such as speech, psychology, English, mathematics, and journalism. In recent years, engineering has made primary contributions to this study. A most basic analysis of the communicative process, "The Mathematical Theory of Communication," was presented by Claude Shannon in *The Bell System Technical Journal* (1948). The following description owes its essential concepts to Dr. Shannon's analysis. See Brooks (1967) for other models.

Communication Systems

A communication system consists of five divisions: source, transmitter channel, receiver, and destination. Each division has a characteristic function, although the details of the function may vary with the nature of any particular communication system.

Information Source

The information source generates the message (or sequence of messages) that is to be transmitted to the destination. Perhaps more accurately, the information source *selects* a message from a constellation of possible messages. This message may consist of ideas, feelings, aesthetic impressions, or other concepts. In interpersonal communication, the brain is the information source.

The Transmitter

The transmitter converts the message to a signal that can be handled by the channel. In human speech the transmitter is the total speech mechanism, the signal a varying sound pressure. Transmission is essentially an encoding process.

The Channel

The channel is the medium by means of which the signal (as opposed to the message) is sent from the transmitter to the receiver. In oral speech the usual channel is the air.

The Receiver

The receiver decodes the signal; its task reverses that of the transmitter. The ear and associated eighth nerve circuits are the receiver for speech.

The Destination

The destination is the mechanism for which the original message was generated. In human speech the brain of the listener is the destination.

This system may be better understood if you now review the essential processes. The message, after selection, is changed into signal form, that is, it is *encoded*. A code is an arbitrary and previously agreed upon (a) set of symbols and (b) rules of usage. Oral language is one particular kind of a code. The basic symbols are sounds and words and the rules of usage are the language structure. The encoded message or signal is transmitted through the channel. After transmission, the signals are decoded for a resultant approximation of the original message. You must remember that meaning is not to be found in the signal. Meaning, in communication, exists at the source and at the destination.

Three Levels of Communication

You should now recognize the existence of three levels of communication. These levels are indicated in the following questions:

Level A. How accurately can the symbols of communication be transmitted? This is the engineering level.

Level B. How precisely do the transmitter symbols convey the desired meaning? This is the semantic level.

Level C. How effectively does the received meaning control behavior? This is the control level.

Efficiency at the semantic and control levels is dependent upon efficiency at the engineering level.

Other concepts relevant to understanding human communication, which depends upon the transmission of symbols but is concerned with meaning and control, will not be introduced.

Noise

Unfortunately, as the message is processed by the system, spurious variations may be introduced into the received signal. Such variations are potentially dangerous because, at best, they modify the signal and, at worst, may destroy it. These unwanted modifications in the signal are referred to by Shannon as *noise.*

In his original use of this term, Shannon was referring primarily to engineering noise, that is, to distortion introduced in the transmission and receiving process. By extension, however, you may refer to another kind of noise, semantic noise, which originates in the language process itself.

In human speech, semantic noise may result from faulty encoding. Examples include the selection of an inappropriate word, an unusual pronunciation, or a misleading grammatical construction. Semantic noise may be introduced in the decoding process by motivational factors, by ambiguities, or by lack of familiarity with the code. Engineering noise may be introduced into the channel by the presence of other acoustical stimuli as in a downtown city street at rush hour (an example, also, of literal noise), by talking in some unusual medium as gas with a high proportion of helium or by electronic distortions as in the telephone.

The clinical fields of audiology and speech and language pathology are concerned with both semantic and engineering noise. The person who uses the wrong sound, the unusual word, the abnormal construction, the exceptional voice, the unusual fluency introduces noise into all he encodes. And the individual whose hearing aid is faulty, or whose neural pathway function abnormally, introduces noise as he decodes.

A Concept of Information

The term *information,* as used by Shannon, has a very special and unusual meaning. In particular, information in this sense has no relationship to meaning or to semantics. As expressed by Weaver (1964):

> To be sure, this word information in communication theory relates not so much to what you do say, as to what you could say. That is, information is a measure of one's freedom of choice when one selects a message. If one is confronted with a very elementary situation where he has to choose one of two alternative messages, then it is arbitrarily said that the information associated with this situation is unity . . . The concept of information applies not to the individual messages (as the concept of meaning would), but rather to the situation as a whole, the unit information indicating that in this situation one has an amount of freedom of choice, in selecting a message, which it is convenient to regard as a standard or unit amount.

Information is here defined, not as meaning, but as capacity, as the capacity of a code. Although a code can be designed with the capacity for any amount of information, certain limitations must always be considered.

If a code has only two signals, and if each may only be used once per second, then the code has a capacity for only one message per second. The unit for such information is the *binit* or *bit*. *Binit* will be used in this discussion, because it is less likely to be confused than is the more common word *bit*. A code with four symbols has a capacity of two binits; one with 8, three binits; one with 16, 4 binits. Thus, as Weaver states, the amount of information in the simplest cases may be conveniently expressed by the "logarithm of the number of available choices," using logarithms to the base 2. If, then, one has a situation in which sixteen alternative messages are *equally* available, one says that this situation is characterized by 4 binits of information, for $16 = 2^4 (2 \cdot 2 \cdot 2 \cdot 2 = 16)$.

Note, however, that the above statement holds only if the freedom of choice remains equal, or, to state this differently, if the probability of one choice is not affected by a previous choice, it can be shown that the value of a choice decreases with the increased probability of its occurrence. Thus, if the probabilty of a particular signal is increased because of the previous signal (or sequence of signals), the amount of information conveyed by the particular signal is reduced. For example, in conventional written English, the letter *u* in the sequence *qu* has a lower binit value than the *u* in the sequence *tu*. In the first instance, the selection of *q* increased the probability of *u's* occurrence to almost 100 per cent; in the second instance, the selection of *t* did not thus heighten the probability of *u's* appearance.

If, then, in a particular code, the information conveyed is reduced because, in the code, freedom of choice is reduced by the normal construction rules of the code, we may say that the system is not being used to capacity. *Redundancy* is the technical name for the difference between the theoretical capacity of any code and the average amount of information in a specific application of the code. Weaver (1964) comments:

> It is most interesting to note that the redundancy of English is just about 50 per cent, so that about half of the letters or words we choose in writing or speaking are under our free choice, and about half (although we are not ordinarily aware of it) are really controlled by the statistical structure of the language.

HUMAN COMMUNICATION

Two types of human communication, verbal and nonverbal, can be differentiated. Although this text is primarily concerned with disorders of verbal communication, nonverbal communication is also vital to the speech and hearing clinician. For, not only must this clinician be able to recognize the existence and effects of nonverbal communication, but, he will need to be able to use it.

Nonverbal Communication

You should be familiar with at least two major types of nonverbal communication. First, as Hayakawa (1949) states:

> There is that vast area of non-verbal communication with children that we accomplish through holding, touching, rocking, caressing, putting food in their mouths and all of the little things that we do. These are all communication, and we do this for a long time before the children even start to talk.

As Hayakawa implies, we continue to use this kind of communication throughout life even after verbal communication has been well established. In psychological terms, this type of nonverbal communication operates close to the level of primary reinforcement, tends to be cross-cultural, and has not been rigorously described. Yet the validity of communication of this type, particularly at the affective level, cannot be ignored.

A second type of nonverbal communication has been emphasized by Birdwhistell (1952) and by Hall (1966). Working from an anthropological viewpoint, Birdwhistell has investigated kinesics, that is, the systematic study of the use and effects of bodily motion, bodily position, and gesture in human communication. Although the rules of this type of communication may not be as rigid as some promulgated by the elocutionists, definite evidence of culturally valid nonverbal codes of communication has been defined. In psychological terms, these kinds of communication operate at the level of secondary or learned reinforcement, are linked to the culture and therefore vary with the culture, and are fairly rigorously held. Unlike true language, however, the rules and, indeed, even the existence of this type of communication are not always recognized. Thus, even if we ignore completely the many differences between certain Latin American languages and spoken English, Hall notes that an American may find it very difficult to talk with his Latin colleagues because the speakers will strongly prefer different "talking distances." The one will want to talk "closer" than will the other. The varying interpretations that each will subconsciously place on his "distance factor" as the one retreats and the other advances may snarl completely the effects of whatever verbal matching they have achieved.

Verbal Communication

Tempting as it is to push the importance of nonverbal communication among humans, the fact remains that the most precise as well as the most human form of communicative behavior is verbal and involves the use of language.

Language may be thought of as *a system of arbitrary vocal symbols which have a somewhat common significance among the humans in a language community and which are used by the members to transmit signals to each other*. This definition emphasizes oral language. But, as Gleason (1955) has stated:

> A written language is typically a reflection, independent in only limited ways, of spoken language. As a picture of actual speech, it is inevitably imperfect and incomplete.

The individual elements of this definition are so important that you will wish to consider each in some detail:

1. *System*. The term *system* implies that you must not think of language as a collection of isolated units but as a process. Viewed functionally, language consists of a series of sounds and a structure for combining these sounds into meaningful units. Not only the order but even the formation of words is determined by the structure of English. Thus we have sound-sequencing rules for a language. In English, for example, we never begin a word with the sound *ng*. With something less than fifty sounds to select from, we begin almost 15 per cent of our words with *t*. The user learns a complete system.

2. *Arbitrary vocal symbols*. As already noted, this statement

implies that language is generically oral. Written languages spring from oral languages. Although written forms may extend, modify, and make more permanent oral forms, oral language has preceded written both in the individual and in the human race. These statements are in no sense a denial of the importance of written language. These statements simply seek to put the two into structural and developmental perspective.

That the symbols are vocal implies that they are made by man's own verbalizing equipment, in particular his respiratory, phonatory, and articulatory apparatus, as commanded by his nervous system.

The existence of visible components is not included in this statement, but the adjunctive value of gesture and expression is freely recognized. Nevertheless, the fact that valid communication is possible in a completely blacked-out room, by radio, by audio recording, and by the blind, demonstrates the primary efficacy of the aural symbol in spoken communication.

Of course, many codes other than those of oral language are used in human communication. Gesture, facial expression, bodily position and movement have already been referred to. Music, painting, sculpture, and mathematics also make use of codes. Codes, and even media may differ, but the process remains essentially the same.

3. *A somewhat common significance among the members of a language community.* This statement emphasizes that the significance of the symbols is limited to the language community that uses the symbols. This limitation is generally recognized even at popular levels, although many an American has attempted to communicate in English with a French or German speaking individual by talking more slowly, more loudly, and in shorter units. An acute need to communicate with another human being may blind us to the limits of our symbols.

The other aspect of this statement, that is *somewhat common significance,* is less clearly recognized even at relatively sophisticated levels. You must always remember that the symbol only *stands for* something but can never *be* the something. Symbols, words, function only as stimuli. As spoken, these stimuli have a speaker-intended meaning; as heard, they have a listener-created meaning. At each end of the communicative process, meaning is within the human and not within the symbol. Inevitably, then, differences will exist in the evaluation of symbols. These differences will vary from person to person, from mood to mood, from context to context, and from time to time.

Differences in evaluation become particularly important with some types of symbols. For example, *cup* can have a very precise meaning because an easily experienced physical referent is available. But other symbols, as *immortality*, do not denote a definite referent.

Each symbol, then, is interpreted or evaluated by its users; this interpretation is individual; the standardization of this evaluation within a language community will vary from symbol to symbol but will always be less than 100 per cent.

4. *Use to transmit signals to each other.* The basic thought here has been somewhat anticipated in statement (3) above, but the present emphasis is somewhat different. As stated in the section on communication systems, the exact message itself is not put in a bag and dropped in somebody else's brain. Communication is not a transfer process. The message itself is first encoded; it is the coded signal that is transmitted; both the coding and the decoding process are subject to error and inexactness.

THE EFFECTIVENESS OF HUMAN COMMUNICATION

As has been developed thus far, communication between humans can never be perfect. At the engineering level, symbols can be changed or lost. At the semantic level, symbols can be variously evaluated. Now a third level of function needs to be discussed; this is the control exercised by human communication.

Oral communication among humans involves social interaction. Risley (1966) has recognized four steps in this interaction:

1. The communicator speaks. His signals serve as a stimulus for the listener (s) and for himself. His encoded message may be analyzed in physical terms after transmission.

2. The listener evaluates the signal. The effect on the listener may be to induce further behavior. Much of this behavior can be described functionally.

3. The listener may respond verbally. This transmission can be described physically and serves as a potential stimulus to the original speaker.

4. Aspects of this verbal response may affect the speaker, and these effects can be described functionally.

Two ways of examining the above sequence of behavior are available. One is to look at the verbal signals or stimuli themselves. This has been a basic approach of the speech scientist and the communications engineer. What is the nature of the acoustic spectra? A second approach has been to look at the effect on the listener. This approach, which was emphasized by the traditional linguist, sought to isolate those elements in the stimuli that had a relatively common effect on a listener who shared the language community of the speaker. Out of such approaches came recognition of the basic sounds of a language, the basic vocabulary, and the basic structure.

But, a third approach is to analyze the interactive verbal behavior in terms of its consequences to the speaker. This last approach is of vital importance to the student of human communication. For, with particular emphasis on the writings of Skinner, if we assume a standard repertoire of responses by the culture to the speakers of a culture, these responses will largely determine the kind of verbal behavior that the speaker learns and continues to use. The normal speaker must not be expected to manifest direct concern with the stimulus value of his speech. Such concern may continue to be the (at times) thankless job of the linguist, the teacher, and the speech correctionist. The speaker who is the natural product of his culture, and not the partial creation of a teacher of the deaf, a speech pathologist, a teacher, or a parent with what Wendell Johnson (1967) has termed ears that are too long, will modify and maintain his verbal responses primarily in terms of their consequences to him. Only those attributes of the stimulus that make a difference in this sense will make a difference to the speaker.

FUNCTIONS OF SPEECH

The most easily recognizable function of speech is that of communication. But, as noted by Eisenson, Auer, and Irwin (1963), speech has many other functions. Among the noncommunicative (or at least pseudocommunicative) functions of speech are oral pleasure and verbal contact. Speech may also be used as a social gesture, to disarm hostility, to ease anxiety, as aggression, and for concealment. Finally, speech may also serve as the indispensable tool for abstract thought. If language is not essential for abstract thinking, it is clearly the prime facilitator.

REFERENCES

Birdwhistell, R.L.: *Introduction to Kinesics.* Washington, Foreign Service Institute, 1952.

Brooks, Keith: *The Communicative Arts and Sciences of Speech.* Columbus, Merrill, 1967.

Eisenson, Jon; Auer, J. Jeffrey, and Irwin, John V.: *The Psychology of Communication.* New York, Appleton-Century-Crofts, 1963.

Gleason, H.A. Jr.: *An Introduction to Descriptive Linguistics.* New York, Holt, 1955.

Hall, Edward T.: *The Silent Languages.* New York, Fawcett World Library, 1966.

Hayakawa, S.I.: *Language in Thought and Action.* New York, Harcourt, Brace and World, 1949.

Johnson, Wendell; Brown, Spencer; Curtis, James; Edney, Clarence, and Keaster, Jacqueline: *Speech Handicapped School Children.* New York, Harper & Row, 1967.

Risley, Todd: *The Establishment of Verbal Behavior in Deviant Children.* Ph.D. Dissertation, University of Washington, 1966.

Shannon, C.E.: A mathematical theory of communication. *Bell System Tech J, 27*:379-423, 623-656, 1948.

Shannon, Claude C., and Weaver, Warren: *The Mathematical Theory of Communication.* Urbana, U. of Illinois Press, 1964.

CHAPTER TWO

AN INTRODUCTION TO SOUND AND THE SPEECH AND HEARING MECHANISMS

HARRY S. COOKER

MATERIAL will be presented in this chapter which is basic to an understanding of the normal function of the mechanisms for producing speech and hearing sound. An adequate foundation in the normal function of these mechanisms is crucial to any real understanding of the disorders of speech or hearing. The presentation of the material is at the introductory level and directed toward the reader who possesses a limited background in mathematics or the physical sciences. In presenting the essential aspects of these very complex human processes, all unnecessary complexities will be avoided. However, if all of the complexities associated with speech and hearing were omitted, understanding would have to be sacrificed and the reader would have to be content with a superficial acquaintance with these functions. Instead, the pace will be slowed and the reader will be led through the more demanding concepts by careful explanation of unfamiliar terms and, on occasion, by the use of analogies. The presentation of the normal function of the speech and hearing mechanisms in this chapter is in no respect intended to supplant a more detailed presentation that one might receive in a course that is devoted mainly to the study of these normal functions. Rather, sufficient information of an essential nature will be provided to make the ensuing chapters more meaningful to readers of varying backgrounds.

Before one can understand the intricacies of the speech mechanism, which is a sound producer, and the hearing mechanism, which is a sound receiver, one must first understand the nature of the phenomenon which we call sound. It is this first hurdle which the typical student finds most difficult to vault. Usually this difficulty may be attributed to exposure to unfamiliar terms, fear of mathematical manipulations, or a consuming belief that physics is actually some poorly disguised subdiscipline of "black magic." In reality, the nature of sound may be adequately explained without resorting to esoteric mathematical formulations, but it is very convenient to be able to employ a limited number of simple mathematical maneuvers. Once the student is convinced that these maneuvers are intended as helpful aids rather than unnecessary obstacles, understanding usually follows at a surprisingly rapid rate. Consequently, the reader is asked to approach the following section of the chapter with an open mind and the conviction that an understanding of the rudiments of the physics of sound is well within the grasp of all who are willing to read.

THE PHYSICS OF SOUND

The perception of sound is a most common human experience. Regardless of the pains we might take to isolate ourselves from unwanted noise, we are constantly bombarded by a wide variety of sound waves. The basic reason for our continuous exposure to these waves is the simple fact that we and our entire earthly environment are bathed in air. The air is composed of several gases in more or less stable proportions, and it possesses certain characteristic physical properties that permit sound propagation. Although sound will travel through steel, water, rubber, glass or any other elastic medium, we are most concerned with air, for man's sound-producing and sound-receiving mechanisms are specifically adapted to function in the atmosphere.

Basic Concepts

The physical properties that make sound propagation possible are *mass* and *elasticity*. Mass or *inertia* is the tendency of a body that is at rest to remain at rest, or the tendency of a body in motion to remain in motion. For example, when it is necessary to push a stalled automobile, considerable effort must be expended to overcome its inertia and set it into motion. However, once it is moving, a considerable amount of effort also is required to overcome its inertia and stop its motion.

Elasticity is that property of a body which resists distortion or compression. For example, if a rubber ball is dropped onto a steel plate it will bounce. Its elastic property produces a *restoring force* which pushes the flattened surface of the ball back to its original shape. If a lead ball were dropped onto the same steel plate, it would probably not bounce at all but remain flattened at the point of contact with the steel plate. The elastic limit of the lead ball was exceeded, for it was unable to return to its original shape. A steel ball dropped on the same plate would bounce even higher than the rubber ball, for it resists distortion much more than does the rubber ball. In general, then, under conditions of constant temperature, all kinds of material exhibit a characteristic mass and a characteristic elasticity. Furthermore, it may be assumed that each *particle** of material will possess the same mass and elasticity characteristics as any other particle of the same material.

The term *force* has been used in connection with the concept of elasticity, but there are many other kinds of forces which act upon us and our environment at any given time. Force is that aspect which tends to produce a change in the position or motion of some mass. When we talk about our weight, we are actually talking about the number of pounds of gravitational force that is pulling on the mass of our body. We can easily see the direct relationship between force and mass by noting the increase or decrease in force (pounds) that accompanies an increase or decrease in mass as we gain or lose weight. However, we can also change the force by holding the mass constant and varying *acceleration* (a change in speed or direction). For instance, if one were to stand on a set of scales in an elevator, a sudden increase in weight would be observed as the elevator accelerated at the beginning of its ascent. Thus, force is dependent on both mass and acceleration and can be varied by changing either one of these attributes.

Another concept that is important for an understanding of the physics of sound is the concept of *work*. Work may be defined

---

*A particle is the smallest unit of a medium which maintains the characteristics of the medium. Thus, a particle of water would be a molecule of water, but a particle of air would be a mixture of molecules of the several gasses present in air.

as a force through a distance. In other words, if a fifty-pound weight is lifted to a height of two feet, 100 ft lbs of work are accomplished. But work is accomplished only if the object actually is moved in the direction in which the force is applied. If the weight were attached to the floor in some manner so that it could not be moved, no work would be performed regardless of the effort put forth. Let us assume, however, that the weight can be lifted but that it takes twice as much time to do so. Although the same amount of work would be performed (100 ft lbs), only half of the *power* would be developed, for the work was accomplished at only half the rate. Power, then, is the rate at which work is accomplished or the rate at which *energy,* the capacity to do work, is expended.

An understanding of these basic concepts will prove useful in the following discussion of particle vibration and wave propagation.

Particle Vibration

The process by which sound waves are propagated is relatively simple but somewhat dicult to visualize. If an elastic body, *e.g.,* a bell, tuning fork, chime, etc., is struck and set into vibration, the body will vibrate or oscillate in such a fashion that the air particles immediately adjacent to the body will be displaced from their resting or neutral positions. This displacement is usually very small but will depend on the *amplitude* or amount of movement of the vibrating body. As the body moves outward in a positive direction, the *inertia* of the adjacent air particles is overcome and they are displaced in that direction. However, the particles of air are so closely packed that they can travel only about one ten-thousandth of a millimeter before striking another particle. Consequently, a "chain reaction" of particle displacement occurs in which each succeeding particle strikes the next which, in turn, is displaced and strikes the next, etc. As was stated previously, the elastic properties of a substance produce a restoring force which allows the substance to return to its original state after being displaced. It is this restoring force that arrests the positive swing of the vibrating body and initiates a swing in the negative direction.

As the negative swing continues, the body's inertia carries it past its neutral position, and it is displaced in the negative direction. Again a restoring force arrests the swing of the vibrating body and initiates a swing back toward the neutral position. This kind of oscillation is called *simple harmonic motion,* and it will continue until external forces or internal friction brings the activity to a halt. Restoring forces similar to those in the vibrating body also are produced as the particles are displaced from their neutral positions. The restoring force of the particle which was first displaced by the positive swing of the vibrating body arrests its positive movement and initiates movement in a negative direction toward the vibrating source. Again because of its inertia, the particle travels past its neutral position until a sufficient restoring force arrests its negative displacement and turns it back in a positive direction. The same type of oscillation takes place for each successive air particle; however, the movement of each sucessive particle lags slightly behind the movement of the preceding particle because of the time required to overcome the particle's inertia.

An analogy which has often been used to illustrate this activity is that of a line of people waiting to purchase tickets for some popular event. If the person at the end of the line is suddenly pushed into the person in front of him (positive displacement), that person in front will push the one in front of him and so forth until the person at the head of the line is pushed against the box office. But long before this happens, the person at the end of the line has recovered his balance and has reacted by stepping backward slightly (negative displacement), and increasing the separation between himself and the person in front of him. The person in front of him reacts in a similar fashion, and the person in front of the next person does the same. This activity continues down through the entire line. If the action is observed from some vantage point, it may be seen that there is an apparent wave of squeezing together (increase in pressure) followed by a wave of separation (decrease in pressure) which travels down the line. This activity is very similar to what happens to the air particles which have been set into motion by the vibrating source. The alternate waves of squeezing together and separation of the particles are known as waves of *condensation* and *rarefaction,* respectively. Waves of this type are called *longitudinal* waves and are produced when the particles of a medium vibrate back and forth in the same direction as the propagating wave.

Longitundinal waves may be contrasted with *transverse* waves in which the particles of a medium vibrate at right angles to the direction of wave propagation. An example of a wave which is approximately transverse is the wave that is produced when the surface of a pond is disturbed. Ripples flow across the surface of the pond in widening circles. Observation of the activity of the individual particles of water reveals that the crests and troughs of the ripples are produced by the alternate up and down movement of these particles. In both types of wave propagation, longitudinal and transverse, it is important to note that *the particles of the medium do not travel an appreciable distance.* Rather it is the *disturbance* which travels through the medium. We may think of sound, then, as a *pressure disturbance* (alternate increases and decreases) which travels through the air (a medium) from some vibrating source (an elastic body) to a listener's ear. The energy in a sound wave decreases as the distance from its vibrating source increases, and it is said to follow the *inverse square law.* Thus, the energy that is present at any point will be *inversely* proportional to the *square* of the distance from its vibrating source. Unlike the disturbance that traveled down the line of people waiting at the box office, sound does not emanate from the source in only one direction. Rather, the sound radiates from the vibrating source in all directions at once, and alternate waves of condensation and rarefaction (high and low density) form ever increasing spheres which continuously expand in size until their energy is dissipated.

The Dimensions of Sound

Although sound may be defined in a very general way as a pressure disturbance, certain physical and psychological dimensions can be identified which will provide more specific descriptions of individual sounds. The physical vibrations which are produced and the psychological effects which result from the physical vibrations are closely but not exactly related. Consequently, it would be inaccurate to refer to a physical attribute of a sound wave by a term which actually indicates the psychological effect of that physical attribute. The interchangeable use of these physical and psychological terms presents no problem to the layman but should be avoided by the professional to eliminate any possible confusion. With this in mind, the physical dimensions of *frequency, intensity, wave composition* or *spectrum,* and *time* will be considered first, and then the psychological effects of *pitch, loudness, tone quality* or *timbre,* and *duration* will be discussed.

Physical Dimensions

Frequency is the rate at which the vibrating particles oscillate, or it may be defined as the number of complete cycles of vibration which take place in one second of time. *Hertz* is the term used to indicate the unit, "cycles per second," and is usually abbreviated *Hz.* Thus, a sound of 100 *Hz* has a frequency of one hundred cycles per second. Two other concepts, *period* and *wave length,* are closely related to frequency. Period is the amount of time that it takes for a particle to execute one complete cycle of vibration. For a 100 Hz tone, the period is one one-hundredth of a second. For a 200 Hz tone, the period is one two-hundredth of a second, etc. The mathematical relationship between frequency (F) and period (T) is simply $T = \frac{1}{F}$; thus, we have an *inverse* relationship in which the period decreases as the frequency increases.

Wave length is the distance that the pressure disturbance will travel in the time of one period. Therefore, wave length also is inversely related to frequency, but in addition it is directly related to the speed of sound. These relationships can be stated mathematically in the formula $WL = \frac{V}{F}$ in which WL is wave length, F is frequency and V is the speed of sound for the medium through which the sound is traveling. It can be seen from these relationships that the wave length of a 100 Hz tone traveling through air with a speed of 1100 feet per second will be eleven feet long. The same 100 Hz tone traveling through water would have a wave length of something more than forty-four feet because the speed of sound in water is a little more than four times the speed of sound in air. It is important to note that sounds of all frequencies travel at the same speed in a given medium and that frequency does not change with a change in medium.

Intensity may be defined as the rate at which energy is radiated through a unit of area which is perpendicular to the plane of propagation. "The rate" at which energy is radiated is another way of talking about power or the amount of work which may be accomplished in a given amount of time (see Basic Concepts). Therefore, intensity may be considered to be a measure of sound power per square centimeter, and it is usually stated in terms of watts/cm² (power per unit of area). Actually the watt is too large a unit to be useful when talking about normal levels of sound. Consequently, the term *microwatt* or millionth of a watt is employed when talking about most sound. Intensity is rather difficult to measure directly, but under certain conditions (a free field) we know that sound intensity is directly proportional to the square of the pressure amplitude. Since our ears and other devices such as microphones, diaphragms, etc., are sensitive to pressure variations, we find it convenient to measure sound pressure (force per unit of area) and infer sound intensity (power per unit of area). The units which are employed to designate sound pressure are dynes/cm.* In our earlier discussion of force, the pound was used as a unit, but the pound, which is equivalent to 445,000 dynes, is far too large for our purposes.*

The *Wave Composition or Spectrum* of a sound establishes the degree of complexity of the sound. Up to this time, only very simple vibratory activity which takes place at only one frequency and produces the simplest of all sounds, *the pure tone,* has been discussed. In reality, the pure tone does not occur frequently in nature. Instead, vibrations of elastic bodies may occur at several frequencies at the same time and produce a complex sound rather than a pure tone. In Figure 2-1 a pure tone and a complex tone are graphically represented. The curve that represents the pure

---

*The decibel (dB), a more convenient unit for discussing intensity and sound pressure, will be presented in the section on the hearing mechanism.

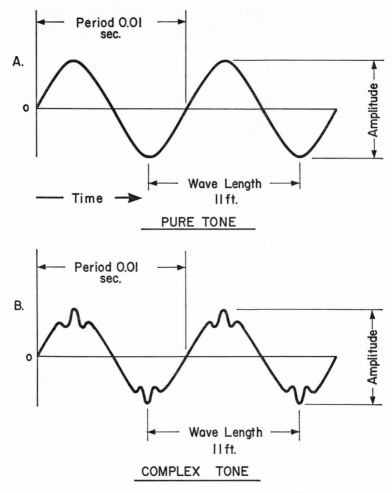

Figure 2-1. A graphic representation of periodic vibrations that are regularly repeated one hundred times per second (100Hz).

tone is called a *sine wave* and is the characteristic shape of all of the simple vibratory activity discussed thus far. The waveform of the complex tone in B of Figure 2-1 is quite different from that of A, but its shape is regularly repeated as in A. Whenever there is regularly repeated vibratory activity, it is termed *periodic* activity. That is, the sound pattern repeats itself at regular intervals in time. Thus, B in Figure 2-1 is actually a complex periodic tone which can be mathematically analyzed* and shown to consist of several pure tones of specific frequencies and amplitudes. Therefore, the wave composition or spectrum of a sound is simply the number of frequencies and their respective amplitudes which comprise the sound. Figure 2-2 presents three waveforms and their

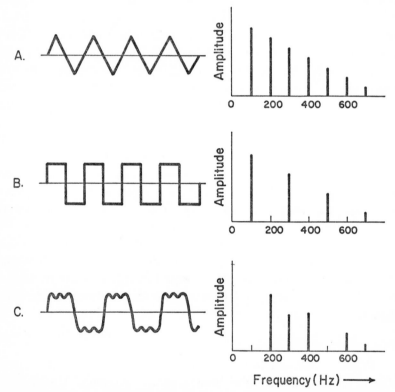

Figure 2-2. Three complex waveforms of 100 Hz with their associated spectral compositions. *A* has energy present at all *whole-number* multiples (harmonic overtones) of the fundamental. *B* has energy present only at the *odd-number* multiples of the fundamental. *C* has energy present at some odd-number and some even-number multiples of the fundamental but *no energy present at the fundamental.*

---

*A complex mathematical procedure devised by Jean Baptiste Joseph **Fourier** and commonly referred to as Fourier analysis.

associated spectral compositions. In A and B of Figure 2-2, energy is present in whole-number multiples of the lowest frequency in the series (100 Hz). This frequency is termed the *fundamental frequency,* and the whole-number multiples of the fundamental are called harmonic overtones.*

It is of interest to note that energy need not actually be present at the fundamental frequency for us to identify it. In C of Figure 2-2 we have a series in which the lowest frequency is 200 Hz, but energy is present at several whole-number multiples of 100 Hz. Consequently the fundamental frequency of the series is 100 Hz rather than 200 Hz. It may be stated, then, that the fundamental frequency of any complex periodic tone will be the least common denominator of the series of frequencies which comprise the tone. In many instances it will be the lowest frequency in the series, but at other times it will not.

From one point of view, *time* is probably the single most important dimension of sound in that our processing system requires a finite amount of time to perceive the effect of the other sound dimensions of frequency, intensity, and spectrum. Sounds which are too brief for us to perceive the psychological effects associated with these dimensions are called *transients.* A detailed discussion of transients is not within the scope of this chapter, but additional information on them will be presented in a later section. Sound, then, is basically temporal in nature, and variations in its other dimensions occur over time.

Psychological Dimensions

Pitch is that psychological dimension of sound which is most closely associated with the fundamental frequency. Under most conditions, we will perceive a higher pitch when presented with a higher frequency and a lower pitch when presented with a lower

---

*The terms *partial* and *harmonic* often are used interchangeably with *harmonic overtone,* but with a slightly different numbering system. In these systems the *first partial* and *first harmonic* are equivalent to the fundamental frequency; the *second partial and the second harmonic* are equivalent to the *first harmonic overtone,* etc.

If energy is present in the complex tone which is not related to the fundamental by some whole number, it is not harmonically related. Consequently, we refer to this energy as an *inharmonic overtone.*

frequency. The normal listener will perceive a range of pitches associated with frequencies of 20 Hz to 20,000 Hz. However, at very low frequencies and very high frequencies the pitch of a sound will change with changes in intensity. Also, different listeners may perceive slightly different pitches for the same frequency/intensity combinations. Consequently, we must be aware that although pitch and frequency are closely related, they are not perfectly correlated.

Loudness and intensity are also closely related. The range of intensity to which the normal ear responds is from 10^{-10} microwatts/cm^2 to 10^3 microwatts/cm^2, and it corresponds approximately to the softest sound that can be perceived through the loudest sound that can be tolerated. However, this range of intensity is applicable only at those frequencies to which the ear is most sensitive (1 kHz–3kHz). At frequencies of less than about 1 kHz or more than about 3 kHz, more intensity than 10^{-10} microwatts/cm^2 is required for the perception of sound by the normal ear. Furthermore, in those frequency ranges loudness tends to increase more rapidly for a given increase in intensity than it does in the middle frequencies. All of this suggests that loudness depends not only on intensity but also on the frequency of the sound that is heard.

Tone quality or timbre is the psychological effect that results from the particular wave composition of a sound. It is that aspect of sound which allows us to differentiate among musical notes of identical frequency and intensity that have been produced on a piano or a violin or a trumpet. Perhaps more importantly, tone quality is that aspect of sound which allows us to differentiate among most speech sounds. Speech can be produced at high or low pitches or in loud or soft voices and still be understood. The reason for this is that speech sounds are the product of a mechanism which varies the spectral characteristics of sound to produce meaningful differences in tone quality. Of course, variations in pitch, loudness and timing are important for meaningful speech, but it is the ability to vary tone quality that is crucial to the speaker.

Duration might be defined as an individual's estimate of the time which transpires between two events. In the special case of sound perception it might be an estimate of the length of a sound, the length of a silent period between two sounds, or just about any other combination which can be constructed. In general, one might say that an estimate of the time duration of any of these sequences will depend on the actual amount of time involved *plus* the frequencies, intensities, and spectra of the various sounds used.

Classes of Sound

Sound may be divided into two general categories: *periodic* and *aperiodic*. Periodic sounds were discussed briefly in a previous section, but for a clear understanding of sound it is necessary to elaborate on the concept of periodicity. In the simplest terms, periodic sounds are tonal in nature and arouse in the listener a definite sensation of pitch; whereas, aperiodic sounds are noisy and arouse no definite sensation of pitch. As has been previously stated, periodic sounds exhibit repetitive waveforms. In contrast to this characteristic, aperiodic sounds exhibit waveforms which do not repeat in time but, rather, fluctuate in a somewhat random fashion. A graphic representation of the spectra of the two classes of sound, such as is presented in Figure 2-3, reveals additional differences. Note that the periodic sound shows concentrations of energy at the fundamental frequency and several of its harmonic overtones, whereas the aperiodic sound exhibits energy over all of the frequencies in a broad frequency band. The spectrum of the aperiodic sound is called a *continuous spectrum,* and that of the periodic sound is called a *line spectrum*. Transients, or sounds of short time duration, present spectra that are continuous and are, therefore, aperiodic. Even though the transient may be a short segment of a sine wave, its abrupt beginning and end produce an aperiodic waveform which results in a noise-like sound.

Both types of sound, noises and tones, are important for speech. The vowels we use are more or less periodic, but the consonants may be periodic, aperiodic, or a combination of both. For example, the word "smooth" contains the letter (s) which stands for an aperiodic consonant sound that is written phonetic-

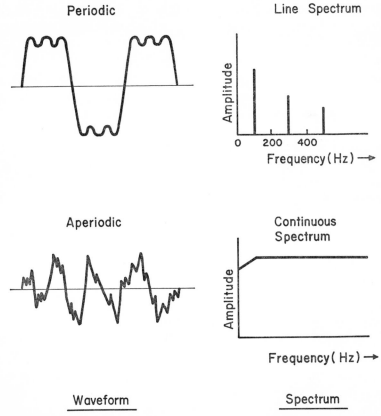

Figure 2-3. Periodic and aperiodic waveforms and their associated spectral compositions.

ally /s/, the letter (m) which stands for the periodic consonant sound /m/, the letters (oo) which stand for the periodic vowel /u/, and the letters (th) which stand for a combination aperiodic-periodic consonant sound /ð/. It should be clear from the foregoing discussion that the use of the term "noise" is purely descriptive and implies no value judgment of the sounds so designated.

Resonance

Resonance is a phenomenon which is common to all elastic systems that are capable of vibration. If such a system is struck, it will oscillate at some frequency which will be determined by the physical properties (mass and elasticity) of the system. The system is said to be set into *free vibration* at its *natural frequency*. The amplitude of the oscillations will diminish at a rate that is determined by the amount of *damping* (losses due to friction) in the system. In highly damped systems the oscillations die out almost immediately. In slightly damped systems (tuning forks, bells, chimes, etc.) free vibration will continue for relatively long periods of time. Instead of striking the elastic system, it may be coupled to a small vibrating source that vibrates at or near the system's natural frequency. In this situation, the system goes into *forced vibration* at its natural frequency (also termed *resonant frequency* under these circumstances) and *resonance* occurs. Often the amplitude of the vibrations will be quite large compared to those of the vibratory source, and the vibrations will continue until the source is removed.

The following example serves as a simple illustration of the difference between free vibration and resonance. If a child on a swing is given one big push, he and the swing (the elastic system) will be set into free vibration at the natural frequency of the system. The vibrations will continue to diminish after the initial push until finally they cease completely. The amount of time that the swing will vibrate may be increased if the friction (damping) in the system is reduced by oiling the bearings which attach the swing to its support. However, a more satisfactory solution would be to allow the system to resonate. Instead of giving the system one big push, it may be given a small initial push followed by another small push on each successive swing at exactly the right time in cycle. Under these conditions, the system will go into forced vibration at its resonant frequency (resonance), and the amplitude will be far greater than the amplitude attained under conditions of free vibration. When the pushing is stopped, the source of vibratory energy is uncoupled from the system, and it reverts to free vibration at its natural frequency.

Many musical instruments employ resonators which transfer the relatively weak vibrations of a reed or string to the surrounding air with increased efficiency and a resultant increase in loudness. It must be understood that a resonator does not add energy to the sound, but simply provides better transmission of the energy being supplied by the vibrator. Often these resonators are in the form of columns (woodwinds) or small enclosures of air (strings). Unlike the child on the swing, some of these columns or enclosures are capable of resonance at many frequencies and are said to be *broadly tuned*. The concept of tuning may be illustrated by examining a piano.

A piano's sounding board is a broadly tuned resonator. The strings of the piano are coupled to the board in a manner that permits it to be excited by the strings' vibrations. Regardless of which piano key is struck, the sounding board resonates the frequencies generated by the vibrating strings associated with that key. Furthermore, it will resonate many different notes at the same time. Of course, it does not transfer the energy from all of the strings to the surrounding air in exactly the same way. Some frequencies will be more efficiently transferred than others because the physical characteristics of the sounding board (mass, elasticity and damping) do not permit a completely linear response across all frequencies. However, the response can be determined for a given sounding board and presented as a graph of frequency versus amplitude. Such a graph can be prepared for any resonant system and is called its *transfer function* or *transmission characteristic*. Figure 2-4 illustrates the transfer functions of several resonators with different degrees of tuning. The resonators which are *broadly tuned* are said to be *highly damped,* and those which are *sharply tuned* are said to be *slightly damped.* It can be seen in D of Figure 2-4 that it is possible to have complex transfer functions which are *multimodal* (several peaks). It is just such a complex, broadly tuned, highly damped, multimodal resonant system that is employed by man when he produces speech sounds. We will find in the next section that it is primarily man's ability to vary the transfer function of his vocal resonant system that allows him to speak.

SPEECH PRODUCTION

Speech may be defined as a process in which sequences of meaningful sounds are generated for transmission through the surrounding medium to a listener who detects the sequences and

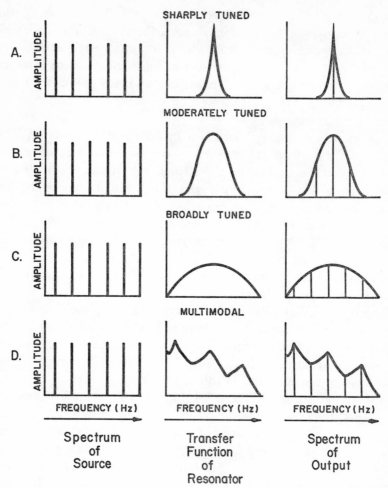

Figure 2-4. The modification of the spectrum of a constant source by various resonators. *A, B,* and *C* illustrate the effect of different degrees of tuning. *D* illustrates the effect of a complex resonant system on the same source.

analyzes them for their meaning. The process is uniquely human, for no other animal is capable of true speech. Although certain birds such as the mina, parrot, crow, etc. can mimic some of the sequences of sound which are detected as speech, the birds function only as a kind of poor quality tape recorder which reproduces with rather low fidelity the sounds that are recorded on it. Other animals, especially the primates, would seem to possess all of the superficial structures which are necessary for the production of speech. Certainly, man shares with these animals such features as a tongue, lips, palate, larynx, breathing mechanism, etc., but the mere presence of such features does not insure the ability to speak. Instead, it is the motility of these structures, their geometrical relationships, and the ability to control them that is vital to the process and unique in man.

The overall process of speech production is sufficiently complex to warrant a rather arbitrary segmentation into three closely related and interdependent functions. These arbitrary segments are *respiration, phonation,* and *articulation.* The total process will be described briefly, and then each of the segments will be considered in some detail. The discussion will center on the function or physiology of the system, and omit detailed anatomical descriptions. However, some anatomical description will be presented where appropriate to help explain the intricacies of function.

The process of speaking usually begins with the inspiration of air into the lungs. This action is accompanied by appropriate muscular adjustments in the laryngeal, thoracic and abdominal regions in preparation for the initiation of a flow of air from the lungs. This flow of air provides the driving force that activates the vocal folds or glottal generator (voice box) which in turn produces the pressure variations that are called vocal sound or phonation. The vocal sound is then transmitted through the vocal tract (throat, mouth, and nose) and radiated into the surrounding air as vocalization. The vocal tract functions as a multimodal resonant system (see D in Fig. 2-4), and it modifies the spectrum of the sound from the glottal generator. Changes in the relative positions of the various elements of the vocal tract (tongue, lips, palate, etc.) produce changes in the transfer function of this resonant system and resultant changes in the spectrum of the phonated sound. In addition to the vocal sound produced by the glottal generator, other sounds may be produced within the vocal tract. These are noise-like sounds that are made by rapidly closing and opening the tract at various points along its length (transients) or by constricting the tract to produce "frictional" sounds. The process of changing the shape of the vocal tract either rapidly or slowly is called articulation, and the elements that execute the change are called articulators. This brief overview of the speaking process provides a framework for the discussion of specific details of respiration, phonation, and articulation.

Respiration

Thoracic Cavity

The primary function of the breathing mechanism is the exchange of oxygen for carbon dioxide to support the life of the individual. This gas exchange is possible because of the particular structural characteristics of the mechanism. The rib cage, consisting of the *vertebral column* (backbone), *sternum* (breastbone), and twelve pairs of *costae* (ribs) is the bony framework of the *thorax* (chest). The framework is connected in such a way that in its normal resting state it is under compression and exerts an outward expanding force. The situation is similar to that of a coiled spring which has been squeezed together and partially compressed (see Fig. 2-5A). There are several layers of thoracic muscles which interconnect the various portions of the rib cage and are capable of increasing and decreasing the dimensions of the thoracic cavity. The floor of the cavity is called the *diaphragm* and is the partition that separates the thoracic cavity from the abdominal cavity. It is a dome-like structure which consists of a large central tendon (a tough, elastic material) and radiating sheets of muscle fibers that connect the central tendon to the sternum, lower ribs, and vertebral column. Contraction of the muscle fibers of the diaphragm tends to flatten the partition, elevate the lower ribs and push the contents of the abdominal cavity downward and forward against a compliant abdominal wall. This action increases the volume of the thoracic cavity during inspiration. According to Campbell (1958) the normal thoracic muscles of inspiration are the *diaphragm,* the *external intercostals,* the *interchondral part of the internal intercostals* (the part that lies between the cartilages of the ribs), and the *scaleni* muscles; whereas

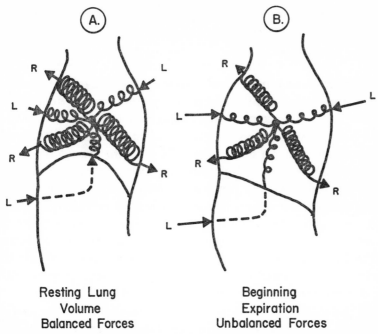

<table>
<tr><td align="center">Resting Lung
Volume
Balanced Forces</td><td align="center">Beginning
Expiration
Unbalanced Forces</td></tr>
</table>

Figure 2-5. An illustration of the interaction of elastic recoil of the lungs (denoted by the L's) and the expanding forces of the rib cage (denoted by the R's). In *A* the two forces are exactly balanced. In *B* the elastic recoil of the lungs has been increased and the expanding forces of the rib cage reduced by the action of the inspiratory muscles.

the *interosseous* (between the bones) part of the *internal intercostals* is the only thoracic muscle of expiration.

Within the thoracic cavity lie the *lungs, heart, esophagus, large nerves,* and *great vessels* of the circulatory system. The cavity is completely filled with these structures and their coverings, and there is no space within the cavity except for the air spaces inside the lungs. The lungs are of major importance for the production of speech and will be examined in some detail. The other structures within the cavity do not have large effects on the respiratory process and will not be discussed.

Lung Structure

The lungs are composed of a spongy material that is highly elastic in nature. Close examination reveals the presence of numerous tiny air sacs called *alveoli*. The alveoli are all connected through a system of small tubes and ducts called *bronchioles* to a series of larger passageways, the bronchial tubes, the bronchi, the trachea (windpipe) the pharynx (throat), the nose and mouth, and finally to the atmosphere outside of the body. The construction of the lungs permits an extremely large surface area (about the size of a tennis court in the average male) to be contained in the relatively small space of the thoracic cavity. Of course this large surface brings a great deal of blood into close contact with the atmosphere for the absorption of oxygen and the elimination of carbon dioxide. The lungs are covered with a smooth membrane called the *pulmonary pleura* which is reflected, or folded back on itself, to form the lining of the thoracic cavity called the *parietal pleura*. These smooth membranes adhere to the surface of the lungs, to each other, to the cavity wall, and to the diaphragm. The importance of these linings will become apparent as the process of normal breathing is discussed further.

In the healthy individual the lungs are under tension and are constantly trying to decrease in size. Each of the alveoli is something like a partially inflated balloon that will deflate and collapse if the air is allowed to escape through its opening. As air flows out of the alveoli, they deflate but do not collapse because of a complex mechanism involving a surface tension reducing agent (soaplike substance) that partially equalizes the elastic tensions among the small and large alveoli (Pattle, R. E. 1963). The overall effect of the elasticity of the tissue is to provide a force that constantly pulls the surface of the lungs toward the middle of the thorax. The lungs may be considered similar to a coiled spring that has been extended past its neutral position and is under tension (see Fig. 2-5A). The lungs do not decrease in size, for the force that tends to pull the surface of the lungs toward the middle of the thorax is exactly counterbalanced by the force of the rib cage (which is trying to expand) pulling on the surface of the lungs in the opposite direction. The forces of the expanding rib cage (under compression) and the collapsing lungs (under tension) are smoothly coupled through the adherent and well-lubricated pleural linings, and changes in dimensions of the thoracic cavity will result in little or no friction between the lung surface and the thoracic wall. This effect of friction reduction is enhanced by the partial vacuum present between the two pleural linings that is due to the opposing forces acting at the pleural interface.

Breathing Function: Ventilation

The volume of air that is present in the internal spaces of the lungs when the forces of compression and tension in the thorax are exactly balanced is known as the *resting lung volume.* It occurs in one's breathing cycle at the end of a quiet expiration in which there is no active breathing muscle contraction. Starting at this point, the breathing activity will be traced through a complete cycle. The initiation of inspiration is accomplished by contracting the muscle fibers of the diaphragm which pushes down on the visceral displacing the abdominal wall and increasing the vertical dimensions of the thoracic cavity. At the same time there is a contraction of the inspiratory muscles of the thorax which increases the lateral and ateroposterior (front to back) dimensions of the cavity. To some extent the diaphragm increases these dimensions also by elevating the lower ribs during contraction.

The pleural linings closely follow the movements of the cavity walls and the diaphragm, for an excessive increase in the intrapleural vacuum would be created if they did not do so. The peripheral surfaces of the lungs also closely follow the movements of the pleural linings for the same reason. As the lung surfaces move to accommodate the increase in cavity size, the pressure of the air within the alveoli drops below the level of the *ambient pressure* (surrounding atmospheric pressure) producing a temporary partial vacuum within the lungs. The end of the inspiratory phase is signalled by that brief moment when the pressure inside and outside the lungs is equal. Shortly after the equalization of pressures, the inspiratory muscles gradually cease their contractions, but they may continue contracting into the beginning of the expiratory phase (Green and Howell, 1959).

At this point in the breathing cycle, the lung volume has increased by approximately 600 ml ($^2/_3$ of a quart), the alveoli have expanded, and the elastic recoil of the lungs has increased.

At the same time, the tendency of the rib cage to expand has been reduced by the amount of expansion that has been accomplished. Figure 2-5B illustrates the directions and relative amplitudes of the forces involved. At this stage of the cycle, the forces due to the elastic recoil of the lungs and the abdominal wall exceed by an appreciable amount the opposing forces of the expanded rib cage and gravitational pull on the abdominal contents. The result is a decrease in the size of the thoracic cavity and a simultaneous increase in the air pressure within the alveoli which rises above the ambient pressure and initiates a flow of air out of the lungs and trachea into the surrounding atmosphere. This is the beginning of the expiration phase, and it continues until the elastic forces of the lungs and rib cage (tension and compression respectively) are again in balance. Thus, a complete cycle of quiet breathing has been described from the point of inspiratory muscle activity to the end of the cycle.

One should note that no expiratory muscle contractions are employed during the normal expiratory phase of the cycle, and that a considerable amount of energy is conserved by eliminating a portion of the muscle effort in the process of quiet breathing. An additional advantage to our counterbalanced double sprung breathing system is that it permits a change in position from upright to supine or prone with no ill effect on breathing performance from the change in the direction of the force of gravity. When an individual assumes a horizontal position, the force of gravity acting on the relatively incompressible contents of the abdominal cavity pushes the viscera against the diaphragm and slightly into the thoracic cavity. Apparently, the counterbalanced forces of rib cage and lungs are of a sufficient magnitude to cope with the added pressure against the diaphragm.

Quiet breathing usually involves no muscle activity during expiration. However, the process of expiration changes from a relatively passive activity to an active one whenever the individual's oxygen requirements increase. The exchange of gas is enhanced by increasing both the depth and rate of breathing. This is accomplished through longer, more forceful contractions of the inspiratory muscles, with the possible enlistment of some accessory postural muscles, *and* the active contraction of expiratory muscles. The most notable of these expiratory muscles are the broad sheet-like muscles of the abdominal wall that connect the pelvic girdle to the rib cage *(external oblique abdominis, internal oblique abdominis, transverse abdominis,* and *rectus abdominis)* and the *interosseous* (between the bones) portion of the *internal intercostal* muscles. During expiration the abdominal muscles squeeze the viscera up against the diaphragm and force the diaphragm into the thoracic cavity to decrease the cavity's vertical dimension. At the same time, the internal intercostals, which are attached to the rib cage, pull downward on the ribs and decrease the lateral and ateroposterior dimensions of the cavity. Thus, ventilation of the lungs is increased to meet the oxygen needs of the individual partially through expiratory muscle contractions that increase the speed and depth of the expiratory phase of the breathing cycle.

Breathing Function: Speech

The activity which occurs during respiration under varying requirements of oxygen demand seems to vary in degree rather than type, but breathing for speech is characterized by an almost opposite function. No longer is the primary goal the ventilation of the alveoli. Instead, *control* of the flow of air from the lungs through the vocal folds and the remainder of the vocal tract is of paramount importance. The emphasis is shifted from the *inspiratory* phase to the *expiratory* phase. Our needs for speech are the following: (a) an adequate supply of air to permit the execution of a reasonable number of syllables, and (b) precise regulation of the flow of air from the supply to operate the glottal generator and provide sufficient intraoral (within the mouth) pressures necessary for the production of the plosive and fricative sounds of the language.

Speech may be initiated from practically any lung volume, but typically, the initiation is signalled by an adjustment of the respiratory muscles which precedes the actual production of sound by as much as 200 to 300 milliseconds (Cooker, 1963). This preparatory activity is probably a postural gesture which facilitates the development by the breathing mechanism of appropriate airflows and pressures associated with speech sounds. It might be considered a kind of shifting point from the quiet breathing mode to the speech mode. Once the individual is in the speech mode, the passive elastic forces of the thorax and the active forces of the respiratory muscles interact to provide an appropriate amount of air flow to the glottal generator. The actual flow of air through the glottis (space between the vocal folds) will be determined by a combination of the subglottal pressure that is developed by the expiratory activity of the breathing mechanism and the valving action of the larynx which presents a variable resistance to the flow of air from the lungs (van den Berg, Zantema, and Doornenbal, 1957).

It has been shown that the pressure developed by the breathing mechanism during expiration in the nonspeech mode will depend in a large part on the particular lung volume attained (Otis, Fenn, and Rahn, 1950). Deep inspirations resulting in high lung volumes produce large recoil forces, whereas shallow inspirations resulting in low lung volumes produce small recoil forces. In the speech mode, it is necessary to control for these differences. Consequently, the flow of air to the glottal generator is regulated by counterbalancing the passive elastic forces of lungs and rib cage with appropriate respiratory muscle contractions (Draper, Ladefoged, and Whitteridge, 1959). At high lung volumes when the recoil forces are appreciable, the inspiratory muscles are contracted to reduce the flow of air to the glottis to an appropriate level. At low lung volumes when the recoil forces are reduced or even reversed, the expiratory muscles may contract to augment the flow of air to the glottis. Of course, as Draper *et al.* found, variations in vocal intensity at different lung volumes will dictate the degree to which the respiratory muscles contract. For example, if a high vocal intensity is desired at a relatively low lung volume, it will be necessary to contract the expiratory muscles with greater force than would be necessary for a moderate vocal intensity. In a similar manner, low vocal intensities at high lung volumes may require rather pronounced contractions of the inspiratory muscles to avoid the build up of inappropriately large subglottal pressures.

Summary

Respiratory function of the breathing mechanism in the speech mode is considerably different from its function in the nonspeech mode. During normal breathing, inspiration seems to be favored over expiration by the geometry of the structures and the number and arrangement of the muscles of the thorax. Whereas inspiration is under active muscle control, expiration seems to be a passive, somewhat uncontrolled activity. The rate at which air flows out of the system varies considerably and depends markedly on the particular lung volume that has been attained. All of these things suggest better regulation of the inspiratory portion of the cycle than the expiratory portion. However, speech is an expiratory function that requires great precision of control, consequently, some compensatory mechanisms or shift in function must be employed to attain this control. We have just such a mechanism in the larynx. Its complex muscle structure and ample neural supply suggests the anatomical capability for fine regulation of a somewhat grossly regulated air reservoir. There is little doubt that the laryngeal mechanism provides a precisely controlled resistance to the flow of air from the lungs to regulate subglottal pressure during speech. However, there is evidence also that respiratory muscle activity is employed to produce high flow rates for the production of certain consonant sounds (Cooker, 1963) and that frequency and intensity of phonation may be influenced by expiratory activity of the breathing mechanism (Isshiki, 1959 and 1964; Ladefoged, 1963; Lieberman, Knudson, and Mead, 1969; van den Berg, 1957). These findings support R. H. Stetson's (1905) original contention that vocal fold valving must be augmented by expiratory muscle activity to account for the variations in stress that occur in a language.

Phonation

It has been shown in the previous section how the respiratory mechanism provides a flow of air to the larynx. The interaction of the larynx with this flow of air will now be examined to determine the manner in which the larynx functions as a vocal sound generator. The most plausible explanation of this function is provided by the modern aerodynamic-myoelastic theory of voice production.* Briefly stated, the theory suggests that airflow from the lungs activates the vocal folds and that their mode of vibration is determined by a combination of laryngeal muscle adjustment and aerodynamic coupling of the folds to the supraglottal spaces, to the subglottal spaces, and to each other (van den Berg, 1968). It is possible for the larynx to generate sound in a number of different ways (van den Berg, 1968), but only two of these modes of vibration or "registers," *modal* (chest) and *falsetto,* will be discussed. Almost all normal speech is produced in the modal register; consequently, it will receive the greater emphasis.

The larynx or glottal generator is located at the top of the trachea, rather high in the anterior neck, and just below the root of the tongue. It may act as a valve to assist in closing off the passages to the lungs, or it may act as a vibratory device that produces the vocal sounds associated with speech. As a valve, it keeps food and other substances out of the trachea, and it works in concert with the respiratory muscles to produce the high rates of airflow associated with such protective activities as coughing and sneezing. Also, it probably is involved in providing tight valving to allow for the development of the high abdominal pressures associated with vomiting, defecation, lifting and other activities requiring more than minimal exertion. However, its function as a sound generator rather than its function as a life support valve is most important for speech, and therefore, its characteristics will be examined from this point of view.

Laryngeal Structure

The structural framework of the larynx is a system of nine cartilages that are interconnected at two pairs of joints by several ligaments and muscles. The four major cartilages are the *thyroid,* the *cricoid,* and a pair of *arytenoids.* The five minor cartilages are a pair of *corniculates,* a pair of *cuneiforms,* and a single *epiglottis.* These structures and their geometrical relationships are illu-

*Another theory of voice production, the neurochronaxic theory, was advanced by R. Husson in 1950. He suggested that each cycle of vocal fold vibration is initiated by a separate neural message from the cetnral nervous system. The theory has not been supported by the bulk of more recent research.

strated in Figure 2-6. The intrinsic muscles of the larynx act on these cartilaginous structures to produce changes in their relative positions and consequent changes in the vibratory activity of the glottal generator. These muscles are the *transverse and oblique arytenoideus,* the *lateral cricoarytenoid,* the *posterior cricoarytenoid,* the *cricothyroid,* the *thyroarytenoid,* and the *vocalis.* With the exception of the transverse arytenoideus, a midline muscle, all of the muscles are paired.

The vocal folds are the vibrating bodies of the glottal generator. Each takes the form of a cushion or shelf of muscular tissue

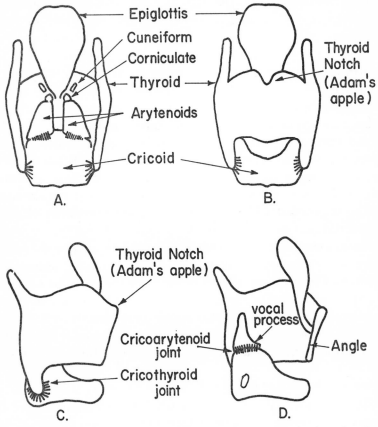

Figure 2-6. Four views of the laryngeal framework illustrating the shapes and relationships of the various cartilages. *A* Posterior, *B* Anterior, *C* Lateral, *D* Lateral with right half of the thyroid cartilage removed.

(vocalis and thyroarytenoid) which is connected between the anterior portion or *vocal process* of the arytenoid cartilage and the inner surface of the anterior portion or *angle* (near Adam's apple) of the thyroid cartilage. At the medial surface of each fold is a tough, elastic covering which is called the *vocal ligament*. It is at this surface that the folds meet both during valving and during vibratory activity.

Regulation of the Glottis

Adjustments to the configuration of the vocal folds and the opening between them (glottis) fall into two major categories which reflect the motions permitted by the two different joints connecting the cartilages: (a) Rotation of the cricoid cartilage with respect to the thyroid cartilage (at the cricothyroid joint) results in a change in the distance from the arytenoid cartilages to the thyroid cartilage and a concomitant change in the *tension and/or length* of the vocal folds; (b) A combination of oblique rocking and gliding of the arytenoid cartilages with respect to the cricoid cartilage (at the crico-arytenoid joint) results in wide separation or close approximation of their medial surfaces (Sonesson, 1960) and a concomitant *abduction* (separation) or *adduction* (closure) of the vocal folds. Of course, any particular vocal fold configuration will be the result of an interaction of all of these activities.

In summary then, the folds may be lengthened or shortened, tensed or relaxed at any of the length adjustments, adducted or abducted with varying degrees of force; or they may be subjected to any combination of these activities through the careful adjustment of the several muscles that act on them directly or indirectly. As will be seen later, these adjustments are essential to the control of both the frequency and intensity of the resultant vocal sound.

Sound Production in the Modal (Chest) Register

With an understanding of the structural configuration of the larynx, the laryngeal activity which produces sound may be described. Figure 2-7 is a diagram of four *coronal sections* (left to right vertical slice) through the middle of the larynx. It shows the

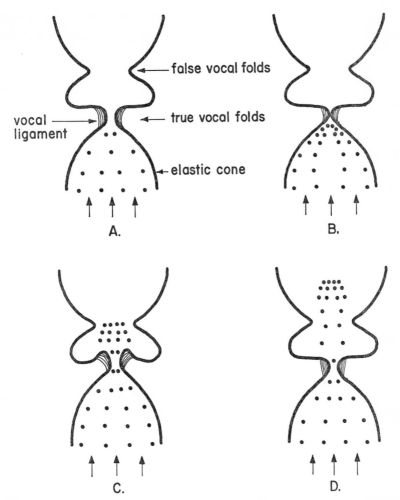

Figure 2-7. Coronal sections through the larynx illustrating four different stages of vocal fold activity during the production of voice. *A* Beginning Subglottal pressure blows folds apart. *D* Vocal fold elasticity forces folds of airflow through the glottis. *B* Bernoulii Effect sucks folds together. *C* back toward midline and cycle of vibratory activity begins to repeat.

pathway that the air from the lungs must take as it flows toward the mouth through the glottis. In A of Figure 2-7, the folds are partially adducted so that they are fairly close together. The air from the lungs encountered the *elastic cone* which is the constriction in the airway that ends at the edges of the folds (vocal ligaments) . The narrowing down of the pathway produces a physical shape that permits the development of Bernoulli pressures. An understanding of the Bernoulli's Effect is essential to an understanding of vocal fold vibration, therefore, a brief explanation of this phenomenon is presented in the following section.

The Bernoulli Effect

The Bernoulli Effect might be thought of as the reduction in the pressure of an incompressible, or nearly incompressible, fluid (in this case air) that is the result of an increase in the fluid's velocity as it flows smoothly (with little friction) through a constriction in a tube. If the fluid is incompressible, the *same volume* must flow through both the *constricted* and *unconstricted* portions of the tube in the *same amount of time*. Consequently, the *velocity* of the fluid *must be greater* through the narrow opening of the constriction than through the wider opening of the rest of the tube. But Bernoulli's equation states that the combined pressure and velocity at the *constriction* must equal the combined pressure and velocity at the *unconstricted portion* of the tube. Therefore, the *pressure* in the constriction *must decrease* in order to offset the increase in velocity.

A carburetor is an example of the practical application of this pressure reducing phenomenon in constricted tubes. The fuel line is introduced at a constriction of the inlet to the engine, and, due to the pressure reduction, the fuel is literally sucked into the engine. Another example of the application of the Bernoulli effect is in the function of an airplane wing. As air flows over the upper and lower surfaces of the wing, the velocity of the air is greater over the upper surface for it must travel a curved path and a greater distance than the air flowing over the lower surface. Again, the increased velocity at the upper surface will result in a decrease in the pressure at that surface. The consequence of this situation is that the relatively greater pressure on the lower surface of the wing pushes it upward into the area of reduced pressure producing "lift." The above examples are somewhat related to the phenomenon described in the following section that occurs at the glottis.

Vibration of the Vocal Folds

As was stated earlier, the air from the lungs flows through the elastic cone and the constricted glottis. Due to the Bernoulli Effect the increased velocity of air through the glottis produces a reduced pressure between the folds. Since the folds are relatively soft and pliable, they are sucked together near the midline of the glottis as is shown in B of Figure 2-7. As the folds meet, airflow through the glottis ceases, and the air particles are impounded by the closed vocal folds. The sudden interruption of the flow results in a piling up of air particles beneath the folds and a simultaneous increase in subglottal pressure (illustrated in B of Fig. 2-7). The pressure increases until it is of a sufficient magnitude to overcome the inertia of the folds. At that point, the folds are blown apart and air begins to flow through the glottis once more (C in Fig. 2-7). The folds will continue to move away from the midline until their elastic properties produce a restoring force that is sufficient to overcome the inertia of the moving folds and snap them back toward the midline once more. As they approach the midline, the physical configuration of the glottis is again appropriate for the development of the Bernoulli Effect (D of Fig. 2-7), and the entire cycle may be repeated. A review of the whole aerodynamic-myoelastic process indicates that the interaction of the elastic vocal folds (myoelastic) with the airflow from the lungs (aerodynamic) has created (a) variations in the area of glottal opening, (b) variations in the velocity of the air particles through the glottis, and (c) concomitant variations in the intraglottal air pressure. Thus, a pressure disturbance has been created and a *pressure disturbance is our definition of sound.** The physical dimensions of the glottal sound will depend mainly on the configuration of the vocal folds and the magntiude of the airflow from the respiratory mechanism. In general, the sound that is produced will be *quasi periodic* (approximately repetitive) and possess a very rich harmonic structure. An acoustic line spectrum of the sound would reveal the fundamental frequency to be the most intense com-

---

*Actually, the volume velocity is the proper correlate of the acoustic output at the glottis (Flanagan, 1958), but to avoid confusion the discussion of sound production will continue in terms of acoustic pressure.

ponent with energy continuously decreasing at higher and higher harmonics.

Frequency Control

The frequency of vibration of the glottal generator is determined by a combination of factors. The folds are the vibrating bodies of the mechanism, and it has been shown that the frequency of a freely vibrating body is determined by its *mass* and *elasticity*. Two factors that participate in the regulation of the frequency of vocal fold vibration, then, are the mass and elasticity of the folds. Another factor that affects frequency is the amount of airflow that is supplied by the respiratory mechanism. Moreover, since the folds are coupled to the airways above and below the glottis and to each other (van den Berg, 1958), the interaction among all of these factors is complex. Nevertheless, there is a substantial amount of evidence which suggests that an increase in fundamental frequency is closely associated with both a *decrease in the thickness* of the folds (Hollien and Curtis, 1960; Hollien, 1962, 1964; Hollien, Coleman, and Moore, 1968; Hollien and Colton, 1969) and an *increase in the length* of the folds (Hollien, 1960; Hollien and Moore, 1960; Hollien, 1962; Damste, Hollien, Moore, and Murray, 1968). The effect on the vocal folds of such changes is a *reduction of mass per unit of length,* and, perhaps a change in the muscle tension or *elasticity* of the folds. Of course, the tension may not necessarily increase with an increase in length, for the folds are longer, and presumably under little or no tension, when they are at rest in the abducted (quiet breathing) configuration than under any condition of phonation (Hollien, 1960; Hollien and Moore, 1960). Changes in the mass and elasticity of the folds produce changes in the glottal resistance to the flow of air from the lungs and concomitant changes in the subglottal pressure. Also, the shape of the folds may change as a result of the length and tension adjustments and add a different aerodynamic component to the vibratory cycle. Therefore, as van den Berg suggests (1968), compensating adjustments of the intrinsic laryngeal musculature to regulate vocal fold adduction may be necessary to maintain phonation in a desired register over a range of frequencies. Furthermore, phonation at very high and very low frequencies may require the activity of extrinsic laryngeal muscles. These muscles change the mass-elasticity characteristics of the vocal folds indirectly by varying the geometrical relationships between the thyroid and cricoid cartilages (Sonninen, 1968).

In summary, we may conclude that in the modal register, the vibratory rate of the glottal generator will be determined by (a) the mass per unit of length of the vocal folds, (b) the elasticity of the folds, (c) the rate of airflow from the lungs, (d) the degree of adduction of the folds, and (e) the aerodynamic configuration of the folds.

Intensity

The intensity of the sound that is produced at the glottis will be determined by the amplitude of the acoustic pressure variations that accompany the opening and closing of the vocal folds. The mechanism that regulates the amplitude of these acoustic pressure variations involves a rather complex interaction between airflow from the lungs and the *glottal resistance* to that flow (Isshiki, 1964). Glottal resistance is closely related to *medial compression* or the force with which the vocal folds are held together by adducting muscle contraction. If we increase medial compression while phonating at a constant frequency we will increase the intensity of the sound that is produced. However, it may be necessary to adjust the mass and elasticity of the body of the folds during this maneuver in order to maintain a constant frequency (Hirano, Ohala, and Vennard, 1969).

The effect of an increase in intensity on the vibratory cycle of the folds has been observed by Timke, Von Leden and Moore (1958). They indicate that at high intensities, the folds remain closed for a greater proportion of the cycle than at low intensities. Also, they indicate that the folds open slowly and close quickly at high intensities and open quickly and close slowly at low intensities. One explanation for these differences in vibratory activity between high and low intensities is that increased medial compression increases the effective inertia and elasticity of the folds which then require a greater subglottal pressure to blow them apart. Thus the folds remain closed for a longer period of time in order to develop the necessary increase in subglottal pressure. Furthermore, the folds open more slowly when the necessary subglottal pressure has been attained because the increase in effective inertia does not permit rapid acceleration of the folds. However, due to the increase in effective elasticity, large restoring forces are built up rapidly as the folds begin to separate, and the folds are snapped back to their adducted positions very quickly to complete the vibratory cycle. As can be seen from the above explanation, the amplitude of the acoustic pressure variations is increased as a result of a change in the ratio of *open time* to the *total time* of the vibratory cycle. This ratio is called the *opening quotient* (O_Q), and it decreases as intensity increases.

In summary, it is important to note that even though the vocal folds are the vibrating bodies of the glottal generator, the *amplitude* of vocal fold vibration is *not* the important determiner of intensity. Rather, it is the amplitude of the pressure disturbance which is determined by the *duty cycle,* or timing characteristics of the vibrating folds, that determines the intensity of the vocal sound. Of course, the duty cycle will depend on (a) the amount of airflow from the lungs and (b) the degree of medial compression acting on the folds.

Falsetto Register

The falsetto register constitutes an entirely different mode of vibration for the glottal generator. Van den Berg (1968) has presented a very clear description of the function of the vocal mechanism in the falsetto mode, and it seems appropriate to introduce the register at this point in our discussion of laryngeal function. The basic difference between the modal register and falsetto is the nature of the vibrating bodies. Whereas the entire shelf of muscular tissue vibrates in modal register, the rather thin *vocal ligaments* are the major vibrating elements in falsetto. This condition is produced by stretching the vocal ligaments and, at the same time, relaxing the muscles within the folds. Much greater tension (elasticity) is developed in the thin, passive ligaments than is possible in the more massive muscles of the body of the folds.

Also, the effective mass of the vibrating body (vocal ligament) is quite small by comparison with the mass of the entire fold. Typically the folds do not completely close during a vibratory cycle, consequently the flow of air through the glottis is not interrupted abruptly, and the resultant pressure disturbance is much smoother than it is in the modal register. The spectrum of the sound that is produced is characterized by a lack of energy in the higher harmonics, and the resultant tone quality is readily perceived as different from that of the modal register in the same individual.

The mechanism for the regulation of frequency and intensity is different in falsetto than in the modal register. Hollien and his colleagues (1960, 1962, 1969) found no close relationships between vocal fold dimensions and frequency of vibration in the falsetto register. A change in either frequency or intensity may be produced by varying the airflow from the lungs (expiratory forces) while maintaining a relatively constant glottal configuration (Isshiki, 1964; Hirano, Ohala, and Vennard, 1969). In order to maintain the appropriate glottal configuration, however, it may be necessary to vary the medial compression on the vocal ligaments through appropriate laryngeal muscle adjustment (van den Berg, 1968).

Articulation

The importance of the articulatory mechanism for the production of speech has been alluded to in a previous section of this chapter. Perhaps its essential contribution to the speech process can be appreciated best if the effects of its dysfunction are compared with the effects of the dysfunction of the mechanisms of phonation and respiration. If the larynx is surgically removed, intelligible speech still is possible through the substitution of some other sound source for the glottal generator (e.g. an artificial larynx). Also, if the respiratory muscles are paralyzed, adequate speech may be produced on the expiratory phase of some artificial breathing device (e.g. an "iron lung"). But if an individual suffers total paralysis or some other major dysfunction of the articulatory mechanism, he may not be able to speak at all.

Fortunately, the mechanism is fairly robust in that it will take considerable insult before speech is affected. It is possible for an individual with a partially dysfunctioning articulatory mechanism to execute many compensatory maneuvers and adjustments to produce acceptable speech. While the major emphasis in the present chapter is on the basic nature of normal articulatory function, further details on disorders of articulation will be presented in another chapter of this book.

Articulatory Structures

The vocal tract extends from the lungs to the mouth and nose, and each portion of the tract contributes to the total resonant effect of the system. It has been general practice to consider the vocal tract as encompassing only those structures that lie above the glottis, but we know that the trachea and lungs contribute to the overall resonant characteristics of the tract, (van den Berg, 1968) and though the effect is relatively constant it should not be ignored. Nevertheless, the major articulatory structures lie above the glottis and form a complex muscular tube that is extremely variable in shape and that functions as a variable acoustic resonator. It is composed of the *pharynx,* the *oral cavity* and the *nasal* passages.

The pharynx lies directly above the larynx and may be divided into three parts: the *laryngopharynx,* the *oropharynx,* and the *nasopharynx.* It connects with both the oral cavity and the nasal passages which are, in effect, extensions of the pharyngeal tube. Its posterior and lateral walls are formed by the cone-like *superior, middle,* and *inferior constrictor* muscles, and the anterior wall is formed by the root of the tongue. Additionally, the posterior and lateral walls contain vertical fibers from the *salpingopharyngeus,* the *stylopharyngeus,* and the *palatopharyngeus* muscles.

The oral cavity contains the upper part of the tongue and the upper and lower teeth; its lateral walls, the cheeks, are formed by the *buccinator* muscles which terminate anteriorly at the lips. The upper and lower lips are composed of a collection of muscle fibers that are called the *orbicularis oris.* Many of these fibers are simple continuations of the fibers of the buccinator muscles and the numerous muscles of facial expression that course toward the lips from the bones of the face and the lower jaw or *mandible.*

The nasal passage are relatively static in shape and have boney walls with shell-like protrusions called *nasal turbinates.* The entire surface of the passages is covered with a thin layer of soft mucous tissue that is continuous with the lining of the pharynx and oral cavity. The nasal passages are separated from the oral cavity by the boney *hard palate* (roof of the mouth and floor of the nasal passages) and the *velum* (soft palate). The velum is a muscular structure consisting of the *palatal levator* and *palatal tensor* which enter its lateral edges from above and to the side, the *palatoglossus* and the *palatopharyngeus* which enter from below, and the *uvular* muscle which courses posteriorly from the hard palate to the uvula. The velum and the walls of the nasopharynx form a muscular valving system, the *velopharyngeal port,* that regulates the degree of communication between the nasal passages and the rest of the vocal tract.

Both the oral cavity and the pharynx are markedly variable in size and shape, for they have flexible muscular walls and share the tongue which is an extremely mobile structure consisting of many sets of muscle fibers that course in several different directions. The extrinsic tongue muscles, *genioglossus, hyoglossus, chondroglossus, styloglossus,* and *palatoglossus,* tend to vary tongue position within the vocal tract, whereas the intrinsic tongue muscles, *superior longitudinalis, inferior longitudinalis, transversus,* and *verticalis,* tend to vary tongue shape. In addition to the variations in cavity configuration produced by the tongue, the lips, which also are very mobile, may be protruded or retracted to elongate or shorten the oral cavity. And finally, the entire cavity may be enlarged or diminished by depressing or elevating the mandible.

Nonspeech Functions

Some of the structures described above form the upper portion of the digestive tract which functions as a food processor. In the oral cavity, food is *masticated* (chewed), mixed with saliva, and squeezed backward and downward by the tongue and constrictor muscles into the pharynx and esophagus through the process of *deglutition* (swallowing). Also, the oral cavity can be used as a pump to force liquid into or out of the mouth. A valve is formed at the rear of the cavity by the tongue and velum to isolate the cavity from the remainder of the tract, and negative or positive pressures are created by changing the position of the mandible.

The nasal passages form the upper portion of the respiratory tract which terminates at the nostrils. Their purpose is to condition the air before it enters the lungs. This function is possible because the surface area of the passages is considerable. The previously mentioned shell-like turbinates increase the surface area appreciably and provide a pretreatment of the air before it enters the lungs by filtering out dust particles and adding heat and moisture.

Although these functions are essential to the maintenance of life, the major emphasis again is on the function of the articulators for speech. Therefore, the remainder of this section will be devoted to the activity of these structures during speech production.

Dual Function of Articulation During Speech

At the beginning of the section on speech production it was stated that the process of articulation encompassed both rapid constrictions of the vocal tract and slower less extreme changes in its configuration. Actually, the slower changes are still fairly rapid, but it is convenient to consider each type separately. The slower, tract shaping changes are associated with vowel-like sounds (some voiced consonants are vowel-like), and the faster, tract constricting changes are associated with certain of the consonant sounds (Fant, 1968).

Tract Shaping Movements

In the section on the physics of sound, it was indicated that the vocal tract was a complex, broadly tuned, highly damped, multimodal resonant system (see D, Fig. 2-4). Consider the fact that this resonant system is coupled to the source of vocal sound, the glottal generator. It will be recalled that the transfer function of such a resonant system is characterized by several peaks and valleys, and that energy present at frequencies near the peaks is more readily transmitted through the system than energy present at frequencies near the valleys. Consequently, the spectrum of the complex sound generated at the glottis is modified by the transfer function of the vocal tract resonator, and the resultant tone quality of the modified sound is dependent upon the particular vocal tract configuration that is employed. In other words, the essential difference between the sound /i/ in *feet* and the sound /ɔ/ in *fought* is one of tone quality. And the tone quality is determined by the transfer function of the resonant system which, in turn, is determined by the geometrical relationships of the articulatory structures (shape of the vocal tract). In the above example the tongue is humped up toward the front of the oral cavity for /i/, and it is humped back toward the pharyngeal wall for /ɔ/. It should be apparent from this that the movements of the articulators produce the particular transfer function that results in a particular speech sound.

Tract Constricting Movements

In addition to the slower, tract shaping articulatory activity that leads to a modification of the glottally generated sound, there is rapid articularory activity that greatly constricts or completely occludes the vocal tract. Rapid articulatory activity also may modify the glottally generated sound, but in addition it produces a source of sound at the point of constriction or occlusion which is noisy and aperiodic. For example, the /s/ at the beginning of the word *sat* is a noisy sound (fricative) that is associated with a frictional flow of air through a constriction of the tract between the *alveolar ridge* (upper gum ridge) and the tongue. The /t/ at the end of the word also is a noisy sound (stopplosive), but it has somewhat different characteristics. It is associated with the sudden complete occlusion of the vocal tract between the tongue and the alveolar ridge followed by an equally sudden opening at the same point in the tract. Acoustically, it is a pulse or transient which follows the brief silent period that occurs during the occlusion or stop phase of the articulatory maneuver. Frequently there is a kind of hissing quality (aspiration) that accompanies the sudden release of air through the narrow opening. Both types of articulatory sound in the examples presented above are resonated by the vocal tract, and the particular vocal tract configurations which accompany their production produce transfer functions that are peculiar to each. Thus, it has been shown that in addition to the glottal sound, there are two types of articulatory sounds, frictional and transient, that are important for the production of speech.

Articulatory Classes of Speech Sounds

Traditionally, all speech sounds have been classified into two broad categories: vowels and consonants. Unfortunately, this classification system is not unambiguous, for some voiced consonants are quite vowel-like. However, the system works fairly well, and it has a certain utility that more complex systems may lack.

Vowels: Glottal vibration or voicing always accompanies the normal production of vowels and diphthongs. (Of course, one may whisper vowel sounds and thereby eliminate the normal voicing aspect by substituting glottal noise, but whispered speech will not be considered in this chapter). *The height of the tongue hump, its relative position toward the front or back of the mouth, the degree of lip rounding (protrusion), and the degree of tension in the articulatory muscles* are used to specify a particular vowel. For example, the /i/ in *feet* is a high, tense, unrounded, front vowel, and the /ɔ/ in *fought* is a low, tense, rounded, back vowel. Diphthongs are produced by changing the configuration of the vocal tract from that of one vowel to that of another vowel at an appropriate rate. The result is the production of a sound that has some of the characteristics of each vowel. However, the combination of characteristics easily distinguishes the diphthong from either of the vowels from which it was constituted. Although the vowel classification system is not precise, it serves as a basis for developing gross vowel categories.

Consonants: The classification of consonant sounds is somewhat more complex than the classification of vowels. In contrast to the vowels, consonants may be either *voiced* or *voiceless*. The glottal generator vibrates during voiced consonants and does not vibrate during voiceless consonants. If they are voiced, they may be either *nasal* or *non-nasal*. Nasal sounds are produced by opening the velopharyngeal port to couple the nasal passages to the remainder of the vocal tract (modifying the overall transfer function of the tract), whereas non-nasal sounds require that the port be closed or nearly closed. Another identifying dimension of consonant sounds is the *place of articulation* which refers to that point along the vocal tract at which the maximum constriction occurs during the production of the sound of interest. It may be *bilabial* (at the two lips), *labiodental* (lower lip and upper teeth), *linguadental* (tongue and upper teeth), *alveolar* (tongue and upper gum ridge), *palatal* (tongue and hard palate), *velar* (tongue and soft palate), or *glottal* (between the two vocal folds.) The *manner of articulation* is another important dimension and refers to the nature of the specific articulatory activity that occurs during the production of the sound of interest. The sound may be a *stopplosive* (occlusion of the tract followed by a sudden release of built up pressure), a *fricative* (a narrowed constriction through which air is forced to produce noise), an *affricative* (an occlusion of the tract followed by a sudden frictional release of built-up pressure through a narrowed constriction), a *semivowel* (vowel-like moderate constriction of the tract), or a *glide* (smooth rapid change in the configuration of the vocal tract from one vowel-like constriction to another).

The classification system that has been presented is extreme in its simplification. It is not intended as a definitive system but as an introductory thrust into the complexities of articulatory detail. Several detailed systems have been proposed, and the reader is directed to the chapters by Gordon E. Peterson, Gunnar Fant, and R. Jakobson and M. Halle in *Manual of Phonetics* (1968) for excellent introductions to three of these systems.

The Essential Nature of Articulation

It should *not* be concluded from the simple classification system which was presented that speech is a series of discrete sounds with invariant acoustical characteristics that are juxtaposed in time. Rather, it must be understood that isolated speech sounds and their associated vocal tract configurations are "ideal" models which do not exist in the real world of connected speech, and that speech is a time-varying phenomenon with few if any, truly steady-state characteristics. The essential nature of articulation, then, is *movement*. We might say that *it is a smoothly flowing series of skilled movements which continuously changes the shape of the vocal tract.** Furthermore, every movement that is performed will affect the movement which precedes and follows it. Consequently, the articulation of one sound is dependent on the articulation of other sounds. This process is called *coarticulation*. The acoustic consequence of coarticulation is that the characteristics of a given speech sound will be determined in part by the sounds that precede and follow it. Moreover, there is some evidence that the third sound in an articulatory sequence may interact with the first to some extent (Ohman, 1966 and 1967).

In general, it may be said that true speech sounds reflect the anatomical and physiological constraints of the human vocal tract and that they are produced only rarely as the isolated "ideal" model would predict. Each sound that precedes or follows another sound presents an obstacle to the attainment by the articulators of the "ideal" or target vocal tract configuration for that sound. Therefore, normal adjustments in the direction and velocity of articulator movements are routinely executed during connected speech and result in permissible departures from target vocal tract configurations. Not only are such departures from the target configurations permissible, they are essential if the speech produced is to sound natural.

A situation that is somewhat analogous to articulator movement is that of the racing skier who is running a slalom course. If he were to try to pass through each slalom gate's exact center in an erect posture (as he might through a single, isolated gate) he would probably not complete the course. Instead of attempting to pass through the gates in some "ideal" manner, the experienced skier determines his course through each gate by anticipating the following gate and plotting the shortest *practical* distance to pass *successfully* through it. At the same time, he monitors his current course and makes adjustments in it to compensate for any changes

---

*This is an elaboration and modification of a statement made by R. H. Stetson in his original 1928 monograph, "Motor Phonetics."

that he might make in his predicted course. Often he is thinking two or three gates ahead of his current position. In certain of the more difficult portions of the course, the gates are very close together, and successful completion of them requires that the skier "coarticulates" these gates. Furthermore, as the skier moves down the course, his posture is continuously adjusted to counter gravity and the inertial forces of his movements. His several parts, shoulders, hips, arms, feet, etc. are continuously moving in different directions and in varying time patterns. At any given instant, his skis will be tracking through the current gate in the course, but his shoulders may be moving toward the position for the next gate, and his arms away from the position for the last gate. Of course, all of the activities are performed in concert and must be appropriate for his current position on the course. The articulatory mechanism behaves similarly in that different portions of the mechanism, jaw, tongue, lips, velum, etc. may function in different temporal patterns in order to produce the appropriate sequence of cavity configurations necessary for speech (Liberman *et al.,* 1967).

The analogy of the skier logically might be extended to include misarticulations. A missed gate could be considered an omitted sound, a dislodged gate, a distortion, and entry from the wrong direction, a substitution. However, an anology may not be carried too far or oversimplification can result. Therefore, the important features of articulation will be reviewed in more general terms. It should be clear that articulation is skilled motor activity involving several interacting articulatory members capable of coordinated movement. The result of these movements is the controlled variation over time in the shape of the vocal tract and a concomitant meaningful variation in the acoustic output of the system. As has been suggested earlier, it is not the particular vocal tract configuration at a given instant in time that is important, but rather it is the *movement from one tract configuration to another* that is crucial to the articulatory process.

Conclusions

It has been shown that the speech process starts with airflow from the lungs and ends with the radiation of meaningful sound from

the speaker's mouth. The neuromuscular activity that transpires
between these two events is enormously complex. No attempt has
been made to explain the neurological aspects of speech production, for the intricacies of central neurol function during speech
are at best not well understood. Emphasis has been on the
mechanical function of the peripheral speech mechanism and the
details of its three interdependent parts. Certainly the division
of the mechanism into three parts is a convenient pedigogical device; however, the whole must be reassembled from its parts if
one is to understand its true function. In addition to the mere
production of a speech sound or series of speech sounds, at least
three *prosodic features* can be observed that are intimately inter-
twined in the process of speech communication. These features
are *intonation* or variations in pitch pattern; *stress,* or variations
in duration, loudness, and pitch; and *tempo,* or variations in the
temporal patterning of speech. It should be quite clear at this
point that such prosodic features can result only from an interaction of all three parts (respiration, phonation, articulation) of
the mechanism. Furthermore, it should be clear also that the
range of prosodic variations and the repertoire of speech sounds
that are available to the speaker are not infinite but are limited
by the physical constraints of the anatomy and physiology of the
human speech mechanism. And finally, one should appreciate the
fact that the production of speech is the most complex and intri-
cate motor activity that the human being ever performs!

THE HEARING MECHANISM

The ear is a delicately balanced system that *transduces* (converts) sound into neural messages in order that they may be perceived by the brain. It is extremely sensitive and functions over a
broad range of both frequency and intensity. Its versatility is obvious when one considers that the highest frequency that the
average listener can perceive is a *thousand times* greater than the
lowest and that the loudest sound he can tolerate is about *ten
trillion times* (10,000,000,000,000) as intense as the softest sound
he can detect. These large ranges are possible because the ear does
not respond linearly to either frequency or intensity. Fortunately,

special scales have been devised that provide us with a convenient method of dealing with the nonlinearity and wide ranges of the ear. Therefore, before the ear is examined in detail, a discussion of the most important of these special scales will be presented.

Sound Measurement

It is probable that you are most familiar with *equal interval scales.* For example, a ruler employs an equal interval scale with one-inch units. When using a ruler one is assured that each of the units is comparable in size to any other one-inch unit on the scale. If an inch-long object is measured it does not matter whether the scale markings between 0 and 1, 1 and 2, or for that matter, 11 and 12 are used. We say the scale is *additive,* i.e. the distance (interval) between 1 and 2 and the distance between 11 and 12 may be added together and will equal a total of two inches. Scales of this type are quite common, are simple to understand, and are convenient to use. However, if one were to use such a scale to measure intensity, it might be too large for practical use. Furthermore, it would not reflect the ear's nonlinear response. Consequently, it is far more convenient to use a *special ratio scale* when dealing with intensity.

This type of special scale employs a *constant multiplier* or *ratio* as a unit rather than a constant interval. For example, if the ratio or multiplier is 2, the scale marks are 2, 4, 8, 16, 32, 64, etc. ($2 \times 1 = 2, 2 \times 2 = 4, 2 \times 4 = 8, 2 \times 8 = 16, 2 \times 16 = 32, 2 \times 32 = 64$, etc.) . It is clear that the *ratios* between scale points are identical but that the intervals between scale points are not. It should be clear also that very large ranges may be handled rather conveniently, for the intervals rapidly become larger with continued application of the constant multiplier (in this case 2). In the example above, the multiplier was first applied to the number 1, but it could have been applied just as easily to 2 or 3 or 1.23 or any other number that was convenient to use. If it had been started with 3, the series would have been 6, 12, 24, 48, 96, etc. Another characteristic of this type of special scale, then, is that the *zero* or *starting point* is arbitrarily defined. This characteristic is very convenient when dealing with the ear, for some universally agreed upon quantity can be defined as zero intensity or zero sound pressure. With an understanding that these special scales employ constant multipliers or ratios as units and some finite quantity that is arbitrarily specified as the zero or starting point, we can proceed to a discussion of the decibel.

The Decibel

In order to discuss the decibel (dB), the *Bel* must first be examined. The Bel is a 10:1 ratio (so named in honor of Alexander Graham Bell), and, as one might suspect from the names employed, the *decibel* is one tenth of a Bel. The ratio or multiplier for the Bel (or 10dB) is used exactly as in the previous example, except that the ratio is now 10:1 instead of 2:1, i.e. $10 \times 1 = 10$, $10 \times 10 = 100$, $10 \times 100 = 1000$, $10 \times 1000 = 10,000$, etc. Each application of the multiplier, 10, increases the amount by one Bel or by ten decibels.* Consequently a sound that is 20 dB higher in intensity than another sound possesses *one hundred times* the intensity of that sound $(10 \times 10 = 100)$, whereas a sound that is 30 dB higher in intensity than another sound possesses *one thousand times* the intensity of that sound $(10 \times 10 \times 10 = 1000)$.

Although the intensity ratio may be determined in dB between any two sounds, the intensity of a sound often is indicated in terms of its relationship to the *standard zero intensity reference of 10^{-10} microwatts/cm²*. This zero point was selected as being close to the softest sound that the normal listener can detect in a quist listening environment. When the intensity of a sound is stated in dB relative to this standard reference, the letters *IL* are included for *intensity level*. For example, a sound that is designated as 30 dB IL has an intensity that is one thousand times greater than the standard reference intensity $(10^{-10}$ microwatts/cm² $\times 1000 = 10^{-7}$ microwatts/cm²), but it is far more convenient to use the designation dBIL than it is to use the absolute amount of intensity in microwatts/cm².

In the section on the physics of sound, it was stated that sound intensity is difficult to measure directly, and that consequently, we

---

*The decibel will be discussed in units of ten in order to simplify the presentation. This simplification yields a 10:1 ratio and eliminates the necessity of dealing with decimals.

measure pressure and *infer* intensity. Of course, this is possible because the intensity is proportional to the square of the pressure. Therefore, if the *sound pressure* of a tone is increased *10 times,* the intensity of the tone is increased by the *square of 10* or *100 times* and is equivalent on the dB scale to an increase of *20 dB.* Even though one might reason that the sound pressure was increased only by a factor of 10, which would correspond to 10 dB, it must be remembered that intensity is inferred from the pressure measurements. Consequently, the simple mathematical expedient of doubling the number of decibels associated with the *measured* ratio of sound pressures yields the exact number of decibels that is associated with the *inferred* ratio of intensities.

There is a *standard zero sound pressure reference* of 0.0002 dynes/cm² that corresponds to the standard zero intensity reference of 10^{-10} microwatts/cm². When the sound pressure of a tone is stated in dB relative to this reference pressure, we say that the sound pressure level or SPL of that tone has been designated. For example, a sound of *40 dB SPL* has a sound pressure that is *100* times greater than the standard reference sound pressure and an intensity that is *10,000* times greater than the standard reference intensity. Several sound pressure and sound intensity ratios and their associated dB are presented in Table 2-I. It should be clear from this discussion that the decibel makes it possible to cope with the extremely wide range of intensities and pressures to which the ear will respond without resorting to the cumbersome manipulation of unwieldy numbers.

TABLE 2-I

SOUND PRESSURE AND SOUND INTENSITY RATIOS AND THEIR ASSOCIATED dB EQUIVALENT

Sound Pressure Ratio	Intensity Ratio	db IL (re:10^{-10}microwatts/cm²) or dB SPL (re: .0002 dynes/cm²)
10:1	100:1	20
100:1	10,000:1	40
1,000:1	1,000,000:1	60
10,000:1	100,000,000:1	80
100,000:1	10,000,000,000:1	100
1,000,000:1	1,000,000,000,000:1	120

Structure and Function of the Ear

As has been previously stated, the ear is a device that converts sound energy into neural messages. In order to understand better this process of conversion, it is convenient to divide the ear on the basis of function into three parts: the *outer ear,* the *middle ear,* and the *inner ear* (see Fig. 2-8) . The pressure disturbances of air-

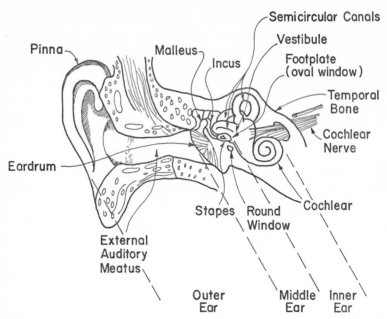

Figure 2-8. The important structures that make up the outer, middle, and inner ear.

borne sound are collected at the outer ear, transformed by the middle ear into mechanical vibrations that are suitable for processing by the liquid filled inner ear, and converted into neural impulses by the hydraulic action of the fluid of the inner ear. In progressing from the outer through the middle to the inner ear, it will become apparent that there is an increase in the complexity of function. However, it is important to remember that the ear functions as a unit and that even slight disruptions of its simpler actions may affect an individual's hearing acuity.

The Outer Ear

The outer ear is made up of the *pinna* or *auricle, external auditory meatus,* and the outer surface of the *tympanic membrane.* The pinna is the external fleshy structure that protrudes from the head in a backward direction and is commonly called the "ear." It assists in directing the sound waves into the external auditory meatus and may be helpful in localizing or identifying the direction from which the sound is emanating. The external auditory meatus is a quarter inch, double curved tube or canal that leads from the pinna to the tympanic membrane or "eardrum." It is about an inch long, and near the pinna its surface is sparsely ringed with hair and special glands. These glands produce the waxy substance, *cerumen,* which together with the sparse hairs keeps insects and other foreign objects from entering the canal. Actually, the canal forms a resonant air column that enhances the transmission of frequencies in the 2000 Hz to 4000 Hz range, and therefore it contributes to the overall frequency response of the ear. The eardrum forms the internal boundary of the external auditory meatus and physically separates the outer ear from the middle ear. It is a light conical diaphragm that is connected to the first of a series of three tiny bones (smallest bones in the body) that are housed in the middle ear.

The Middle Ear

The middle ear is a small cavity that lies within a portion of the *temporal bone* (one of the skull bones). It houses the *ossicular chain* which is the series of three small bones referred to above. Each of the *ossicles* has a distinctive shape for which it has been named. Starting at the tympanic membrane and proceeding inward toward the inner ear, they are the *malleus* (hammer), *incus* (anvil), and *stapes* (stirrup). The interconnected ossicles are delicately suspended from the walls of the middle ear cavity by a system of ligaments and tendons. This moveable boney chain links the outer ear to the inner ear through its attachment to the eardrum at the malleus and the *oval window* at the stapes. There are two muscles, the *tensor tympani* and *stapedius,* that emanate from the walls of the middle ear cavity and attach via their tendons to the malleus and stapes respectively. They appear to help fixate the ossicular chain and prevent the pointed ossicles from separating during large vibratory excursions (Bekesy, 1960). Under certain conditions they may help also in the protection of the hearing mechanism against loud sounds.

The middle ear cavity is filled with air which is maintained at atmospheric pressure through a connection with the air in the nasal passages. This connection is made through the *Eustachian tube,* a canal of bone and cartilage that is normally closed at the cartilagenous end. During swallowing or yawning, muscular contractions open the flattened end of the tube producing a brief communication between the middle ear and the nasal passages. These brief instances of communication eliminate any pressure differences between the outer ear and the middle ear. It is important for the pressure to be equal on both sides of the eardrum, or the drum will not vibrate properly, and the sensitivity of the ear will be reduced. At one time or another, most of us have experienced a temporary reduction in hearing acuity as the result of such minor pressure differences. For example, when traveling in a car down a long hill, one may notice that a sudden increase in road noise accompanies the act of swallowing. Swallowing opens the closed Eustachian tube and eliminates the pressure differential between the outer ear and middle ear that has been increasing gradually during the drive down the hill. Balancing the pressure across the eardrum restores its normal function and results in an apparent increase in hearing acuity. Of course, large pressure differences associated with some pathological condition may produce discomfort or pain and may require the services of a physician to restore the balance of pressures.

It is the function of the middle ear to transmit sound energy from the air in the external auditory meatus to the fluid of the inner ear. The geometry of the middle ear structures and the lever action of its parts interact to carry out this function very efficiently. The system transforms the sound pressure variations that impinge upon the eardrum into mechanical vibrations at the oval window and increases the effective sound pressure at the oval window by 25 to 30 dB. The middle ear functions also to protect the inner ear from excessively loud sounds. This is accomplished by a change in the vibratory pattern of the ossicular chain that accompanies an increase in the intensity of a sound.*

The Inner Ear

The inner ear is a complicated system of liquid filled tunnels and canals that are channeled into the *petrous* (rock hard) portion of the temporal bone. Because of its complexity, it is often referred to as the *bony labyrinth*. It contains the end organs for both the sense of hearing and the sense of balance. These end organs form another complex system, the *membraneous labyrinth*, that roughly approximates the course of the bony labyrinth. As can be seen in Figure 2-8, the bony labyrinth may be divided into three parts: the *semi-circular canals,* the *vestibule,* and the *cochlea.* The semicircular canals and the vestibule contain the end organs for the sense of balance (vestibular mechanism) while the cochlea houses the organ of hearing.

The cochlea is a snail-like spiraling canal of two and one-half turns that is divided longitudinally into three chambers: the upper, *scala vestibuli;* the lower, *scala tympani;* and the middle, *scala media* or *cochlear duct.* It has a central bony core, the *modiolus,* in which there is a channel that passes the neural fibers of the cochlear branch of the acoustic nerve (VIIIth Cranial Nerve). A cross-section of a portion of the cochlea which reveals the minute structures of the hearing end organ is presented in Figure 2-9. The two larger chambers, the scala vestibuli and the scala tympani, are separated partly by the *osseous spiral lamina,* a bony shelf that emanates from the inner cochlear wall, and partly by the cochlear duct. Both large chambers communicate with the middle ear through small openings at their basal ends: the scala vestibuli at the *oval window,* and the scala tympani at the *round* window (see Fig. 2-8).

---

*The footplate of the stapes normally moves in a piston-like fashion in and out at the oval window to transmit the vibratory activity to the fluid of the inner ear. However, when the sound becomes intense, the stapes pivots back and forth around the long axis of the footplate displacing a smaller quantity of fluid at the oval window and preventing excessively large displacement amplitudes of delicate inner ear structures (Bekesy, 1960).

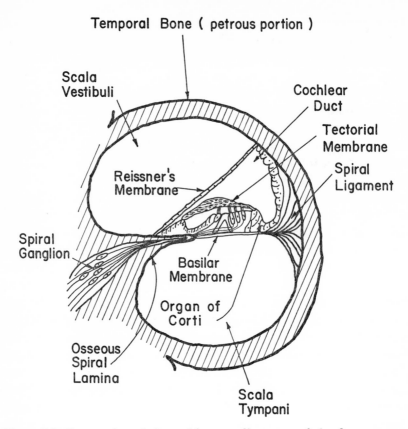

Figure 2-9. Cross-section of the cochlea revealing some of the fine structure of the cochlear duct.

The floor of the cochlear duct is formed by the *basilar membrane,* an elastic strip that connects the edge of the osseous spiral lamina to the outer wall of the cochlea (at the *spiral ligament*). The basilar membrane is relatively narrow and stiff at the base of the cochlea near the oval window, but becomes continuously wider and more flexible as it nears the apex of the cochlea. The ceiling of the duct is formed by *Reissner's membrane,* a very delicate flexible membrane that separates the cochlear duct from the scala vistibuli. Together with the outer wall of the cochlea, these two structures produce a triangularly shaped closed end tube that courses from the vestibule to a point just short of the apex of the cochlea. This leaves the *helicotrema,* a space at the cochlear apex through which the scala vestibuli and the scala tympani may communicate. The cochlear duct and the remainder (vestibular portion) of the membraneous labyrinth are filled with *endolymph,* while the scala vestibuli, the scala tympani, and the remainder of the bony labyrinth are filled with *perilymph.* Both of these fluids are physically similar watery liquids that bathe the membraneous structures, but they are quite different in their chemical compositions.

All of the hearing end organ structures are contained within the cochlear duct. The floor of the duct or basilar membrane supports the *organ of Corti,* a complex structure which contains four rows of *hair cells* (the sensory cells for hearing) . The cilia or hairs of these cells are imbedded in, or otherwise attached to, the *tectorial membrane* which is anchored at its inner edge to the soft tissue covering of the spiral lamina and at its outer edge to some of the support cells of the organ of Corti. The cilia are mechanical receptors which respond to bending or shearing forces by producing electrochemical changes at the base of the hair cells. The cell bodies of the cochlear branch of the acoustic nerve are located in the modiolus and form a collection of nuclei called the *spiral ganglion.* Their bipolar (two-ended) nerve fibers interconnect the base of the sensory hair cells with the brain stem. The neural pathway then becomes a complex of multiple synapses from the brain stem to the auditory cortex where the neural messages from the ear are processed and perceived as sound.

The Hearing Process

The structures and the isolated functions of the three divisions of the ear have been examined rather briefly. During normal hearing, each of these divisions must function as part of a coordinated unit. Consequently, we will trace the pathway of sound energy from its source through the entire peripheral hearing mechanism and examine the interrelationships of its parts.

Air Conduction

Since man lives in an atmosphere of air, his hearing mechanism is specifically adapted to receive airborne sound. The longitudinal waves that emanate from a sound source impinge on the general area of the head and are directed by the pinna toward the external auditory meatus. The particles of the air within the external auditory meatus transmit the sound pressure variations to the eardrum and set it into mechanical vibration. The whole eardrum moves in a piston-like fashion and imparts its movement to the ossicular chain. At the footplate of the stapes, the same piston-like movements faithfully transmit the sound pressure variations through the oval window to the perilymph of the scale vestibuli. Normally, when sound passes from air to water, most of the energy (99.9%) is reflected back into the air from the air/water interface. However, the middle ear mechanism of eardrum and ossicles transforms the airborne pressure variations so that they are transmitted efficiently to the fluid of the inner ear.

The nearly incompressible perilymph is displaced toward the scala tympani, and as the footplate of the stapes is pushed inward, the membrane of the round window bulges outward into the middle ear cavity. The flexible cochlear duct also is displaced toward the scala tympani as the stapes moves inward. When the stapes moves outward away from the oval window, the round window bulges inward toward the scala tympani, and the cochlear duct is displaced toward the scala vestibuli. Since the basilar membrane is stiffer and narrower at the base of the cochlea and more flexible and wider at the apex of the cochlea, high frequencies will result in a maximum displacement of the cochlear duct near the basal end, and low frequencies will result in maximum displacement of the cochlear duct near the apical end.

As the cochlear duct is displaced upward and downward, the basilar membrane pivots at its attachment to the osseous spiral lamina and tilts the organ of Corti upward and downward. The sensory hair cells are supported by the organ of Corti, but their cilia are attached to the tectorial membrane. Since the tectorial membrane has a different pivot point than the basilar membrane, the tilting of the organ of Corti results in a bending or shearing of the cilia (Davis, 1970). This action is represented in Figure 2-10. The shearing forces exerted on the cilia produce an electrochemical change in the base of the hair cells that leads to the

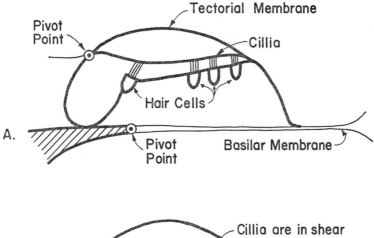

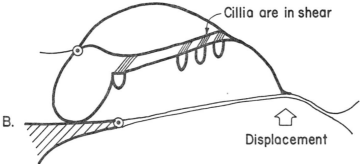

Figure 2-10. Schematic representation of the movement of the basilar membrane and the resultant shearing of the hair cell cillia.

transmission of neural impulses via the spiral ganglion to the brain.

Bone Conduction

In addition to the transmission of sound through the normal airborne route, the ear may receive sound pressure disturbances directly through the bones of the skull. Of course, this is not a very efficient pathway, for the transformer action of the middle ear is bypassed. However, if some vibrating source is placed against the skull (e.g. a ticking watch held tightly between the teeth) the pressure disturbances will be transmitted through the bone directly to the inner ear and then processed in exactly the same manner as the airborne pressure disturbances. At relatively low frequencies (below 800 Hz), the skull vibrates as a whole, but the ossicles lag behind in their movement because of their inertia (Bekesy, 1960). This results in movements of the footplate of the stapes relative to the oval window, and a consequent up and down displacement of the cochlear duct. At higher frequencies (above 1500 Hz) the skull vibrates in sections rather than as a whole, and waves of condensation and rarefaction alternately squeeze and expand the entire bony labyrinth. The fluid of the inner ear is forced against both the round and oval windows, and both of them bulge outward into the middle ear cavity. The membrane of the round window is more flexible than the oval window with its attached ossicular chain, and therefore its excursions into the middle ear cavity are of greater amplitude than those of the oval window. The result is an asymmetrical movement of the perilymph in the two scali and a displacement of the cochlear duct toward the scala tympani during condensation and toward the scala vestibuli during rarefaction.

The two types of bone transmission described above are *inertial bone conduction* (below 800 Hz and *compressional bone conduction* (above 1500 Hz). At frequencies between 800 Hz and 1500 Hz a combination of both actions seems to occur. It should be clear, then, that sounds that are transmitted through inertial and compressional bone conduction produce the *same type of cochlear activity* as do air-conducted sounds; and it should be clear also that all of these sounds are processed by the neural system in exactly the same manner.

Cochlear Processing

The mechanical movement of the cochlear duct has been described above as a displacement in an up and down manner. Actually, this is a simplification of a rather complex wave pattern that is propagated within the cochlea. Bekesy (1960) has shown that displacement of the cochlear duct is in the form of a *traveling wave*. This is, displacement of the basilar membrane begins at the basal end of the cochlear duct as the footplate of the stapes begins its inward movement. This displacement travels toward the apex and increases in amplitude until it reaches a maximum at some point between the base and the helicotrema. For pure tones, the envelope of such displacements is shaped like a teardrop with its widest portion toward the apical end of the membrane. The point at which the maximum occurs depends on the vibratory rate of the stapes which is determined by the frequency of the sound that is being received. Higher frequencies produce maximal displacement amplitudes toward the stiffer base and lower frequencies produce maximal displacement amplitudes toward the more flexible apex. Thus, the pitch that a listener hears will be determined at least in part by the location along the basilar membrane of maximum displacement. It should be clear, then, that the processing of frequency information begins in the cochlea by the hydromechanical selection of specific groups of hair cells for maximal stimulation.

The processing of intensity also is begun in the cochlea. Sounds of greater intensity produce wider overall excursions of the basilar membrane and result in larger traveling wave displacement envelopes. One can see that the larger the displacement envelope, the greater the number of stimulated hair cells. Recently, Davis (1970) has suggested that each *"auditory sensory unit"* (described by Davis as an afferent auditory neuron and its associated hair cell or cells) responds most readily to stimulation at a "best frequency" but will respond to an increasing band of frequencies as the intensity of stimulation for these frequencies increases. Consequently, it may be stated that an increase in loudness probably results from an increase in the number of "neighboring" auditory sensory units that are activated as a consequence of an increase in the amplitude of the overall displacement envelope. Furthermore, it is possible that the different rows of hair cells have "graded thresholds" at a given frequency and may respond differentially to different levels of sound intensity. In addition, the firing rate of each auditory unit may increase with increased sound intensity and present a greater initial density of neural impulses to the central auditory system.

Neural Processing

The extreme complexity of the processing of the neural impulses by the central auditory system is beyond the scope of this introductory chapter. However, some general comments may be made concerning the nature of the auditory pathways. The pathways divide and branch at several points, and a portion of the neural fibers cross to the opposite side of the brain stem for further branching and crossing. At each of these junctions there may be crucial ongoing processes that contribute to the eventual perception of both simple and complex sounds. The activities that occur at these junctions are being studied by many researchers, but a clear picture of the specific processes involved must await further investigation.

REFERENCES

von Bekesy, G.: In E. G. Weaver (Ed.) : *Experiments in Hearing.* New York, McGraw-Hill, 1960.

Campbell, E.J.M.: *The Respiratory Muscles and the Mechanics of Breathing.* London, Lloyd-Luke, 1958.

Cooker, H.S.: Time relationships of chest wall movements and intra-oral pressures during speech. Ph.D. Dissertation, State U of Iowa, Iowa City, Iowa, 1963.

Damste, P.H.; Hollien, H.; Moore, P., and Murray, T.: An x-ray study of vocal fold length. *Folia Phoniat, 20:*349, 1968.

Davis, H.: In Davis, H., and Silverman, S. R. (Eds.) : *Hearing and Deafness.* New York, Holt, Rinehart and Winston, 1970.

Draper, M.H.; Ladefoged, P., and Whitteridge, D.: Respiratory muscles in speech. *J Speech Hearing Res, 2:*16, 1959.

Fant, G.: Analysis and synthesis of speech processes. In Malmberg, B. (Ed.) : *Manual of Phonetics.* Amsterdam, North Holland, 1968.

Flanagan, J.L.: Some properties of the glottal sound source. *J Speech Hearing Res, 1:*99, 1958.

Green, J. H., and Howell, J. B. L.: The correlation of intercostal muscle activity with respiratory airflow in conscious human subjects. *J Physiol, 194:*471, 1959.

Hirano, M.; Ohala, J., and Vennard, W.: The function of laryngeal muscles in regulating .fundamental frequency and intensity of phonation. *J Speech Hearing Res, 12:*616, 1969.

Hollien, H.: Vocal pitch variation related to changes in vocal fold length. *J Speech Hearing Res, 3:*150, 1960.

Hollien, H.: The relationship of vocal fold length to vocal pitch for female subjects. *Proc. XII Int Speech Voice Therap Conf, Padua, 38,* 1962.

Hollien, H.: Vocal fold thickness and fundamental frequency of phonation. *J Speech Hearing Res, 5:*237, 1962.

Hollien, H.: Laryngeal research by means of laminography. *Arch Otolaryng, 80:*303, 1964.

Hollien, H.; Coleman, R., and Moore, P.: Stroboscopic laminography of the larynx during phonation. *Acta Otolaryng, 65:*209, 1968.

Hollien, H., and Colton, R.H.: Four laminographic studies of vocal fold thickness. *Folia Phoniat, 21:*179, 1969.

Hollien, H., and Curtis, J.F.: A laminographic study of vocal pitch. *J Speech Hearing Res, 3:*361, 1960.

Hollien, H., and Moore, P. G.: Measurements of the vocal folds during changes in pitch. *J Speech Hearing Res, 3:*157, 1960.

Husson, R.: Etude des phenomemes physiologiques et acoustiques fondamentaux de la voix chantee. Thesis, Universite de Paris, Paris, France, 1950.

Isshiki, N. Regulatory mechanism of pitch and volume of voice. *Otorhinolaryng (Kyoto), 52:*1065, 1959.

Isshiki, N.: Regulatory mechanism of voice intensity variation. *J Speech Hearing Res, 7:*17, 1964.

Jakobson, R., and Halle, M.: Phonology in relation to phonetics. In Malmberg, B. (Ed.) : *Manual of Phonetics.* Amsterdam, North-Holland, 1968.

Ladefoged, P.: Some physiological parameters in speech. *Lang Speech, 6:*109, 1963.

Liberman, A.M.; Cooper, F.S.; Shankweiler, D.P., and Studdert-Kennedy, M.: Perception of the speech code. *Psychol Rev, 74:*431, 1967.

Lieberman, P.; Knudson, R., and Mead, J.: Determination of the rate of change of fundamental frequency with respect to subglottal air pressure during sustained phonation. *J Acoust Soc Amer, 45:*1537, 1969.

Ohman, S.E.G.: Coarticulation in VCV utterances: Spectrographic measurements. *J Acoust Soc Amer, 39:*151, 1966.

Ohman, S.E.G.: Numerical model of coarticulation. *J Acoust Soc Amer, 41:*310, 1967.

Otis, A.B.; Fenn, W.O., and Rahn, H.: Mechanics of breathing in man. *J Appl Physiol, 2:*592, 1950.

Pattle, R.E.: The lining layer of the lung alveoli. *Brit Med Bull, 19:*41, 1963.

Peterson, G.E.: The speech communication process. In Malmberg, B. (Ed.) : *Manual of Phonetics.* Amsterdam, North-Holland, 1968.

Sonesson, B.: On the anatomy and vibratory pattern of the human vocal folds. *Acta Otolaryng* (Stockholm) , *52* (suppl.) :156, 1960.

Sonninen, A.: The external frame function in the control of pitch in the human voice. In Sound Production in Man. *Ann N Y Acad Sci, 155:*68, 1968.

Stetson, R.H.: Motor phonetics. *Arch Neurol Phyisol, 13:*179, 1928.

Stetson, R.H.: A motor theory of rhythm and discrete succession II. *Psychol Rev, 12:*293, 1905.

Timcke, R.; von Leden, H., and Moore, P.: Laryngeal vibrations: Measurements of the glottic curve. *Arch Otolaryng, 68:*1, 1958.

van den Berg, J.: Subglottic pressure and vibration of the vocal folds. *Folia Phoniat, 9:*65, 1957.

van den Berg, J.: Myoelastic-aerodynamic theory of voice production. *J Speech Hearing Res, 1:*227, 1958.

van den Berg, J.: Register problems. In Sound Production in Man. *Ann NY Acad Sci, 155:*129, 1968.

van den Berg, J.: Mechanism of the larynx and laryngeal vibrations. In Malmberg, B. (Ed.) : *Manual of Phonetics.* Amsterdam, North-Holland, 1968.

van den Berg, J.; Zantema, J. T., and Doornenbal, P., Jr.: On the air resistance and the Bernoulli effect of the human larynx. *J Acoust Soc Amer, 29:*626-, 1957.

CHAPTER THREE

CHILDREN'S LANGUAGE

ROBERT D. HUBBELL

MAN IS CONSTANTLY involved in communication. While there are many definitions of communication, I prefer the approach of Watzlawick, Beavin and Jackson (1967), defined simply as transfer of information. Such a definition implies that not only speech and language, but virtually all behavior has message character. More accurately, perhaps, all behavior is potentially communicative. The phrase, *potentially communicative,* is used to indicate that the receiver must know the code the sender is using in order to "read" the message. Note, however, that *transfer of information* does not imply any particular level of accuracy or truth, or even intent to communicate. Stated differently, it is impossible not to communicate. The refusal to communicate still involves behavior, even if it is only sitting still and keeping a poker-face, and this behavior carries the message, "I am not interacting with you."

Further, any particular communication situation may include simultaneous messages at various levels of meaning. First of all, there is the purposeful communication of ideas, thoughts and feelings, the things we typically think of when we consider communication.

Another level of communication involves the definition of the relationship between the participants in an interaction: the professor stands, the students sit; the professor wears a suit, the students dress casually; the professor talks, the students write. All of these behaviors help identify the relative positions of the professor and the students, their roles and status.

Another level involves the type of relationship between the participants. The professor and the students work out what kind of a relationship they will have, relaxed, formal, or whatever. This process is related to still another level, which consists of messages about how messages should be taken, or metacommunication (Haley, 1963). For example, the professor tells the students he is going to give them all D's, but he laughs and smiles as he says it, thus sending the metamessage that his remark is not to be taken seriously. Much of this multilevel communication is going on without the explicit awareness of the participants.

Language is one subset of this totality of communicative behavior. Language is a particular means of communication, consisting of an arbitrary set of symbols or lexical items and a set of rules for their combination transmitted and received primarily through the auditory-vocal channel. Much of the great power of language stems from the fact that it is made up of symbols, things that stand for other things. Thus, we can talk about things out of sight, in the past, in the future, and so on. These symbols are arbitrary, that is, they have no direct relation with what they refer to but simply are used to refer to roughly the same thing by the speakers of any particular language. The rules for their combination allow us to string words together to construct, manipulate and communicate complex ideas and thoughts. Language is primarily auditory-vocal. That is, it is based on speaking and listening. Writing is a relatively recent development.

This chapter contains two major sections. The first section will deal with children's language as it occurs in the communicative milieu described above. After discussing children's language and family interaction, I will discuss some ideas about therapy with children who are not using language as normal children do. The second section will consider children's language from a linguistic point of view.

LANGUAGE DEVELOPMENT AND FAMILY INTERACTION

Language acquisition is an interactive process, involving conjointly the child who is acquiring language and the speakers of that language who comprise his immediate environment, typically his family. In more general terms, the child learns to communicate by participating in the communication system his family has already developed. In turn, his participation in the system alters the system somewhat, so that the overall picture of language acquisition is one of a complex, multiply determined, reciprocal process.

In order to understand the family's role in language learning it is necessary to understand something about how families function. The family may be viewed as a social system in which all members of a family affect each other in a complex, dynamic balance. This concept is quite different from viewing the family as an environment in which things happen to a child, or focusing on particular dyadic relationships within the family.

The essence of a social system is interaction, which in turn is comprised of communicative behaviors. The major emphasis in considering a family as a social system is on how the family communicates, their rules for behaving toward each other.

Rules of this kind are everywhere, not just in families. Consider the rules governing the behavior of strangers in an elevator. It is not permissible to look at anyone's face for very long—it's better to throw your eyes slightly out of focus and stare at the neck in front of you, or concentrate mightily on the numbers flashing what floor is next. It is not permissible to touch anyone else. If someone backs into you, you move away, but not so far that you touch anyone else—it's better to suck everything in, think thin. There are strict rules governing what you can say—remarks must remain in the "social gesture" category, or be clearly humorous.

Usually we are not too aware of these rules. In fact, rules such as these do not come to strong awareness unless they are broken. If someone stares at you or leans on you in an elevator you become intensely aware of it. This paradoxical situation in which we follow these rules carefully but are not consciously aware of them stems from at least two factors. First, these rules are so ubiquitous, so omnipresent, that we don't think about them or recognize them as rules: *That's just the way people are.* Second, for the most part rules such as these are not taught directly as a child is taught to tie his shoes or write his name; we just pick them up.

The same ideas apply to many of the rules families develop for behaving toward each other. The result is a very subtle but well-developed and deeply entrenched pattern of behavior in a family: a communication system.

An important part of a family theory is the idea of *family homeostasis* (Satir, 1964). This term is used analogously to its meaning in biology, where it refers to the tendency of an organism to maintain some sort of equilibrium. Family members work out a balance with each other that maintains the system. Thus, if there is change in one family member others must change too in order to restore the balance of the system.

The regular, routinized, stabilized characteristics of a family may be referred to as family structure. Murrell and Stachowiak (1965) have described this structure in terms of three interrelated dimensions. The first is family style. This dimension involves the characteristic manner of relating that family members use. Some families are always jovial, some argumentative, some very intellectual, and so forth. To a great extent, family style determines the atmosphere in which a child learns to talk.

The second dimension is the pattern of interactions. These patterns involve such things as who talks to whom, who talks the most, and so on. The pattern of interaction in a family will control how much opportunity the child has to talk and what responses he gets. Interestingly enough, family members are usually unaware of these patterns.

The third dimension is the distribution of power and influence among family members. While the parents typically hold the power, deviant children, such as a child who does not talk, may have considerable control over the family. Again, family members may not be conscious of this situation.

Having briefly reviewed some aspects of how families function, let us now return to the subject of language development and interaction. The human infant begins communicating with people in his environment at a very early age. At one month he quiets down when picked up; soon afterwards he starts smiling and cooing; between six months and a year he's imitating, gesturing, and using many other communicative behaviors.

Most descriptions of children's preverbal development have focused on the child's behavior only (e.g. Lewis, 1951; Eisenson,

Auer and Irwin, 1963). However, Schiefelbusch (1967) has described this same period in the child's development in terms that include interaction with the environment. The first stage is *sensory stimulating and smiling.* This stage occurs during roughly the same time period as the crying and cooing stages of traditional descriptions. The infant seeks out stimulation and spends much of his time looking at things. He learns early to turn toward the bottle at feeding time. At approximately one month of age he begins to smile. Soon it becomes apparent that he smiles in response to environmental stimulation. His smiles, in turn, elicit more stimulation. In general, he seeks stimulation everywhere in his environment.

The second stage is *attachment.* This stage corresponds to the period of babbling and echolalia in traditional descriptions. The child continues seeking stimulation, but particularly from other human beings. Gradually an attachment forms between the child and the principle caretaker, usually the mother in our society. This attachment involves many social exchanges, such as smiling, babbling, and echolalia.

It is apparent, then, that when first words begin to appear, at about one year of age, the child has already developed considerable communicative ability. More specifically, in terms of speech development, the child has developed considerable skill in using his voice as an instrument of expression before he uses his voice to produce speech. In one sense, then, the development of speech can be seen, not as the development of a new mode of communicating, but as an enhancement of an already existing mode, vocalization. In fact speech may be considered an "overlayed" means of communication in the child (and sometimes in adults as well). Young children only use speech when they are relatively calm. When they are excited or emotional they express themselves through crying, laughing, jumping, gesturing, and so on.

From the family perspective, speech gradually develops in a context of relationships maintained by other modes of communication. The acquisition of speech provides the child a powerful tool, not only for ordering his environment through the use of symbols, but for extending his participation in relationships.

Research in Children's Language and Interaction

While the importance of the environment in the study of language acquisition has been recognized for a long time, the bulk of the literature has focused on the individual language learner, the child. In the past few years, however, interest in the interactive aspects of language acquisition has increased.

Of particular interest is a paper by Brown and Bellugi (1964) discussing some processes in the acquisition of syntax. This paper was part of a larger project, a study of syntactic development in two-year-olds. One of the processes they described was *imitation with reduction:* the child imitates utterances of the mother but reduces them to telegraphic form. For example, the mother's remark, *The car is blue,* might be reduced by the child to "Car blue."

Another process was *imitation with expansion.* In this case the mother imitates the child's utterances, but at the same time expands them to the nearest grammatical statement. The child's remark, *See truck,* might be expanded by the mother to *You see the truck,* or *Yes, I see the truck,* or some similar grammatically complete statement. Thus, according to Brown and Bellugi, much of the interaction between mother and child is a series of reductions and expansions. In addition they note that mothers appear to adjust the level of their language to be equal to or just a little above the level of the child.

Brown and Bellugi's discussion was based on the longitudinal study of two highly verbal children. Therefore, their descriptions of these processes are perhaps best considered only working hypotheses.

The significance of the observations of Brown and Bellugi in the present context is twofold. First, it is immediately obvious that language learning is very much an interactive process rather than simple imitation of a model. Second, the general picture that emerges is a reciprocal one in which the child's language usage affects the language in his environment at the same time that his language environment is affecting the language he uses.

McNeill (1966a, 1966b) has proposed that language is innate in man; the child is "prewired" for language learning with a "universal grammar," an abstract set of rules for how languages are formed. The function of the child's interaction with speakers in his environment, then, is to discover how the abstract set of rules is manifested in his particular language environment. For example, the universal grammar the child brings with him may include a rule that sentences are divided into subject and predicates. As he interacts with his language environment, the child's task is to find the rules for the formation of subjects and predicates in that particular language.

McNeill has suggested that this process is one of hypothesis testing by the child. The child hypothesizes how to form a particular utterance, and then tries it out. Feedback from more mature speakers in his environment gives him information about the accuracy of his hypothesized form. McNeill suggested that imitation with expansion may be a major avenue of this syntactic feedback. He points out that up to 30 per cent of the mother's remarks may be expansions in middle class families, although the percentage was much lower in the one more proletarian family for which data are available.

Cazden (1965) explored the phenomenon of imitation with expansion in a project in which she systematically expanded the remarks of a group of children in a Headstart program. Her findings did not support the notion that imitation with expansion was important in language learning.

It is worth emphasizing that the focus of research in this area has been on syntactic development, not on the communication of meaning. It seems probable that, whatever its effects on syntax, imitation both with expansion and reduction is a powerful semantic tool for both the child and his parents.

John and Goldstein (1964) presented a more semantically oriented view in their discussion of parental factors influencing the acquisition of labels. In particular, they emphasized the importance of corrective feedback from the parents as the child is learning a new label.

However, the functions and mechanisms of feedback in language learning are poorly understood and not all the evidence supports the idea that children use feedback when they receive it.

Braine (1968) argued that children who are learning language do not seem to be very influenced by corrective feedback at the level of syntactic learning. Further, Glucksberg and Kraus (1966) have demonstrated that, at least in their experimental situation, children of five years of age or younger are limited in their ability to make use of feedback at the referential level. A more basic question that has not even been approached yet concerns the relationships between the learning of the linguistic levels of language and the semantic and referential levels of language.

The emphasis in the discussion so far has been on how parents affect children's language behavior. In light of the interactive frame of reference being developed, it is necessary to ask also how children might affect their parents' language behavior.

While this area has not been explored experimentally, some findings are available concerning interaction between adults and retarded children. Siegel (1963a, 1963b; Siegel and Harkins, 1963) has studied verbal behavior between adults and retarded children by observing adults in interaction with retardates of high verbal and low verbal level in various structured situations. His general finding indicated that the adults' language behavior was different with the high verbal level children than with the low level children. With the high verbal level children the adults made more statements, demonstrated a longer mean length of response, and a higher type-token ratio (ratio of number of different words used to total number of words used, a measure of vocabulary) ; with the low level children the adults asked more questions and spent a greater portion of the total time talking. In general, these differences held constant whether or not the adults knew the verbal level of the child and even when they were told they were with a high level child when they were actually with a low level child and vice versa.

It is interesting to compare Siegel's findings with the suggestion by Jaffe (1958) that when communication is difficult, type-token ratios go down, because more repetition and simplification are necessary. Conversely, when communication is proceeding easily, type-token ratios get relatively higher, because a larger vocabulary and more elaborate statements can be used.

Returning again to the family perspective, O'Connor (1967) found that in families with one retarded child the whole family appears to "take care" of the retarded member, speaking for him and so forth. The retarded child takes on the corresponding role of the perpetual youngest child.

While empirical evidence is lacking, it would seem reasonable to extend the findings of Brown and Bellugi, Siegel, and O'Connor to include the family constellation of any child who is learning language, at least in middle class families. This general frame of reference has considerable import for the study of speech and language disorders.

Consider, as a hypothetical example, the child who is delayed in using language or whose speech is unintelligible. It seems possible that the whole family might compensate for this child's lack of speech, talking for him and so forth. At the same time the child, through his impoverished language behavior, limits the amount and level of language that other family members use with him, thus limiting his opportunities for learning more language. Looking at this process from a somewhat different viewpoint, the child's language behavior structures a situation which minimizes those responses in other family members which would, in Satir's (1964) terms, validate those attempts at language the child does make. The problem is even further complicated if the child is relatively successful at nonverbal communication (and most children are).

An important point in discussing this whole, reciprocal, homeostatic pattern is that it is not necessarily pathological. In a family in which the child's language delay is due to hearing loss or mental retardation, for example, this kind of pattern might be a relatively healthy way for the family to deal with that child, as opposed to such patterns as scapegoating or strong rejection. Nevertheless, the family militates against change in the child.

The point is that the family must communicate with the child, however he communicates, simply because they live together. The parents have to feed him, clothe him, get him to bed, toilet train him, and so on. If he doesn't talk, or if his language usage is limited, the family and child will work out ways of communicating that don't require much language on his part.

Again, this is not to be regarded as "sick" or poor parenting, although, of course, some speech and language disorders may be related to pathological family functioning. The problem is that the communication pattern the family works out won't do much to encourage more language from the child. In fact, the pattern may resist increased language development from the child. Further, the parents are not aware of much of this pattern, or its consequences for the child.

A good example of this resistance is *spokesmanship* or *mind-reading* (Watzlawick, 1963). I have had the following general experience a number of times. I will talk with a parent, and suggest that they give the child as many opportunities to talk as possible. We discuss this thoroughly, and I'm quite sure they understand. The next time I see them in the clinic waiting room, I will speak directly to the child, but the parent will answer for him. Therapist: "Hello, Johnny, I see you've got some new shoes." Parent: "Yes, we got them yesterday . . ." The parent understood my suggestion intellectually, but he wasn't applying it. Further, he probably isn't aware that he's shutting the child off.

In summary, children's language development and pathological language functioning are multiply determined, reciprocal processes. They are deeply enmeshed in family processes. The implications of this view are obvious: we must involve family members in the therapeutic process.

THERAPY

Therapy is a form of interaction. The reciprocal nature of interaction has previously been discussed. Each participant in an interaction is affecting the other participants; conversely, each is modifying his behavior according to how the other behaves. Siegel (1967) has discussed this phenomenon as it appears in therapy. As he suggested, the verbal behavior of the clinician is influenced by the verbal behavior of the client. Try tape-recording a therapy session with a child who doesn't talk much. You will be surprised (and possibly embarrassed) at how much of the total time was taken up by your verbalizations, even though the goal of the session was to encourage the child to talk. With a more verbal child, the picture may be quite different.

Therapy with children who are delayed in language usage should take cognizance of the fact that talking is an interactional process, and that most of the interaction influencing early language development takes place in the home. The child spends a few hours a week at most with the clinician. He is at home many times that amount.

Wyatt (1969) has mothers and children talk together every day. They discuss pictures, tell stories, and so on. No direct speech exercises are involved. She guides the mothers in providing verbal stimulation and feedback to the child. An important point is that she demonstrates what she wants the mothers to do, rather than relying on explanations alone. It is important also to follow up the next week, discussing with the parents in considerable detail how things went, so that you know how the parents are following your suggestions, and what changes need to be made, if any.

Wyatt teaches the mothers to use simple vocabulary, slow rate, and careful articulation during their daily sessions with their children. She also has them keep a notebook, so that they always use the same word for the same thing. Along similar lines, I have had parents put printed labels on various items around the house, so so that everyone, including the child, is constantly reminded that each item has a name, and what that name is. In addition to reminding family members to say the word, this procedure helps to minimize the confusion caused by using different words for the same referent. Thus the child always hears *water,* rather than such things as *Are you thirsty?, How 'bout a drink?* and *Want some water?*

Along with Wyatt, I suggest making home visits. Parents (and therapists) are often quite different people in their home environment. They're on their home ground, their fortress, rather than our fortress, the clinic.

Make sure you schedule your visits when both father and mother are home, and at least meet all the siblings. The tendency in speech pathology has been to work only with mothers, partly because they're more readily available, and partly because they often spend more time with the children than the fathers do. However there are many other factors that enter into the picture. For example, in a study in which both parents together were involved in a teaching task with each of their children, one at a time, I found that fathers were more active with younger siblings and male siblings, while mothers were more active with older siblings and female siblings (Hubbell, 1969). Thus it appears that sibling position and sex of the child may be instrumental in determining which parent would work best with a particular child. Further, from the perspective of family theory, it would seem most effective to work with both parents together, and perhaps with other family members as well.

The approach being suggested here is not parent counseling in a psychotherapeutic sense, although that may sometimes be necessary. Wyatt (1969) has pointed out that if a mother seems to be a poor language "teacher," it does not necessarily follow that she is a poor mother or that there is a poor relationship between mother and child. I approach parents with the attitude of "How can I help you?," rather than "Here's what I want you to do." This approach recognizes that they have the primary responsibility for the child, rather than relegating them to the position of "junior therapist," or amateur ancillary personnel. The approach is one of problem solving, of helping them find ways of enhancing their child's communicative performance.

For example, if you know that the child can vocalize or say a word for some particular thing, but he usually gestures for it, you might suggest that the parents ignore or "act dumb" to the gestures. Along the same lines, parents can hold out for a word or vocalization before giving some payoff, such as a snack or toy. Occasionally a parent will go overboard with this kind of thing, but this tendency can be minimized by demonstrating what you're talking about, making clear when and how much they should do it, and by following up soon afterward to see how it's going. Some clinicians formalize tactics such as these into operant conditioning programs. Further, some clinicians train parents to use operant conditioning techniques with the child as a regular part of the therapy program (Sloane and MacAulay, 1968).

One further point about having parents require some sort of verbalization from the child: it is important that parents understand that they need not expect nor demand full sentences from the child if he is not capable of them. For some children, single words, even if they are misarticulated, or just vocalizing, might be fine.

As you recall from the earlier discussion of family interaction, parents may not be aware of many of the things they're doing, many of the patterns they're following that operate against the child talking more. In working with the family you try to bring these things to awareness. One technique used by some family therapists is as follows. Have the family members agree on some specific behavior they want to change, spokesmanship for example. Then have them count and keep an accurate record of the number of times this behavior occurs for you to see next time. Often, the behavior will change with no other treatment. Apparently, two factors are involved. First, the behavior is brought to awareness. Second, the consequences of that behavior are changed.

I began this section on therapy with some discussion about how the child affects what the therapist does. I would like to close by mentioning another factor which influences the therapist's behavior. Rosenthal and Jacobson (1968) carried out the following experiment in a public school setting. Without telling the teachers, he randomly selected a few children in each classroom. Early in the school year he casually mentioned to the teachers that on the basis of some testing he had done these children could be expected to make a big spurt in achievement during the coming year. At the end of the school year he tested and found that these children had indeed accelerated beyond their peers, particularly in grades one and two. However, the only thing different about these children was that their teachers were told they were going to accelerate! This phenomenon has been called the self-fulfilling prophecy: as a child is labeled, so shall he be. Think on this as you approach children in therapy. Assume that the child can do more than he is now doing.

Linguistic Approaches to Children's Language

Grammar may be defined as the rules for combining words and morphemes into sentences. To the linguist, grammar does not refer to what we are taught in school about how to write a "proper" sentence. Rather, a grammar of a language is based on observations of how people talk, and their ideas about what is permissible and what is not in their language. The study of grammar is based on distributional evidence. In other words, the primary focus is on the privileges of occurrence of various elements in sentences, that is, discovering which elements (words, phrases, etc.) can occur in which positions in sentences.

Recent studies (Bellugi and Brown, 1964) of children's syntactic development have differed in a fundamental way from earlier studies (Templin, 1957). In the earlier approach the adult grammar was taken as the model, and the children's language was studied from that viewpoint. The current approach is to study children's utterances as if they were a foreign language, without references to adult grammar.

The first thing a linguist might do would be to gather a "corpus," i.e. a sampling of utterances. While in the case of a "real" foreign language the collection of this sample would be organized in various ways to obtain as much information as possible, with young children all one can do is record everything they say.

For example, suppose we wanted to describe all the multiple-unit vehicles on a freeway. We might station ourselves on an overpass over the freeway where we can easily watch. In a short time we might observe examples of the following combinations:

car	—	cargo trailer
truck	—	cargo trailer
car	—	house trailer
truck	—	house trailer
car	—	boat trailer
truck	—	boat trailer

The units in the left-hand column always precede those in the right as they go down the freeway.

In describing the privileges of occurrence of these combinations, we note first that there are two units in each combination, two positions to fill. Call these positions *slots*. Next we note that the first position can be filled by either a car or a truck, and the second by any of the three types of trailers. Thus there are two classes of vehicles, one for each slot.

Inspection of the corpus reveals that the fillers of the class in the left-hand slot can be interchanged. That is, it is permissible to have either a car or a truck in front of a cargo trailer, etc. Similarly, the fillers of the right-hand class are interchangeable. However, there are no instances of a trailer preceding a car or a truck. That is, the two classes are not interchangeable.

Let us now write these observations as a series of rules:

1. Multiple-vehicle $\longrightarrow$ $C_1 + C_2$
2. $C_1 \longrightarrow$ car, truck
3. $C_2 \longrightarrow$ cargo trailer, house trailer, boat trailer

These rules may be stated in words as follows:

1. A multiple-vehicle is composed of a class-one vehicle followed by a class-two vehicle.
2. A class-one vehicle is a car or a truck.
3. A class-two vehicle is a cargo trailer or a house trailer or a boat trailer.

By following these rules we could produce or *generate* all the combinations we say on the freeway, but no others. This same kind of procedure would be followed in writing a grammar of children's utterances.

The positions of the two classes are ultimately related to their function. That is, C_1 vehicles supply the motive power, whereas C_2 vehicles merely roll along. Exceptions to the rules can occur if these functions are not followed. For example, if we watch long enough, we will see one C_1 vehicle pulling another C_1 vehicle. At this point we invoke another practice of the linguist who is exploring the grammar of a language: we flag down the driver of one of these $C_1 - C_1$ combinations and ask him why one C_1 vehicle is pulling another C_1 vehicle. When he has recovered from the shock, he answers that the second vehicle threw a rod, or is out of gas, or is in some way not acting as a C_1 vehicle should, that is, it is not supplying motive power.

Stated more formally, we found an informant (a person who is a native speaker of the language we are studying, although in this example I suppose he would be a "native driver"). We asked our informant for information about a part of the grammar we did not understand. We could also ask him what kinds of combinations are possible and what aren't, etc. From the informant we learned that $C_1 - C_1$ combinations are permissible in certain situations.

Let us now expand our *grammar* to include single vehicles also, that is, cars and trucks by themselves. We may conceptualize this situation in the following way: the use of a trailer is optional. You may drive a car or truck, with or without a trailer. This is written into the rules by placing parentheses around the class that is optional (note that the other rules do not change):

$$\text{Vehicle} \longrightarrow C_1 + (C_2)$$
$$C_1 \longrightarrow \text{car, truck}$$
$$C_2 \longrightarrow \text{cargo trailer, house trailer, boat trailer}$$

This set of rules will generate all the multiple vehicles in the original corpus, plus individual cars and trucks.

We also notice that there are some combinations with three vehicles, for example a car, house trailer and boat trailer in a row. We look, but do not find, any instances of the order, car, boat trailer, house trailer. An informant tells us that this order is dangerous, and is not used. From this evidence, we can take the boat trailers out of C_2 to form a separate class, C_3. We now have three classes, two of which are optional. The order is not optional.

$$\text{Vehicle} \longrightarrow C_1 + (C_2) + (C_3)$$
$$C_1 \longrightarrow \text{car, truck}$$
$$C_2 \longrightarrow \text{cargo trailer, house trailer}$$
$$C_3 \longrightarrow \text{boat trailer}$$

This set of rules will generate all permissible single vehicles, two-unit vehicles, and three-unit vehicles.

Note that we now have three slots, although they are not always filled. In combinations such as car + house trailer, the driver has elected not to fill the third slot. In combinations such as car + boat trailer, the driver has elected not to fill the second slot. The filler of the third slot (the boat trailer) is moved over next to the first slot, but only because the second slot is not filled. It is necessary to think in terms of the maximum number of slots possible in order to number the classes properly, even when all slots are not filled.

The procedures outlined above are not intended to provide a fully developed method of grammatical analysis. They are intended merely as a brief introduction to one such method, based on the work of Kenneth Pike (Elson and Pickett, 1965). In summary, the method is based on distributional evidence. The slots, the classes that go in those slots, and the fillers that make up each slot are identified. Then rules which specify the relationships between these elements are worked out.

This same general approach has been used in the study of children's grammatical development. The first step is the gathering of a corpus. This is most easily done by tape-recording a child while he is talking in normal situations, such as play and interaction with parents and siblings. Sometimes a verbatim record of what the child says is taken down as a complement to the recording. In order to reveal the regularities of children's early language usage, this corpus should be extensive, probably five hundred utterances or more. The corpus is then organized to facilitate the study of the grammar involved.

From the very first it appears that children's word combinations are rule governed (Menyuk, 1969). That is, they are regular, rather than haphazard or random. At around one and a half years of age, the child starts combining words. These two-word combinations have been studied in considerable detail (Braine, 1963; Brown and Bellugi, 1964). The following examples are typical of these combinations (all examples are hypothetical data):

> daddy car
> daddy book
> daddy pipe

big car
big book
big pipe

We note that there are two slots and two classes. The rules to generate these sentences are as follows:

$$S \quad C_1 + C_2$$
$$C_1 \quad \text{daddy, big}$$
$$C_2 \quad \text{car, book, pipe}$$

(My use of the symbol "S", implying sentence, is somewhat arbitrary. Lee (1966) labels utterances such as these *constructions,* to indicate that they are regular and grammatical for the child, but are not fully grammatical from the adult's point of view) .

Suppose the child also made remarks such as:

car
book
pipe

We can amend our rules to generate these remarks also by indicating that C_1 is optional:

$$S \longrightarrow (C_1) + C_2$$
$$C_1 \longrightarrow \text{daddy, big}$$
$$C_2 \longrightarrow \text{car, book, pipe}$$

Thus, there is no remark that does not contain a C_2 word, but there are some remarks that do not contain a C_1 word. So far our development has closely paralleled the motor vehicle example.

Up till now we have said nothing about the functions of these two classes. In fact, by labeling them simply as C_1 and C_2 we have carefully avoided making any statement about function, but have restricted ourselves to indicating privileges of occurrence. It turns out, in real life, that children use a relatively large number of C_2 words, but relatively few C_1 words. The C_2 class has been called the *Open* class, because many different words can go in that class. The C_1 class acts somewhat as modifiers. They have been called the *Pivot* class. Thus this construction has been called the Pivot-Open construction, although more recently Menyuk (1969) has used the terms *Topic* for Open, and *Modifier* for Pivot. These labels represent judgments about the functions of these classes, about what they do in sentences. We can indicate these functions in our rules by substituting Pivot for C_1, and Open for C_2:

$$S \longrightarrow (P) + O$$
$$P \longrightarrow daddy, big$$
$$O \longrightarrow car, book, pipe$$

Now, suppose the child also uttered remarks such as the following (all the previously presented remarks are included also, to bring the entire corpus together) :

> see daddy car
> see big pipe
> see big book
> see daddy pipe
> see car
> see book
> daddy car
> daddy book
> daddy pipe
> big car
> big pipe
> big book
> car
> book
> pipe

These three-word constructions present no problem as long as we use our purely descriptive symbols. There are now three slots and three classes. We can label the new class (the word, "see") as C_1 and indicate that it is optional:

$$S \longrightarrow (C_1) + (C_2) + C_3$$
$$C_1 \longrightarrow see$$
$$C_2 \longrightarrow car, book, pipe$$
$$C_3 \longrightarrow daddy, big$$

(Note that I have renumbered the three classes, so that the numbers reflect the word order) .

This set of rules will generate all the utterances in the corpus and some others as well. While there is some debate about this, it is a common practice to permit the generation of such additional utterances because the distributions of the classes suggest that these utterances would be possible.

In considering function, it appears that C_1 is also a Pivot class, or modifier, particularly in the constructions *see book* and *see car*. We can indicate the function of this class by identifying it as "P_1" and adding it to our rules:

$$S \longrightarrow (P_1) + (P_2) + O$$
$$P_1 \longrightarrow \text{see}$$
$$P_2 \longrightarrow \text{daddy, big}$$
$$O \longrightarrow \text{car, book, pipe}$$

Another interpretation would be to describe the functions of these classes in terms of adult grammatical classes where possible. The Open class consists entirely of words adults would call nouns. The two Pivot classes contain a variety of adult classes, and therefore are best left as Pivots. We can rewrite our rules to reflect the fact that all Open class words in this corpus are Nouns very simply:

$$S \longrightarrow (P_1) + (P_2) + O$$
$$P_1 \longrightarrow \text{see}$$
$$P_2 \longrightarrow \text{daddy, big}$$
$$N \longrightarrow \text{car, book, pipe}$$

As a further step in considering function in the three-word combinations, we can assume that the second two words, e.g. *daddy car*, are treated as a unit by the child, and that this unit, in turn, is *modified* by another Pivot. *Daddy car* would then be considered as a Noun Phrase (NP), consisting of a Pivot plus a noun. This interpretation will require an extra step in our rules:

$$S \longrightarrow (P_1) + NP$$
$$NP \longrightarrow (P_2) + N$$
$$P \longrightarrow \text{see}$$
$$P_2 \longrightarrow \text{daddy, big}$$
$$N \longrightarrow \text{car, book, pipe}$$

It is important to point out that, in the last three statements of our rules, the utterances that can be generated are the same.

What has changed is our interpretation of how the child organizes these utterances. These changes in interpretation are reflected in changes in the forms of the rules. In the first instance we made no interpretation and labeled the classes simply as C_1, C_2, and C_3. In the second instance, we judged that the child was organizing the classes as Pivots and Nouns, and labeled them accordingly. In the final case we judged that the child was organizing the same classes as Noun Phrases, Nouns, and Pivots, and constructed our rules accordingly.

The reader should be reminded again that the above corpus consists of hypothetical data. In actual experience the corpus would be much larger and contain a much greater variety of utterances, including various syntactic forms, and doubtless some unintelligible material. One can see how quickly this kind of analysis gets complex.

Interpretations of Children's Grammatical Structures

Brown and Bellugi (1964) have described the early utterances of children as *telegraphic speech*. Children seem to form their utterances in the same way adults form telegrams. They retain the contentives, or content words, such as *book* and *go*. At the same time, they omit the functors, or function words, such as *to* and *is*. It is possible that, in using telegraphic speech, children are reducing what they hear adults say to a level they can handle. However, some authors (e.g. McNeill, 1966b) believe that the child is producing sentences with his own grammar, albeit limited, and that telegraphic speech has little to do with imitation of adult models.

McNeill (1966b) has interpreted the expansion of children's grammatical constructions to more than two words as the differentiation of the Pivot and Open classes. Neither the Pivot nor the Open class is equivalent to an adult class. According to McNeill, as the child expands his utterances, he is breaking down these two classes into classes more nearly approximating adult classes, such as nouns and verbs.

In the last several years, the theory of generative grammar has been proposed and developed (Chomsky, 1957, 1965; Fodor and

Katz, 1964; Bach and Harms, 1968, and many others). A generative grammar is one that will generate all of the sentences possible in a language, and no utterances which are not permissible. Thus the generative grammarian ic concerned with discovering a finite set of rules (a grammar), that will generate the infinite number of sentences possible in a language (Postal, 1968). The generative model is the basis of much of the work being done in the area of children's language.

In simplified form, this model posits three components to a grammar. The first is the *base*. This component contains the lexicon, or listing of words and the restrictions on their use, and the set of phrase-structure rules necessary to construct logical statements. The output of the base is called the deep structure. The deep structure may be roughly interpreted as the meaning level of a sentence. It seems to take a form somewhat similar to that of formal logic (McCawley, 1968).

Next is the *syntactic* component. This component transforms the deep structure representation of a sentence into a grammatically acceptable statement. This process is carried out through the mechanism of *transformations*. Transformations are rules for performing such operations as changing word order, deleting certain items, adding certain items, and so forth. They do not affect the meaning of the sentence. The output of the syntactic component is called the surface structure.

For example, consider the two sentences, *Bill painted the barn* and *The barn was painted by Bill*. Both of these sentences mean about the same thing. Thus, they are two different surface structures with essentially the same deep structure. They are produced by applying different transformations to the deep structure. Menyuk (1969) has discussed transformations in children's language in considerable detail.

The third component of a generative grammar is called the *phonological* component. This component provides a phonological representation of the deep structure. That is, it converts the surface structure into the sequence of sounds that we would use to say that sentence, according to the rules governing the usage of sounds in the language.

The theory of generative grammar is in considerable flux, with much debate on all sides. For example, it was originally thought that semantics and syntax could be considered as separate entities. However, there has been considerable argument to the contrary (e.g. McCawley, 1968). McCawley has also argued that there exists no compelling reason for positing a level of deep structure. Rather, the establishment of this level is an arbitrary decision. The point I would like to emphasize in this connection is that, while it may be useful in grammatical analysis, we do not know whether or not deep structure has a psychological reality. That is, we don't know if people actually use a deep structure in processing language. This concept needs further clarification before we devise therapeutic strategies that assume the existence of deep structure.

Another theme in generative grammar is the distinction between *competence* and *performance*. Competence refers to all one's understanding and intuitions about his language. Performance refers to what he actually does: what kinds of sentences an individual produces, and what kinds of sentences he comprehends. For example, we know the rules (have the competence) to construct a sentence so long and complicated that we couldn't possibly say or comprehend it, because performance is affected by memory and other psycholinguistic skills (Postal, 1968).

The distinction between competence and performance is related to an important problem in research in children's language: most of the work has concentrated on the child's output, his overt performance. The primary reason for this situation is that young children do not make good informants for linguistic analysis. They are unable to discuss such things as the grammaticalness of various utterances, or their intuitions about their language in general. Therefore, the investigator is forced to study how the child uses language, particularly his expressive behavior. However, it seems clear that the child's grammatical skills are greater in handling sentences that he hears than those he produces. Linguists assume that there is only one grammar for both expressive and receptive functions. Because this grammar is more fully demonstrated in receptive functions, this is clearly an area that warrants considerable study.

A case in point is the evidence Shipley, Smith and Gleitman

(1969) have presented that children do not always respond best to remarks couched in the grammar they use for expression. Specifically, children at the level of two-word combinations responded more frequently to remarks directed to them in simple declarative sentences than in two-word combinations. This finding strongly supports the notion that studying the syntax of children's productions will not fully illuminate their grammatical performance, much less their competence.

Some attempts have been made to explore children's receptive language skills (e.g. Fraser, Bellugi and Brown, 1963; Carrow, 1968; Berko, 1958). The general method has been to show the child pictures that differ in ways that can be represented in sentences through primarily syntactic, rather than semantic features. For example, two stimulus sentences might be, *The sheep is jumping* and *The sheep are jumping,* or *The boy hits the girl* and *The girl hits the boy.* The child would point to an appropriate picture, depending on which sentence he heard. One of the problems with this kind of approach is that there are only so many syntactic features that can be pictured in contrasting forms.

REFERENCES

Bach, E., and Harms, R.: *Universals in Linguistic Theory.* New York, Holt, Rinehart and Winston, 1968.

Bellugi, V., and Brown, R.: *The Acquisition of Language. Monog Soc Res Child Develop, 29:*43. Yellow Springs, Antioch Press, 1964.

Berko, J.: The child's learning of english morphology. *Word, 14:*150, 1958.

Braine, M.: Lecture delivered at the University of Kansas, 1968.

Braine, M.: The ontogeny of english phrase structure: The first phase. *Language, 39:*1, 1963.

Brown, R., and Bellugi, U.: Three processes in the child's acquisition of syntax. *Harvard Educ Rev, 34:*131, 1964.

Carrow, M.: The development of auditory comprehension of language structure in children. *J Speech Hearing Dis, 33:*99, 1968.

Cazden, C.: *Environmental Assistance to the Child's Acquisition of Grammar.* Doctoral thesis, Harvard University, 1965.

Chomsky, N.: *Aspects of the Theory of Syntax.* Cambridge, MIT Press, 1965.

Chomsky, N.: *Syntactic Structures.* The Hague, Mouton, 1957.

Eisenson, J.; Auer, J., and Irwin, J.: *The Psychology of Communication.* New York, Appleton-Century-Crofts, 1963.

Elson, B., and Pickett, V.: *An Introduction to Morphology and Syntax.* Santa Ana, Summer Institute of Linguistics, 1965.

Fodor, J., and Katz, J.: *The Structure of Language.* Englewood Cliffs, Prentice-Hall, 1964.

Fraser, C.; Bellugi, U., and Brown, R.: Control of grammar in imitation, comprehension, and production. *J Verb Learn Verb Behav, 2:*121, 1963.

Glucksberg, S.; Krauss, R., and Weisberg, R.: Verbal communication processes in children: Method and some preliminary findings. *J Exp Child Psychol, 3:*333, 1966.

Haley, J.: *Strategies of Psychotherapy.* New York, Grune and Stratton, 1963.

Hubbell, R.: *An Exploratory Study of Selected Aspects of the Relationship Between Family Interaction and Language Development in Children.* Unpublished doctoral dissertation, Kansas University, 1969.

Jaffee, J.: Language of the dyad: A method of analysis of interaction in psychiatric interviews. *Psychiatry, 21:*294, 1958.

John, V., and Goldstein, L.: The social context of language acquisition. *Merrill-Palmer Quarterly, 10:*265, 1964.

Lee, L.: Developmental sentence types: A method for comparing normal and deviant syntactic development. *J Speech Hearing Dis, 31:*311, 1966.

Lewis, M.: *Infant Speech,* 2d ed. New York, Humanities Press, 1951.

McCawley, J.: The role of semantics in a grammar. In Back, E., and Harms, R.: *Universals in Linguistic Theory.* New York, Holt.

McNeill, D.: The capacity for language acquisition. *Volta Review, 68:*17, 1966a.

McNeill, D.: Developmental psycholinguistics. In Smith, F., and Miller, G.: *The Genesis of Language.* Cambridge, MIT Press, 1966b.

Menyuk, P.: *Sentences Children Use.* Cambridge, MIT Press, 1969.

Murrell, S., and Stachowiak, J.: The family group: Development, structure, and therapy. *J Marriage Family, 27:*13, 1965.

O'Connor, W.: *Patterns of Interaction in Families with High Adjusted, Low Adjusted, and Retarded Members.* Unpublished doctoral dissertation, Kansas University, 1967.

Postal, P.: Epilogue. In Jacobs, R., and Rosenbaum, P.: *English Transformational Grammar.* Waltham, Blaisdell, 1968.

Rosenthal, R., and Jacobson, L.: Teacher expectations for the disadvantaged. *Sci Amer, 218:*19, 1968.

Satir, V.: *Conjoint Family Therapy.* Palo Alto, Science and Behavior Books, 1964.

Schiefelbusch, R.; Copeland, R., and Smith, J.: *Language and Mental Retardation.* New York, Holt, Rinehart and Winston, 1967.

Shipley, E.; Smith, C., and Gleitman, L.: A study in the acquisition of language. *Language, 45:*322, 1969.

Siegel, G.: Adult verbal behavior in play therapy sessions with retarded children. *J Speech Hearing Dis Monogr Suppl, 34* (No. 10) 1963a.

Siegel, G.: Interpersonal approaches to the study of communication. *J Speech Hearing Dis., 34:*112, 1967.

Siegel, G.: Verbal behavior of retarded children assembled with pre-instructed adults. *J Speech Hearing Dis, Monogr Suppl, 42 (No. 10)*:1963b.

Siegel, G., and Harkins, J.: Verbal behavior of adults in two conditions with institutionalized retarded children. *J Speech Hearing Dis, Monogr Suppl., 39 (No. 10)*, 1963.

Sloane, H., and MacAulay, B.: *Operant Procedures in Remedial Speech and Language Training*. New York, Houghton Mifflin, 1968.

Templin, M.C.: Certain language skills in children, their development and interrelationships. *Inst Child Welf (Monogr Ser)*, No. 26. Minneapolis, University Minneapolis Press, 1957.

Watzlawick, P.: *An Anthology of Human Communication*. Palo Alto, Science & Behavior Books, 1963.

Watzlawick, P.; Beavin, J., and Jackson, D.: *Pragmatics of Human Communication*. New York, Norton, 1967.

Wyatt, G.: *Language Learning and Communication Disorders in Children*. New York, Free Press, 1969.

CHAPTER FOUR

VOICE DISORDERS

JAY W. LERMAN

T HE DISCUSSION of voice and voice pathologies can be a very complex issue. Chapter Two demonstrated that the production of a sound consists of more than the simple abduction-adduction of the vocal folds, encompassing the action and interaction of large groups of muscles propelling a puff of air through a series of chambers (trachea, larynx, resonators) in a specific manner so as to produce an acceptable sound. Although much research has been conducted the entire process of sound production is not yet completely understood.

There will be no attempt in this chapter to discuss in detail the anatomy and physiology of voice production, except as they relate to specific vocal disorders.

It is impossible in the limited space available to discuss the many types of voice pathologies which exist. Several excellent books can be consulted for additional knowledge (Greene, 1964; Murphy, 1964; Levin, 1962; Luchsinger and Arnold, 1965; Brodnitz, 1959; and Van Riper and Irwin, 1958). This chapter will attempt to introduce the student to those voice disorders which are most often seen in clinics and schools, and to discuss the possible etiology, symptomatology, and course of treatment in relation to recent research in voice.

It is well to keep in mind that phonation is only one function of the larynx, the two primary ones being respiration and protection. A disruption in any one of these, however, can have negative consequences for the others; improper breathing patterns may have an effect on phonatory habits, and poor phonatory habits can result in pathologies of the vocal folds and associated laryngeal structures.

In voice production the function of the larynx is complex, but it is this very complexity that allows for its variety of movement.

However, like all complex devices, the larynx is subject to break-down. When sound production is disrupted, the whole life of the person is affected. We are concerned with the cause (more likely causes) of the dysfunction and with the restoration of the entire system (Damste and Lerman, 1970).

Normal or Abnormal

The question may not only be when is a voice *abnormal,* but also, when is it normal. Normality in voice as it relates to those aspects that make up an acceptable voice pattern (quality, pitch, loudness) has a wide range (Curtis, 1967), varying according to age and sex (Van Riper and Irwin, 1958) and from listener to listener (Dreher and Bragg, 1953).

Curtis (1967) has set up certain criteria for an adequate voice; the voice must be appropriately loud; pitch level must be adequate; voice quality must be reasonably pleasant; and flexibility must be adequate. Berry and Eisenson (1956) on the other hand, view voice in terms of abnormality. They state that a voice is defective:

> (a) when a defective structure or organic disorder of the vocal organs produces patterns of pitch, loudness, or quality which are sufficiently atypical to interfere with communication; (b) when voice production *results* in organic disorders of the vocal organs; or (c) when the habitual manner of voice production results in atypical patterns of pitch, loudness, or quality which are not appropriate to the sex and chronological age of the speaker or which detract markedly from the meaning or feeling that he wishes to communicate (p. 188).

The Diagnostic Examination

Like any other communication disorder voice problems require as complete an evaluation as possible. *Any individual with a voice problem should receive an examination from a laryngologist.*

Regardless of who sees the patient first, larynologist or speech pathologist, a case history should be taken. In most instances this will be done by the speech pathologist, since laryngologists generally pursue only the medical aspects of the problem. It should not be assumed by the speech pathologist that because the patient has had a laryngoscopic examination a case history has also been obtained. In many instances a second "going over" of the history may reveal previously overlooked factors and provide new insights into the disorder and its etiology.

Although the basic aspects of interview technique will not be discussed here it is important to note several things. Certain areas must be included such as family relationships, medical history, previous history of voice disorders, and a self-evaluation by the patient. Second, it is necessary to be very observant. Too often interviews get bogged down in the complexity (or ease) of their forms and are not really attentive to the patient's behavior. It is an important skill to interview for information while simultaneously analyzing the pitch, quality and loudness of the patient's voice. Third, it is strongly suggested that the entire diagnostic evaluation be recorded. This will enable the interviewer to reevaluate statements made by the patient, listen more carefully to the voice quality without interference of data gathering, and preserve permanently the interview so that it can be used later for comparison, for therapy, and for research.

As in any diagnostic evaluation the disorder itself must be analyzed. It is incumbent upon the speech pathologist (a) to determine if the vocal quailty, pitch, and loudness are truly abnormal; (b) to give an adequate description of the presenting voice; (c) to check the ability of the individual to produce a more normal vocal quality, which can be accomplished by observing closely what happens to the vocal quality under different methods of phonation.

In attempting to determine if the vocal quality is abnormal, the investigator may have to depend on those definitions of normal and/or abnormal presented earlier or any other criteria or standards with which he is familiar. In the final analysis, however, in most clinical situations the determination of normal or abnormal will be dependent upon the subjective analysis of the listener.

VOICE DISORDERS

Harshness

The distinguishing feature of harshness, as defined by Fairbanks (1960) is "irregular aperiodic noise in the vocal fold spectrum. . . .such speakers often overuse the extremely low pitches in their vocal areas, where maximum intensity is relatively low. Harsh speakers tend to initiate phonation abruptly with obtrusive glottal attacks." Other characteristics found in individuals with harsh voices may be rapid articulation, monotony, reduced pitch range, and in some instances, glottal or vocal fry.

Rees (1958a) indicated that perceived harshness changes in relation to a number of variables, such as the type of vowel being produced, height of tongue position in relation to vowel being produced, vowel environment (voiced, voiceless). In a later study (1958b) she found nonstatistically significant evidence "of a relationship between abruptness of vowel initiation and degree of perceived harshness." She did, however, present enough conclusive evidence to support the thesis that the obtrusive glottal attack is associated with harshness.

In the past, vocal fry has been viewed as a disorder of the voice either by itself or in conjunction with harshness. However, Hollien (1966) and others point out that "Vocal fry involves a physiologically normal mode of laryngeal operation that results in a distinctive acoustic signal." The fundamental frequency of the vocal fry is extremely low, far below that of the modal phonatory register. The study by Hollien and Michel (1968) indicated that the frequency range for male subjects producing vocal fry was from 7 to 78 Hz, while that for females was from 2 to 78 Hz. The many studies dealing with this phenomenon (Wendahl, Moore and Hollien, 1963; Coleman, 1963; Michel and Hollien, 1968; and Hollien and Michel, 1968) would suggest that it is indeed a separate phonational register resulting from periodic repetition rates, but it can also be present in vocal pathology, such as harshness.

Zemlin (1968) proposes that:

> The feature which differentiates the normal from the harsh voice is aperiodic noise, or irregular vocal fold vibration, which is often due to excessive tension of the folds (p. 209).

This concept of "aperiodicity" or roughness of the voice was investigated by Wendahl (1966) who used the terms "jitter" and "shimmer." Jitter is defined as the "abrupt cycle-to-cycle frequency variation," or "the rapid random variations in fundamental frequency." When the amplitude levels of adjacent pulses were alternately attenuated their resulting amplitude varying signal was termed "shimmer." It should be noted that the larynx and its concomitant structures are not perfectly symmetrical, so there may be some normal cycle-to-cycle variation in the vocal cord vibration (jitter), as well as in the amplitude levels (shimmer).

Wendahl (1966) and Coleman and Wendahl (1967) indicated that there is a proportionate increase between this cycle-to-cycle frequency variation and the listeners' judgments of roughness. Wendahl's work also shows "a systematic relationship between auditory roughness generated by the two procedures (jitter and shimmer) suggesting that the stimuli exist in the same auditory continuum. . . " The results of these studies, together with Fairbanks' definition, would suggest that the greater the extent of this aperiodic component in the vocal output, the more likely will be a judgment of harshness and/or hoarseness.

Harshness can be associated with organic and/or nonorganic voice problems, but it is the latter which is of main interest in this section. Generally speaking, excessive force due to tension in the various laryngeal muscle groups may be considered the prime cause of harshness not associated with organicity. Hypotheses have been made regarding relationships between voice quality and personality (Markel, 1964, 1969; Barbara, 1958; Moses, 1954; Muma *et al.*, 1968). Van Riper and Irwin (1958) state, "Our own impression is that in many instances the users of harsh voices are aggressive and antagonistic individuals, highly competitive and hypertense."

Hoarseness

Descriptive terms such as "strained, coarse, raspy" have often been used with hoarseness. A somewhat more sophisticated description is Fairbanks' (1960) approach that, ". . . .hoarseness combines the features of harshness and breathiness. . . . " (p. 182). Too often, usually, it is viewed simply as a symptom of severe colds or laryngitis. However, it may also be one of the very early signs of carcinoma, or even related to tuberculosis and syphilis; hence it is of special importance that a laryngological examination be done whenever prolonged hoarseness is the presenting symptom (Chew, 1966).

As with harshness, one of the most common causes of hoarseness is excessive muscular tension in the laryngeal area. This type of vocal disorder can result in, or be the result of, organic deviations of the laryngeal mechanism. Both physiological and acoustic studies have indicated that there are acoustic disturbances (noise components) within the fundamental frequency, as well as the higher formant ranges (particularly the third), that give this particular characteristic to the voice (Moore and Thompson, 1965; Yanaghiara, 1964, 1967a, 1967b). Von Leden (1968) has developed aerodynamic and acoustic measures of laryngeal function that have allowed him to recognize four types of hoarseness (Types I, II, III, and IV).

When seen in children (Baynes, 1966), hoarseness may be due to laryngitis, to abuse and misuse of the voice, together with excessive tension, or to the mutation period in the male adolescent (which will be discussed further in the section on pitch problems).

Breathiness

"Breathy quality is almost invariably accompanied by limited vocal intensity . . . Vocal attacks tend to be aspirate, in contrast with the glottal attacks of harshness" (Fairbanks, 1960:179). Breathiness is an escape of air through the glottis due to lack of proper closure which, in most instances, is organic in nature, but the familiar breathy voice of the "sexy" female is undoubtedly, in many respects, functional in origin.

Breathiness as opposed to hoarseness and harshness may be due to hypotension rather than hypertension. There is another point of view, however, suggesting that it is not strictly "either-or," but perhaps a combination that ultimately results in the disorder. In all likelihood the breathy voice, with no organic deviation, is learned. Since it is generally associated with females who are attempting to exhit a certain concept of femininity, and because of its general acceptance by the public, such a nonorganic vocal dysfunction rarely comes to the attention of the speech patholo-gist.

Resonance

Here we are referring primarily to hypernasality. In most cases, hypernasality is organic, due to clefts of the hard and/or soft palate, submucous clefts, and generally insufficient velopharyngeal closure. Among many children, hypernasality often occurs follow-ing the removal of tonsil and adenoid tissue, but in most instances it is temporary (Wallner *et al.*, 1968). Brodnitz (1959) states:

> Functional hyperrhinolalia occurs after tonsillectomy. Due to the postoperative pains, the patient 'splits' his soft palate, and hyper-rhinolalia results. After the pain has disappeared, the pattern of speaking with relaxed velum may persist and become permanent (p. 95).

Although a one-to-one correlation does not exist between the degree of closure and the perceived rating of hypernasality, the degree of velopharyngeal closure has a great effect on the amount of nasal resonance. The literature in cleft palate abounds with methods of determining adequate velopharyngeal closure and ways of measuring "objectively" the degree of nasal resonance. However, in the final analysis, it will be the examiner who makes the decision.

While there may indeed be other nonorganic and organic reasons for hypernasality, they are rarer ones or those more dif-ficult to observe or detect. The causes presented here are the most common and most normally seen.

Pitch

We have long used the terms *habitual* and *optimal* (natural) pitch. The former refers to that pitch level presently used by the speaker; this will vary but will be easily understood if we refer to Fairbanks (1960) who stated, "The central tendency of the pitches actually used by the individual will be termed the *habit-ual level*" (p. 123). By optimal or natural pitch we refer not to one note on the scale, but to a range of notes that allows for the most efficiency and least effort in the production of voice.

One of the most widely used methods of determining pitch level is that of Fairbanks (1960:169) who states, "The most satisfactory method that has been devised thus far for the calculation of the *natural* pitch level of an individual involves the determination of that pitch which lies 25 per cent of the way up that individual's total singing range including falsetto." (Both Fairbanks, 1960, and the revised edition of *Speech Handicapped School Children*, 1967:538-541, give examples of this method of estimating natural pitch.) Another way of measuring habitual pitch level is to have the speaker read a passage over and over, reducing the inflection pattern until a monotone is obtained, then matching this monotone with a musical device (piano, electronic organ, pitch pipe). But, because of the "musical ear" that is necessary for such an evaluation, this may not be a suitable method for all speech pathologists. Determining the difference between the individual's habitual and optimal pitches should be a routine investigation in almost all cases of voice disorder. It must be remembered, however, that with any of the methods used to determine pitch the examiner should not be influenced by a single note or pitch, but rather by a more well-defined range of notes or pitches.

Among the most common disorders are high pitch and falsetto. Physiologically and acoustically there are definite differences between normal high pitch and falsetto. When viewed in terms of registers, normal high-pitch is within the modal register, while falsetto is in the falsetto register (see Chap. Two and also Damste, 1968). Excellent descriptions of the mechanism of falsetto are given by Van den Berg (1968) and in a film by Rubin and Hirt (1960). In a study by Lerman and Duffy (1970) listeners were able to distinguish between falsetto and normal high-pitch at least 70 per cent of the time.

The Falsetto Voice. Prior to puberty the voice of the male child is generally perceived as of "high-pitch." With the onset of puberty (12 to 15 years of age) certain physiological as well as psychological changes take place. Some of the normal aspects of voice change in the male adolescent are hoarseness (Curry, 1949; Naidr *et al.*, 1965), or breaks or fluctuations of the voice between the newer voice quality (chest register) and the falsetto register.

Usually falsetto voice quality cannot be traced to organic deviation. True, there may be certain endocrinological disorders (eunuchoidism, castration, Klienfelter's syndrome) that affect voice quality in such a way that it remains high-pitched, but these are rare. Laryngoscopic examination is generally negative; in fact, some authorities feel that falsetto voice quality can be produced only by a mature laryngeal mechanism. In most instances the examining physician can obtain a lower voice in the patient "by pressing the thyroid cartilage inward" which counteracts the excessive contraction of the cricothyroid muscle (Arnold, 1964a).

The adult male with a falsetto voice, or *mutation falsetto,* as sometimes referred to, has already gone through the period of normal laryngeal growth; in other words, he is producing this vocal quality with a normal larynx. In such cases, with no organic deviation, possible etiologies can only be hypothesized: (a) inability of the individual to accept the responsibilities that come with maturity (Murphy, 1964), (b) a substitute, which has become habitual, for the embarrassing voice breaks that occurred naturally, and (c) premature voice change perhaps causing that child to maintain the "high" voice in order not to call attention to himself. Voice therapy may be difficult because of habitual use of the falsetto voice and the possible psychological variable involved. Therefore, counseling or psychotherapy in conjunction with direct voice therapy may be indicated (with such a disorder).

Other areas relating to pitch and mutation are *prolonged mutation,* and *incomplete mutation.*

In prolonged mutation, the voice quality is not one of high pitch alone, but rather a continuation of pitch breaks to the degree that it is noticeable and may interfere with adequate communication. The voice fluctuates between high and low, although in some instances the dominating pitch will be high, with the voice going to a lower pitch on those syllables that are accentuated. This certainly differs from the mutation falsetto, in which the use of this pitch has become habitual. Etiology here is considered psychogenic.

The individual with incomplete mutation "has failed to develop normal adult male pitch, although the physical mutation seems to have been completed and sexual development is normal. The voice lacks normal chest resonance, is somewhat dull, high-pitched, but not falsetto" (Damste, 1970). Etiology of this is still unknown.

Among other deviations in this classification are low pitch, mon-opitch (usually associated with congenitally deaf), and abnormal inflection (occurring mostly in foregin dialect). Van Riper and Irwin (1958) and Murphy (1964) also include tremulous speech and disorders of vibrato and tremulo, respectively.

ETIOLOGIES OF VOICE DISORDERS
Vocal Nodules

Vocal nodules are benign growths on the true vocal folds, varying in size from pin points to large polyp-like growths. They are located in the anterior and middle one-third of the true vocal folds and are bilateral and symmetrical. The cause of these benign epithelial neoplasms, which Van Riper and Irwin (1958) point out as resembling corns or callouses, is misuse or abuse of the voice.

It is felt by some that the highly tensed vocal folds tend to collide with each other with great impact, and at this point of impact a hyperplasia of epithelium arises as a source of protection for the folds. Luchsinger and Arnold (1965) and Arnold (1962) present excellent discussions related to the pathology, histology and laryngoscopic appearance of vocal nodules, which are probably the most frequently occurring organic voice disturbance.

Although they are seen in both children and adults, clinical evidence suggests they occur more frequently among middle-aged individuals and in those people who, by reason of their profession, are required to do a great deal of speaking, e.g. politicians, teachers, preachers, singers. Fitz-hugh (1958) stated that nodules are more prevalent in males (68.3%) than in females (31.7%), while in contrast Arnold's research (1962) indicates that the incidence varies within each sex group as a function of age, in women tending to increase with age, but decreasing with men. Ash and Schwartz (1944) report that there are more whites than blacks suffering from this disorder, reasoning that "The disproportion between whites and colored might be presumed to be based on the roomier, more relaxed and deeper pitched larynx of the Negro" (a point which merits further investigation).

Rubin and Lehroff (1962) feel that vocal nodules result in definite changes in vocal quality, such as breathiness and poor chest resonance and overtones. This is supported by Van Riper and Irwin (1958), who feel that the voice becomes weak, husky and breathy. This vocal quality may be due to the weighting of the cords by the nodules, which would interfere with the normal vibratory pattern. Other possible symptoms are voice fatigue, irritation, lowering of pitch.

The treatment of nodules is dependent upon many factors: age of the patient, motivation, size of the nodules, and length of time they have existed. Vocal rest, if practiced long enough, may result in complete disappearance of the nodes. However, a person who has had a long-standing problem is still left with the poor habits of phonation that originally contributed to the development of the nodes; hence, there is a greater chance that the disorder might recur. Vocal rest alone, therefore, is not the best form of treatment, but would be more beneficial in conjunction with voice therapy.

At times the surgical removal of nodules is necessary. This is usual in cases of long-standing nodules and when the patient is an adult. Brodnitz (1959) warns against the surgical removal of nodules in children because of the delicate nature of their laryngeal mechanism and also because children seem to respond well to voice therapy.

Polyps

Polyps can be unilateral or bilateral and occur almost anywhere along the vocal folds (but most commonly seen close to the anterior commissure) and, like nodules, vary in size and shape. "They may be pedunculated, projecting into the glottis, or they may hang down and become difficult to visualize" (Brodnitz, 1959).

Polyps have been said to be due to overstrain and abuse of the voice, or may also develop as a result of vocal fold edema if the accumulation of tissue fluid (effusion) is concentrated in one area and if the epithelium is thereby pushed forward. It is also felt that the polyp growth is not caused by vocal abuse but, due to its impeding of normal fold vibration, causes vocal abuse and voice quality dysfunction. The history of patients with polyps is very similar to that of patients with vocal nodules. The voice quality usually associated with a polyp is hoarseness, but other factors such as pitch and loudness may be affected, depending upon how the polyp interferes with the vibration of the folds.

The usual therapeutic treatment for polyps is surgical intervention. After removal, however, it is necessary that voice therapy begin in cases where poor phonatory habits have been established.

Vocal Fold Edema

Vocal fold edema means a swelling of the vocal folds.

> The epithelium which covers the muscles and the ligament of the vocal fold is attached to the underlying tissues by a loose connective tissue. The space between the vocal fold and this epithelial layer is called the subepithelial space of Reincke. Accumulation of tissue fluid in this space is called vocal fold edema (Damste, 1970).

This swelling of the folds is usually symmetrical. Although etiology is unknown it is thought to be caused, at least in part, by abuse and misuse of the voice by overtaxation, or by excessive use of the voice during throat infection. Because of the heaviness of the vocal folds, due to swelling, the pitch of the individual is low in frequency. This, of course, is caused by the reduced rate of vibration of the folds. In some instances glottal fry is noted.

Voice rest, in mild cases of edema, may reduce the swelling. When this is not successful, surgical procedures must be performed. This consists of *stripping* the cords in order to remove the swollen mass. Voice therapy should be initiated soon after surgery.

Contact Ulcers

Chevalier Jackson (1928) was among the first to use the term *contact ulcer,* and one of the best descriptions has been formulated by Peacher (1947):

> On indirect laryngoscopy, a tiny point denoting the ulcer is seen on the edge, involving the almost perpendicular internal surface of

the arytenoid cartilage. The lesion is exposed to view during respiration, but on phonation its internal surface is in contact with the inernal surface of the opposite arytenoid eminence which may or may not be ulcerated. The bordering mucosa is inflamed. Sometimes the edges of the ulcer are the same color as the surrounding mucosa. Granulomas formed from the granulation material are sometimes seen in the bed of the ulcer though, in most cases, it is only epithelialized.

These lesions, then, are located in the area of the arytenoid cartilage, usually at the point where the vocal cords attach to the vocal process. They differ from nodules or polyps in that they are not projections from the cord, but rather indentations in the cord. Contact ulcer is apparently an uncommon anomaly, Jackson (1935) reporting 127 cases in forty years, and Brodnitz (1961) claiming treatment for twenty-six persons in a period of eight years. The exact cause or causes of contact ulcer is unknown, although vocal abuse is still thought to be the main one. Peacher (1947) suggests that the disorder may be associated with age and sex; in her sample the average was fifty years, and the sex ratio was fifteen males to every one female.

In the same study, Peacher found the following deviations from accepted vocal usage:

1. Extreme tension of the speech musculature as well as generalized bodily tension;
2. Forcing the pitch far below the average pitch of male or female voices;
3. Glottal plosive attack;
4. Explosive speech;
5. Hoarse quality (p. 189).

The problem of treatment is still a confusing issue. Some feel that surgery may be necessary, while others rely mainly on vocal rest. However, all agree that whatever is done must be done in conjunction with vocal reeducation (Peacher, 1947).

Laryngeal Paralysis

There are many etiologies of vocal fold paralysis, but they are not all (in detail) relevant here. In brief, the problem is generally concerned with some lesion of the nerve tracts relating to the laryngeal mechanism, and for the most part due to involvement of the recurrent laryngeal nerve. Brodnitz (1959) feels that "the most frequent cause of vocal cord paralysis is damage to the nerve during a thyroid operation," which would seem to be borne out by Clerf (1953) who reported that fifty-nine of sixty-eight patients with unilateral paralysis became afflicted following a thyroid operation.

Paralysis can include the adductor and abductor functions. When there is an adductor paralysis, those nerve fibers that innervate the cricothyroid, the thyroarytenoid, and the lateral cricothyroid are damaged. These are the muscles responsible for adducting (closing) the vocal folds. The vocal symptomatology in this type of disorder is breathiness, weak voice, and constant or intermittent aphonia. Individuals suffering from such a disorder are seen to have a speech pattern that is strained, labored, tense. Such individuals often find it necessary to resort to whispering frequently. Certainly functions other than speech are affected, particularly respiration and protection of the larynx.

In contrast, abductor paralysis is characterized by a failure of the glottis to open. This is due to the lack of motor impulses transmited via the recurrent laryngeal nerve to those structures involved in the abduction of the vocal folds. The particular symptoms for this type of disorder are sudden spasm and inability to breathe.

Recent literature has been extensive with regard to the use of Teflon injection in the vocal fold (in unilateral paralysis) to bring it closer to the median position. (Arnold, 1964; Rubin, 1965a, 1965b; Kirchner *et al.*, 1966; von Leden and others, 1967). In general, the use of Teflon has been most advantageous in unilateral laryngeal paralysis when the affected cord has been immobilized in a position away from the midline. Other beneficial applications, as pointed out by Arnold (1964b), have been in chordectomy, vocal cord defects arising from surgical intervention (excessive removal of tissue), and "cases of congenital vocal cord deficiency, when the presenting hoarseness is due to bowling glottis . . ." Contraindications are also spelled out by Arnold. In those instances where Teflon may be contraindicated (bilateral laryngeal paralysis), surgical intervention may be necessary. A number of surgical methods have been devised, but the main objective is not to improve voice function, but to establish an adequate airway for purposes of respiration.

Carcinoma of the Larynx

The term laryngectomy means complete surgical removal of the larynx. The reason for such a drastic procedure, in most instances, is cancer of the larynx. When such an operation occurs phonation is no longer possible through the normal phonating mechanism.

The etiology of laryngeal carcinoma is still unknown. However, evidence suggests a link to excessive smoking and excessive use of alcohol and it has been further indicated that such disorders as leukoplakia, keratosis, and recurring papillomas may be precursors of laryngeal carcinoma. Although hoarseness is an early symptom of this disorder, it is also a symptom for many other types of disorders, including the common cold. As such, it is often ignored and consequently may serve to conceal, rather than reveal, the disorder. A thorough laryngeal examination is strongly recommended if the problem of hoarseness has existed for six weeks or longer. The late symptoms of this disorder are dyspnea, ear pain, aphonia and possible hemorrhaging.

Prognosis for laryngeal carcinoma is good, in fact, more so than for some other forms of cancer. Approximately 5 per cent of cancerous disease can be found in the larynx, but only "$1\frac{1}{2}$ per cent of mortality by malignancy is due to laryngeal cancer" (Damste, 1958). Reports on sex ratio have varied from as many as nine to fourteen males to every one female, and occurrence in most instances is in the forty-five to sixty-five year age group. In at least 50 to 60 per cent of the cases (all factors taken into consideration), there will be a survival rate of five years or more.

Various treatments have been attempted: radiotherapy (x-ray or radioactive cobalt), laryngo-fissures, and hemilaryngectomy. The latter two are not performed now as frequently as they were in the past. In the majority of cases either a narrow field or wide field laryngectomy is performed. Basically, the surgical procedure consists of the separation and removal of the larynx from the other structures (narrow field), but in some instances the hyoid bone and/or strap muscles (extrinsic laryngeal musculature) are also removed (wide field). Depending upon the extensiveness of the malignancy, a radical neck dissection may also be necessary. Snidecor (1967) in his book *Speech Rehabilitation of the Laryngectomized* supplies the reader with a comprehensive discussion of the surgical procedures involved in laryngeal cancer, including a discussion of the more recent Asai technique.

The removal of the larynx results in more than just a loss in voice. This leaves the individual without the socalled "voice-box" (the phonatory mechanism) and with a new airway (the tracheostoma). Because of the elimination of the normal airway, there will no longer be any concern about choking, but this is perhaps only a minor advantage, considering all the possible adverse effects of such a drastic surgical procedure. Since the laryngectomee now breathes through the "hole in his neck" (the tracheostoma), care must be taken so that no foreign objects enter this area, as it has no protection (other than being covered with some material), and leads directly to the lungs. He is no longer able to blow his nose or bring up phlegm in the normal manner; all this must be done via the tracheostoma. Extreme care must be taken during bathing and/or showering so that water will not intrude into the trachea, and various other physiological changes take place, affecting taste, smell, heavy lifting, etc.

Other Disorders Affecting Voice

Two other disorders of concern to the speech pathologist are spastic dysphonia and aphonia. While these problems occur relatively infrequently they are probably seen more often by the speech pathologist than the other disorders to be discussed in this section. Therefore, it behooves the reader to refer to other sources for a more complete understanding of the etiological and therapeutic aspects of these problems (Van Riper and Irwin, 1958; Murphy, 1964; Luchsinger and Arnold, 1965).

Spastic Dysphonia

This has also been referred to as "vocal stuttering." The individual with such a disorder usually exhibits the following voice symptomotology: (a) excessive strain in attempting to phonate; (b) actual stopping of phonation at times due to the great amount of tension in the laryngeal mechanism; (c) a tremendous amount of labor and effort in uttering a sentence of a few words, and (d) complete fatigue and aphonia after speaking only a short while. For many years the etiology of spastic dysphonia was thought to be of psychogenic origin (Bloch, 1965; Heaver, 1958; Cornut, 1965), but in recent years various researchers (Robe *et al.*, 1960; Aronson *et al.*, 1968a, 1968b) have proposed the possibility of neurological involvement.

Hysterical Aphonia

In this disorder no organic dysfunction is present. Aphonia literally means "no voice," but in the majority of such cases whispering is present. "When aphonia occurs in the absence of such physical factors, we look to the emotions" (Murphy, 1964). The onset of such a disorder may be very sudden, with the patient awakening one morning unable "to talk." In other cases, the patient may report that there has been loss of voice previously, but that it has always returned. Since the term "hysterical" historically refers to women, it would be obvious that more women than men have this "malady." "Therapy in almost all cases of hysterical aphonia must be at least partially psychiatric; usually a combination of psycho-therapy and voice therapy is effective" (Murphy, 1964).

Some voice disorders are congenital in origin; congenital asymmetry, laryngeal webs, laxity of the vocal ligaments, hypoplasia of the vocal folds, and even more exotic congenital disorders can be found in *Voice, Speech, and Language* (Luchsinger and Arnold, 1965).

Disturbances of the voice due to endocrine dysfunction may be hypogonadism (eunuchoidism), hyperthyroidism, hypothyroidism, and virilization of voice in women (Damste, 1964a, 1964b, 1967). Although the latter has not generally been familiar to the speech pathologist it is of considerable interest and one that suggests a great deal of further research.

Of the other organic disturbances, the most common, though

still infrequent, would be laryngeal trauma. Such disorders as tuberculosis and syphilis of the larynx, cysts of the vocal folds, granulomas, and papillomatosis of the larynx are relatively rare and infrequently encountered by the speech pathologist.

THERAPY

Voice therapy, be it for organic or nonorganic voice disorders, has as its major goal the use of more proper methods of phonation and the reduction or elimination of the original causes and maintaining factors. Certainly the methods for the elimination of organically caused voice disorders may differ from nonorganic ones, but usually only in terms of surgical intervention.

Moore (1957) states:

> The therapeutic approach . . . . recognizes the individual nature of voice defects and the need for planning each remedial program specifically for the person and his voice problem. Certain principles of therapy, however, are applicable to many kinds of voice problems, which makes it possible to offer some generalization about treatment (p. 689).

The goal of therapy is to obtain the best possible voice, utilizing the least possible effort, in relation to the existing anatomical situation (In some instances compensatory efforts must be made, as in the case of laryngeal paralysis where the functioning fold must exercise greater movement to take over some of the function of the paralyzed fold). Therapy involves more than vocal exercises, relaxation, and improvement in breathing, although these are all very important. Therapy also involves the person, his motivation, willingness to change, to learn new and more adequate methods of phonation. In general, however, there are certain therapeutic areas of importance in dealing with most voice quality disorders, these being relaxation, breathing and voice exercises.

Most individuals undergoing voice therapy find it difficult to relax. "Tension and vocal strain are recognized by speech pathologists as causes of numerous vocal difficulties. It is easier to achieve efficient, effective voice production if you can relax your entire body to a level of tension just adequate to the job at hand"

(Hanley and Thurman, 1963). Moore (1957) express it very well in his statement that "relaxation is a dynamic balance, in which the opposing groups of muscles exert just enough reciprocating tension upon each other to accomplish the desired movement with perfect control."

It would appear, from the previous discussion, that excessive tension is associated with some voice quality disorders, and if this tension could be reduced (or controlled) better habits of phonation could be established. Most therapists have tended to use the concept of "differential relaxation" suggested by Jacobson (1938, 1957). In using this approach the therapist is attempting to make the patient more acutely aware of the specific tension areas and then teaching him techniques to relax these muscles. Since the laryngeal area is the one primarily involved in voice disorders the patient may be asked to intentionally tense these muscles and then relax them so as to become more aware of the differences. Once the patient has attained this awareness and develops the techniques of relaxation the purposeful contraction of these muscles is no longer necessary prior to relaxation.

Greene (1964) states that relaxation of tension in any one part of the body "tends to overflow" to other parts and suggests working on relaxing the body initially while in the supine position. She also speaks of relaxation through suggestion. Fisher (1966) suggests specific exercises for the relaxation of neck and laryngeal muscles. She states that the purpose of these relaxation exercises is to learn how your throat feels when your laryngeal muscles are more relaxed so you control the degree of muscle tension in the future (p. 67-68).

Relaxation is not instantaneous. It does not alter the emotional attitude of the patient, but may have some minor psychological value in that in a more relaxed state the patient may be able to approach his problem(s) more realistically. However, in order to be truly effective, in regard to voice quality, relaxation must work in harmony with breathing and phonation.

Breathing exercises have long been advocated for individuals with voice disorders, indeed often stressed to such an extent that they are given to patients indiscriminately. It should first be determined whether or not a patient is breathing well enough to produce speech; then for those who do present improper breathing patterns, such exercises and training are a necessity. Differences may exist among voice therapists as to the efficiency of diaphragmatic breathing versus thoracic breathing, but almost all are in agreement that clavicular breathing is inefficient and unwanted. If poor breathing patterns exist then change must occur. The patient must be taught to make more efficient use of the breath, to learn to maintain a steady pressure without forcing or tensing, which requires a synchrony of movement of the muscles of respiration. Breathing exercises vary from therapist to therapist, but some excellent examples are suggested by Fisher (1966) and Greene (1964).

Vocal exercises will vary according to the particular disorders of pitch, quality, resonance, etc. (Greene, 1964; Murphy, 1964; Moore, 1957; Hanley and Thurman, 1963). In remembering that these exercises are utilized to establish a "new voice" with patients, it must be recognized that it is usually the therapist's voice which serves as the model. This means we may be asking the patient to produce a sound that may not be feasible, with his laryngeal mechanism, without forcing or tensing; in brief, the therapist's efficient voice may not be the most efficient for the patient. His new voice must come from his own repertoire.

One therapeutic methodology respecting this concept has been developed by Svend Smith of Hamburg, Germany (Unfortunately, there seems to be nothing written to describe it, hence the limited discussion to follow is based only on this author's discussions with, and observation of, various European logopedists using this method).

Smith feels, and rightly so, that phonation is concerned with more than just the adequacy of the laryngeal structure. Factors such as body position, breath control, and tension all play an important role in voice production. Although the patient will, of course, imitate the therapist, he will be simulating rhythmical pattern more than a voice model. It is this rhythmical pattern, with accompanying bodily movement—first in breathing, then phonation—that is the nucleus of the Smith method. Through this, tension is reduced and aspects of relaxation, breathing, and voice exercises are improved without undue therapeutic attention to each area separately. Since phonation must be effortless and easy to produce, exercises in the initial stage commence with a soft breathy sound and progress to louder less breathy vocalization (this is similar to one point in the five point program suggested by Moore, 1958). Smith does nothing to change pitch, feeling that during the vocal exercise it will change spontaneously as the poor stress and tension positions used by the patient are altered. The Smith approach neither lends itself easily, nor is done justice by written "instructionalization." Considerable observation and practice are indicated both for the therapist, who must become thoroughly familiar and at ease with the methodology, and for the patient, who must engage in very active participation.

Methods are avaliable so that the laryngectomized individual may speak again. While buccal speech, pharyngeal speech and the artificial larynx are still used by some, esophageal speech is generally considered the most adequate and preferable. Certainly, though, some of the clinical evidence (Diedrich and Youngstrom, 1966) would suggest that the artificial larynx be considered as a tool for immediate communication following the larngectomy.

Esophageal speech has been defined by Diedrich and Youngstrom (1966) as that type of speech:

> . . . . in which the vicarious air chamber is located within the lumen of esophagus and the neoglottis is located above (cephaled) the air chamber. The site of the neoglottis is the pharyno-esophageal segment or junction and may contain fibers of the inferior constrictor, cricopharyngeus, and/or the superior esophageal sphincter which are predominantly located at C5 and C6 (p. 108).

Most authorities agree with Diedrich as to the site of the neoglottis (Robe *et al.*, 1956; Damste, 1958; Snidecor, 1967) but one dissenting opinion can be found in the work of Micheli-Pelligrini (1957).

The process of speech rehabilitation has been very well presented by Diedrich (1966) and in the book *The Laryngectomized Individual and His Communication Problems,* edited by Lerman and Rigrodsky (1970). The following excerpt, taken from Lerman (1966), presents very basically therapeutic approach to teaching esophageal speech to a laryngectomee:

> The initial step in developing esophageal speech is the intake of air. There are basically three methods of trapping air: 1) inhalation, 2) injection, 3) swallowing. Any of these methods is satisfactory, provided the air is not completely 'swallowed' and stored in the stomach. Once the air has been taken in, the next step is the expulsion of the air.
>
> The terms 'belch' and 'burp' have often been used in referring to and describing esophageal speech. While many people, both the laryngectomized individuals and speech pathologists, have reacted negatively to such terminology, the use of these terms can prove invaluable as a therapeutic tool. The universal familiarity with burping or belching makes it a quick, unambiguous, vivid reference for the patient, and in the primary stages of therapy can be an excellent starting point. Although the approach is a very simple one, it can be met with early success and give reassurance, confidence and optimism. For the individual who has belched naturally since his operation, the prognosis for eventual speech would probably be very good. With others for whom the production of a 'belch' will be difficult to obtain, the speech pathologist will have to resort to other therapeutic techniques. However, once the 'belch' can be produced voluntarily on command, it should then be referred to as the esophageal sound or esophageal speech. When the sound can be produced at will, the next step is to attempt production of vowel sounds. Following a period of practice and success on the vowels, they may be combined with voiceless consonants, which do not require esophageal sound but rather the air already in the oral cavity (particularly the p, t, k and s) to form short words and syllables. From words the individual will go to short phrases, sentences and conversation.
>
> It must be noted that esophageal speech is not an easy process to learn. The simplicity with which it is explained here is not indicative of the difficulties which can be encountered in the therapeutic process (p. 272).

The reader should take special note that the system described above does not profess to be the entire therapeutic methodology. A description of the entire methodology would involve a discussion of all the psychological and physiological problems that the therapist may encounter, as well as a discussion of such factors as articulation, phrasing, air intake, prosody, etc. The previously stated reference should serve as beginning reading for the person interested in therapy with the laryngectomee.

Approximately 30 to 35 per cent of the individuals who undergo a laryngectomy do not learn, for psychological and/or physiological reasons, how to produce adequate esophageal speech. Studies concerned with this inability have been completed by Stoll (1958), Shames *et al.* (1963) and Gardner (1966). Recently changes in surgical procedures, such as the Asai operation and the procedure described by Taub (1970), as well as the laryngeal transplant done in Ghent, Belgium in 1969 (Kluyskens, 1970), may eventually eliminate or greatly reduce the need for esophageal speech. Indeed, it is hoped that continued research in the whole area of cancer may eliminate altogether the need for such types of speech rehabilitation.

Voice therapy, like others, must take into account the individuality of the patient. Usually, by the time the individual is seen for therapy, he has established a very set vocal pattern; he has become associated with his voice and vice versa, and to change to a "new way" of speaking often meets with resistance. The psychological components involved in dealing with individuals with vocal disorders will vary. They may be relieved with symptomatic management of the disorder or may require deeper consideration (It is hoped that the learning principles now being applied to problems such as stuttering and articulation may soon be applied successfully to voice disorders). The maturity and ability of the therapist will dictate whether these psychological components can be approached within the voice therapy situation, or whether a referral to an outside source is necessary.

SUMMARY

This chapter has covered disorders of the voice in relation to the following: (a) abnormality or normality; (b) voice quality; (c) diagnostic procedures; (d) voice disorders; (e) etiologies of voice disorders, and (f) therapy. The discussion was limited in scope, but attempted to emphasize clinical aspects and their research backgrounds. The function of the laryngeal mechanism is very complex indeed. Many factors involved in the causes of voice disorders are still unknown but further research and changes in therapeutic methodologies continue to increase our knowledge and provide answers to many questions.

REFERENCES

Arnold, G.E.: Vocal nodules and polyps: Laryngeal tissue reaction to habitual hyperkinetic dysphonia. *J Speech Hearing Dis, 26*:296-317, 1962.

Arnold, G.E.: Clinical application of recent advances in laryngeal physiology. *Ann Otol, 73*:426, 1964 (a).

Arnold, G.E.: Further experiences with intra-chordal Teflon injection. *Laryngoscope, 74*:802-815, 1964 (b).

Aronson, A.E. *et al.*: Spastic dysphonia. I. Voice, neurologic and psychiatric aspects. *J Speech Hearing Dis, 33*:203-218, 1968 (a).

Aronson, A.E. *et al:* II. Comparison with essential (voice) tremor and other neurological and psychogenic dysphonias. *J Speech Hearing Dis, 33*:219-231, 1968 (b).

Ash, J., and Schwartz, L.: The laryngeal node. *Amer Acad Ophthal Otolaryng, 48*:323-332, 1944.

Barbara, D.A.: *Your Speech Reveals Your Personality.* Springfield, Thomas, 1958.

Baynes, R.A.: An incidence study of chronic hoarseness among children. *J Speech Hearing Dis, 31*:172-176, 1966.

Berry, M., and Eisenson, J.: *Speech Disorders: Principles and Practices of Therapy.* New York, Appleton-Century-Crofts, 1956.

Bloch, P.: Neuro-psychiatric aspects of spastic dysphonia. *Folia Phoniat, 17*:301-364, 1965.

Brodnitz, F.S.: *Vocal Rehabilitation.* Rochester, Minnesota, *Amer Acad Opthamol Otolaryng,* 1959.

Brodnitz, F.S.: Contact ulcers of the larynx. *Arch Otoloryng, 74*:70, 1961.

Chew, W.: Importance of early diagnosis of hoarseness and its management. *EENT Digest, 28*:63-69, 1966.

Clerf, L.H.: Unilateral vocal cord paralysis. *JAMA,* 1953.

Coleman, R.F.: Decay characteristics of vocal fry. *Folia Phoniat, 15*:256-263, 1963.

Coleman, R.F., and Wendahl, R.W.: Vocal roughness and stimulus duration. *Speech Monogr, 34*:85-92, 1967.

Cornut, G.: Contribution a l'etude clinique et acoustique des dysphonies spastiques. *J Franc Otorhinolaryng, 14*:439-445, 1965.

Curry, E.T.: Hoarseness and voice changes in male adolescents. *J Speech Hearing Dis, 14*:25, 1949.

Curtis, J.F.: In Johnson, W.; Brown, S.F.; Curtis, J.F.; Edney, C.W., and Keaster, J.: *Speech Handicapped School Children,* revised ed. New York, Harper and Bros, 1967.

Damste, P.H.: *Esophageal Speech.* Thesis, print, Gronigen; Gebr: Hoitsema, 1958.

Damste, P.M.: Virile changes in the voice by androgens. Boerhaave Postgrad Course on Side Effects of Drugs. University of Leiden, Netherlands, 1964 (a).

Damste, P.H.: Virilization of the voice due to anabolic stereoids. *Folia Phoniat, 16:*10-18, 1964 (b).

Damste, P.H.: Voice change in adult women caused by virilizing agents. *J Speech Hearing Dis, 32:*126-132, 1967.

Damste, P.: X-ray study of phonation. *Folia Phoniat, 20:*65-88, 1968.

Damste, P.H.: De Pathologische Stembandfunctie. Leiden, Netherlands, 1970.

Damste, P.H., and Lerman, J.W.: Unpublished Manuscript, 1970.

Diedrich, W.D., and Youngstrom, K.A.: *Alaryngeal Speech.* Springfield, Thomas, 1966.

Dreher, J.J., and Bragg, V.C.: Evaluation of voice normality. *Speech Monogr, 20:*74-74, 1953.

Fairbanks, G.: *Voice and Articulation Drillbook.* New York, Harper and Bros, 1960.

Fisher, H.B.: *Improving Voice and Articulation.* New York, Houghton Mifflin, 1966.

Fitz-hugh, G. *et al.:* Pathology of 300 clinically benign lesions of vocal cords. *Laryngoscope, 68:*855-875, 1958.

Gardner, W.H.: Adjustment problems of laryngectomized women. *Arch Otolaryng, 83,* 1966.

Greene, M.: *The Voice and Its Disorders,* 2nd ed. Philadelphia, Lippincott, 1964.

Hanley, T., and Thurman, W.L.: *Developing Vocal Skills.* New York, Holt, Rinehart and Winston, 1963.

Heaver, L.: Psychiatric observation of the personality structure of patients with habitual dysphonia. *Logos, 1:*21, 1958.

Hollien, H., and Michel, J.F.: Vocal fry as a phonational register. *J Speech Hearing Res, 11:*600, 1968.

Hollien, H. *et al.:* On the nature of vocal fry. *JSHR, 9:*245-247, 1966.

Jackson, C.: Contact ulcer of the larynx. *Ann Otolaryng, 37:*227, 1928.

Jackson, C.: Contact ulcers of the larynx. *Arch Otolaryng, 22:*1-15, 1935.

Jacobson, E.: *Progressive Relaxation.* Chicago, U. of Chicago Press, 1938.

Jacobson, E.: *You Must Relax,* 4th Ed. New York, McGraw-Hill, 1957.

Kirchner, F.R. *et al.:* Studies of the larynx after Teflon injection. *Arch Otolaryng, 83:*350-354, 1966.

Kluyskens, P., and Ringoir, S.: Follow-up of a larynx transplantation. *Laryngoscope, LXXX:*1244-1250, 1970.

Lerman, J.W.: Laryngeal voice production. *Conn Med, 30:*271-273, 1966.

Lerman, J.W., and Duffy, R.: Recognition of falsetto voice quality. *Folia Phoniat, 22:*21-27, 1970.

Lerman, J.W., and Rigrodsky, S.: (Eds.): *The Laryngectomized Individual and His Communication Problems,* 1970 (in press).

Levin, N.M. (Ed.): *Voice and Speech Disorders: Medical Aspects.* Springfield, Thomas, 1962.

Luchsinger, R., and Arnold, G.E.: *Voice, Speech, and Language.* Belmont, Wadsworth, 1965.

Markel, N.M.; Meisels, M., and Houck, J.F.: Judging personality from voice quality. *J Abnorm Soc Psychol, 69:*458-463, 1964.

Markel, N.M.: Relationship between voice quality profiles and MMPI profiles in psychiatric patients. *J Abnorm Psychol, 74:*61-66, 1969.

Michel, J.F., and Hollien, H.: Perceptual Differentiation of Vocal Fry and Harshness. *J Speech Hearing Res, 11:*439-443, 1968.

Michel, J.F.: Fundamental frequency investigation of vocal fry and harshness. *J Speech and Hearing Res, 11:*590, 1968.

Micheli-Pellegrini, V.: On the so-called pseudo-glottis in laryngectomized persons. *J Laryng, 71:*405, 1957.

Moore, G.P.: Organic voice disorders. In Travis, L.E. (Ed.) : *Handbook of Speech Pathology.* New York, Appleton-Century-Crofts, 1957.

Moore, G.P., and Thompson, C.L.: Comments on physiology of hoarseness. *Arch Otolaryng, 81:*97-102, 1965.

Moses, P.J.: *The Voice of Neurosis.* New York, Grune & Stratton, 1954.

Muma, J.R.; Laeder, R.J., and Webb, C.E.: Adolescent voice quality aberrationals: Personality and social status. *J Speech Hearing Res., 11:*576-582, 1968.

Murphy, A.T.: *Functional Voice Disorders.* Englewood Cliffs, N.J., Prentice-Hall, 1964.

Naidr, von J.; Zboril, M., and Sevcik, K.: Die Pubertalen Veranderungen der Stimme bei Jungen in Verlauf von 5 Jahren. *Folia Phoniat, 17:*1-18, 1965.

Peacher, G.: Contact ulcer of the larynx. I. History, IV. A clinical study of vocal re-education. *J Speech Hearing Dis,* 67-77; 179-190, 1947.

Rees, M.: Some variables affecting perceived harshness. *J Speech Hearing Res, 1:*155-168, 1958a.

Rees, M.: Harshness and glottal attack. *J Speech Hearing Res, 1:*344-349, 1958b.

Robe, E.Y. et al.: Study of the role of certain factors in the development of speech after laryngectomy. I. Type of Operation. *Laryngoscope, 66:*173-186, 156. II. Site of Pseudoglottis. *Laryngoscope, 66:*382-401, 1956.

Robe, E. et al.: A study of spastic dysphonia: Neurological and electroencephalographic abnormalities. *Laryngoscope, LXX:*219-245, 1960.

Rubin, H.J., and Hirt, C.C.: The falsetto: A high speed photographic study. *Laryngoscope, LXX:*1305-1324, 1960.

Rubin, H.J., and Lehroff, H.: Pathogenesis and treatment of vocal nodules. *J Speech Hearing Dis, 27:*150-161, 1962.

Rubin, H.J.: Intracordal injection of silicone in selected dysphonia. *Arch Otolaryng, 81:*604, 1965 (a).

Rubin, H.J.: Pitfalls in treatment of dysphonia by intracordal injection of synthetics. *Laryngoscope, 75:*1381, 1965b.

Shames, G. et al.: Factors related to speech proficiency of the laryngectomized. *J Speech Hearing Dis, 28:*273-287, 1963.

Snidecor, J.C.: *Speech Rehabilitation of the Laryngectomized.* Springfield, Thomas, 1967.

Stoll, B.: Psychological factors determining the success or failure of the rehabilitation program of laryngectomized patients. *Ann Otolaryng, 67:* 550-557, 1958.

Taub, S.: New Prosthetic larynx. *Roche Medical Image and Commentary,* 1970.

van den Berg, J.W.: Register problems. Bouhuys, A. (Ed) : Sound production in man. *Ann Acad Sci, 155:*1968.

Van Riper, C., and Irwin, J.: *Voice and Articulation.* Englewood Cliffs, N.J., Prentice-Hall, 1958.

Von Leden, H. *et al.:* Teflon in unilateral laryngeal paralysis. *Arch Otolaryng, 85:*666-674, 1967.

Von Leden, H.: Objective measures of laryngeal function and phonation. Bouhuys, A. (Ed.) : Sound production in man. *Ann NY Acad Sci, 155:* 1968.

Wallner, L.J. *et al.:* Voice changes following adenotonsillectomy. *Laryngoscope, 78:*1410-1418, 1968.

Wendahl, R.W.: Laryngeal analog synthesis of harsh voice quality. *Folia Phoniat, 15:*241-250, 1963.

Wendahl, R.W.; Moore, P., and Hollien, H.: Comments on vocal fry. *Folia Phoniat, 15:*251-255, 1963.

Wendahl, R.W.: Laryngeal analog synthesis of filter and shimmer auditory parameter of harshness. *Folia Phoniat, 18* (2), 98-108, 1966.

Yanaghihara, N.: Experimental observations on the noisy quality of hoarseness. *Studia Phonolog, III:*46-57, 1964.

Yanagihara, N.: Hoarseness: Investigations of the physiological mechanisms. *Ann Otolaryng, 76:*472-488, 1967a.

Yanaghihara, N.: Significance of harmonic changes and noise components in hoarseness. *J Speech Hearing Res, 10:*531-541, 1967b.

Zemlin, W.R.: *Speech and Hearing Science: Anatomy and Physiology.* Englewood Cliffs, N.J, Prentice-Hall, 1968.

CHAPTER FIVE

CLEFT PALATE

HUGHLETT L. MORRIS

T HE PURPOSE of this chapter is to provide information about the problem of cleft palate, a description of the communication problems which the individual with cleft palate may demonstrate, a discussion of the etiological bases for those communication problems, information about diagnosis and treatment for those communication problems, and some comments about the role of the speech pathologist in the management of cleft palate. In addition, there is limited discussion about some unanswered questions concerning the speech pathology of cleft palate.

The chapter is written for the student of speech pathology in the intermediate stages of training. The material is not intended to be cursory nor is it intended to explore the various topics in great depth. A relatively detailed consideration of the effect of cleft palate on communication is presented by Spriestersbach and Sherman (1968). The reader who wants additional material or additional references should refer to that text.

THE CLEFT PALATE PROBLEM

Cleft lip and palate is a birth defect which results from the lack of fusion of the various parts of the upper lip and of the roof of the mouth. There is great variance in the extent to which the cleft can be demonstrated: incomplete cleft lip, cleft lip only, soft palate cleft only, cleft uvula only, celft of the hard and soft palate, cleft lip and palate, etc.

The birth defect occurs approximately once in every seven hundred births. While there are still many questions to be answered about etiology, many clefts are apparently the result of a genetic trait. Others appear to be the result of *in utero* factors which seem to interfere with fusion of the lip or palate or both. In general, the heredity factor appears to be closely related to the etiology of the cleft lip only or cleft lip and palate, while the *in utero* factors are associated with cleft palate only. There seem to be exceptions to that dichotomy, however. Whatever the etiology, it seems clear that the interruption in the growth-fusion process takes place between the sixth and twelfth week of pregnancy because, by the end of the first trimester, the lip and palate structures are "complete."

There are a number of effects of the cleft on the individual, some direct, some indirect. Certainly the individual with cleft lip looks different. Even after surgery, the remnants (some use the word *stigmata*) of the cleft lip scar remain. In addition, there is frequently distortion of the nose that is somewhat visible. The cleft lip has no effect on speech, however.

Usually, there is no effect in cosmetic appearance from a cleft palate only. The individual with the cleft palate, with or without cleft lip, can be expected to have problems with speech. Certainly he will have speech problems before the cleft palate is physically managed, and sometimes even after it is managed.

The individual with a cleft that extends through the alveolar ridge can be expected to have dental problems, usually related to malposed or missing teeth in the area of the cleft or adjacent to the cleft. Frequently, there are also problems of facial growth deformities. Sometimes these deformities may be related to tissue deficiencies, but more often they may be the result of interference with the growth process by the surgical procedures used to manage the cleft (lip or palate).

The individual with cleft palate can be expected to have more middle ear disease and associated loss of hearing sensitivity than is demonstrated by the normal individual. Although there is some disagreement about the cause of this otological-audiological problem, the etiology is probably related to the effect of the cleft on the function of the eustachian tube and/or the normal nasopharyngeal sepsis.

The cleft probably has an effect on the psychosocial aspects of the individual or on his family, although there is not much research evidence to support that contention. One explanation of the negative results of this kind of research is that in cleft lip and palate the emotional stress on the individual and/or his family occurs at highly specific times, such as at birth, when physical management is conducted, when the child starts to talk, when he starts school, and when he begins to show interest in the opposite sex. None of the available research has been designed to assess emotional status of the individual and/or his family at such times, and so the matter is still somewhat conjectural.

There is substantial evidence, however, to indicate that as a group cleft lip and palate individuals obtain scores on IQ tests which are a little lower (between 94 and 96) than the "normal" IQ. The slight reduction in IQ is probably related to the communication problems which these individuals demonstrate although that relationship has never been substantiated by research data.

Finally, the probabilities are somewhat higher that the cleft palate individual will have some other birth defect (in addition to the cleft) than they are for the noncleft individual. Within the group, individuals with cleft palate only have more defects than individuals with both cleft lip and palate. Certainly, the other birth defects are not caused by the cleft but are probably a part of the "syndrome" of cleft palate.

The management of cleft lip and palate is a highly complex procedure and requires the efforts of workers from a number of professions. It is difficult to describe a typical program of management because of the range of severity of the defect and because different emphases are placed on different aspects of the problem by different treatment centers. In general, the cleft lip is surgically repaired when the infant is about six weeks of age. The cleft palate may be surgically repaired, usually between the ages of one year to three years, or the cleft palate may be obturated with a prosthetic appliance. If an obturator is used, the prosthodontist will usually wait until the child has a sufficient number of teeth to enable the appliance to be secured. A major problem after initial (primary) management of the cleft palate is to decide whether the patient, child or adult, can obtain adequate separation of the nasal cavity from the mouth in speech (velopharyngeal competence) with the new structural arrangement, or whether additional physical management will be needed before velopharyngeal competence is possible.

The patient will usually need speech therapy for the purpose of modifying inappropriate patterns of speech behavior. Frequently, many of the inappropriate speech patterns stem from the fact that the child originally learned speech before palate management and so he had to compensate as best he could for the nasal escape of oral air pressure and excessive nasal resonance during speech.

The child with cleft palate will need various kinds of dental management: restorative, orthodontic, and prosthetic. Typically, the program of dental management is not completed until the patient is in his early teens. The adult with a cleft may need restorative and prosthetic dental care, also.

There are several kinds of medical treatment that an individual with cleft palate may need. As an infant and young child he may have repeated ear infections and will probably need treatment by an otolaryngologist. As he grows into the teen years, he may also need plastic surgery to revise orofacial structures, usually for cosmetic purposes.

Finally, he and his parents may need counseling from a clinical psychologist and social worker in order to work through problems of emotional stress which arise from time to time.

DESCRIPTION OF THE COMMUNICATION PROBLEMS OF THE INDIVIDUAL WITH CLEFT PALATE

There are three kinds of communication problems which the individual with cleft palate may demonstrate: articulation, voice, and language. A fourth communication problem, hearing loss, must be considered in clinical planning and management. However, the impact of hearing loss on the communication ability of cleft palate individuals is the same as that for individual without cleft palate. Since that material is presented elsewhere in this text (Chapt. Two), it will not be repeated here. One possible difference is that, in the main, the hearing loss shown by the cleft palate patient is conductive in type, not sensori-neural. Another possible difference is that as a child the cleft palate patient may demonstrate that type of hearing loss more frequently than the normal child.

A. Articulation Problems

Some of the articulation errors that children with cleft palate demonstrate are pretty typical of most children's speech. They show distortions of /r/ and /l/. They substitute front consonants for back consonants. They demonstrate interdental productions of sibilants or distortions of sibilants related to problems of tongue placement or a lack of an adequate dental cutting edge.

There are some articulation errors, however, that are unique to the patient with cleft palate or other kinds of palatal problems. The major characteristic of those errors is the audible nasal emission of oral air pressure during the production of plosives, fricatives, and affricates. The nasal emission may be "overlaid" on an otherwise normally-produced speech sound, in which case the type of error is usually referred to as a nasal distortion. Or the nasal emission may be "overlaid" on the substitution of another speech sound; such an error is referred to as a nasal substitution. There is great intersubject variability in the amount of nasal emission demonstrated. Some patients have so much nasal escape that it becomes difficult to recognize the speech sound. Other patients demonstrate so little that the leak of air is barely detectable. There is also considerable intrasubject variability in the amount of nasal emission during speech, particularly for the individual with a relatively small amount of escape. Typically, such an individual may be able to minimize the amount of nasal escape during the production of isolated words or in very slow speech. Maximal nasal escape (for the individual) may become more evident in rapid-fire connected speech.

Frequently, the individual who demonstrates nasal emission of oral air pressure during the production of the so-called pressure consonants also shows another typical feature of cleft palate speech: nares constriction. Nares constriction is an attempt to decrease the size of the nares by movement of the upper lip or the nose. The logical explanation for the behavior is that the speaker is trying to prevent the nasal escape of oral air pressure *anteriorly* that he cannot prevent in the velopharynx.

There are two other types of articulation errors that are relatively unique to the cleft palate patient: glottal stop substitutions and pharyngeal fricative substitutions. The glottal stop is a plosive-like sound produced at the level of the larynx and typically is used as a substitution for plosives, specifically /k/ and /g/. The pharyngeal fricative is a fricative-like sound produced by the constriction of the air stream by the walls of the pharynx. Both articulation activities are used apparently in an attempt to block or restrict the air stream at a level closer to the lungs than the velopharynx. The mechanics of these activities will be discussed in further detail later in this chapter.

B. Voice Problems

The major voice problem shown by cleft palate speakers is hypernasality. However, one can expect to hear other kinds of voice disorders, such as hoarseness, at least as often in the cleft palate population as in the normal population.

There is relatively great intersubject variability in degree of hypernasality, ranging from very slight to very severe. The intrasubject variability is less great for the group. However, speakers who demonstrate slight nasality are often very inconsistent; sometimes their voice quality is quite normal.

C. Language

Apparently, children with cleft palate demonstrate language which is less well developed than that of normal children, although the evidence is rather sketchy. What little data there is indicates that this "retardation" obtains only in early childhood and that, by the age of eight, the cleft palate child has developed language skills within the normal range.

CAUSES FOR CLEFT PALATE COMMUNICATION PROBLEM

Articulation errors characterized by nasal emission are caused by the inability to obtain closure of the velopharyngeal port. This difficulty is usually referred to as velopharyngeal incompetence.

The cause-effect relationship between velopharyngeal incompetence and hypernasal voice quality is somewhat less clear. Clearly, there is a relationship: coupling the nasal cavity to the oral tract results in hypernasality. But the question of whether there *must* be velopharyngeal opening for hypernasality to be perceived is unsettled. One recent research report (Carney and Morris, in press) indicates that listeners identified some very short samples of speech as hypernasal even though x-ray films taken simultaneously with the speech sample showed velopharyngeal closure. Additional research is needed to support that single finding before it can be viewed as conclusive. However, it may be true and, if it is, it would indicate that hypernasality is a very complex phenomenon, dependent on a number of factors other than velopharyngeal incompetence.

In any event, current information indicates that velopharyngeal incompetence is a major etiological factor in the speech problems of individuals with cleft palate.

The other major etiological factor in cleft palate speech is inappropriate learning. This factor is very difficult to define for this population, yet there are a few generalizations which can be made.

1. Some articulation errors are as clearly *functional* for the cleft palate individual as for the normal individual, notably such errors as distorted /r/ and distorted /l/. The cleft palate individual is surely as subject to factors which lead to the adoption of inappropriate articulation patterns as is the normal individual. Indeed, there is evidence that the cleft palate individual may be more likely to show these kinds of errors. Pitzner and Morris (1966) found that cleft palate children with velopharyngeal incompetence showed more errors on /r/ and /l/ than did children with velopharyngeal competence or than had been reported for normal children.

2. There is substantial clinical evidence that cleft palate speakers may adopt (learn) inappropriate articulation patterns in an attempt to compensate for oral structural defects. It is not difficult to understand how this can happen because, except in highly unusual instances, the cleft palate child must learn speech before he has all the necessary equipment! That is, he learns speech before the cleft palate is physically managed. The major equipment

problem he has is the inability mechanically to direct the air stream orally because of the opening between the nasal and oral cavities. Attempts to compensate for this inability may take many forms, usually having to do with tongue placement. Two very good examples of inappropriate articulation placement are the use of the glottal stop and the pharyngeal fricative. Clearly, these reflect learned behavior yet the two articulation gestures seem logically to be compensatory for the inability to direct the air stream orally (the result of velopharyngeal incompetence). That is, the individual is attempting to produce the plosive or fricative by valving the air stream in a location along the tract closer to the lungs than the velopharyngeal port. Apparently, he recognizes that if he tries to impede the release of the air stream at the level of the velopharyngeal port, nasal emission will occur. Consequently, he tries to do it "before" the level of the velopharyngeal port.

That the glottal stop and the pharyngeal fricative are learned is demonstrated by the fact that many cleft palate speakers continue to use them after velopharyngeal competence (and hence oral direction of the air stream) is possible.

Another example of a compensatory articulation pattern is the distortion of sibilants resulting from inappropriate tongue placement adopted to compensate for an inadequate dental cutting edge. The effect of the tongue placement is an oral distortion of the sibilant. (There may also be nasal escape, of course, unrelated to the tongue placement.) A variety of distortion can occur: interdental, lateral, and so forth. Again, that such distortions are learned is demonstrated by the fact that many cleft palate speakers continue to use them after an adequate cutting edge has been provided by means of newly-erupted teeth or a new dental prosthesis.

There is essentially no difference in the mechanics of this kind of compensatory articulation pattern between the cleft palate speaker with dental problems and the normal (noncleft) speaker with dental problems. Both must adjust articulation patterns to the lack of an adequate cutting edge. The difference is in frequency of occurrence and the duration of the dental problem. The normal child may have a relatively short period of time, around the age of six, in which the deciduous teeth are missing and the permanent teeth not yet erupted. By the age of eight, the probabilities are high that he will have adequate dentition. In contrast, if the cleft palate child's defect extends through the alveolus, he may not have an adequate cutting edge for a number of years, from infancy until perhaps age ten, at which time a prosthesis may be provided to supply the missing teeth. In the case of a cleft palate child, then, the process of speech learning will take place before he has adequate dentition and the problem of producing speech without adequate dentition frequently is extended over a considerable number of years.

There has been considerable speculation about the effects on articulation learning of other structural deficits which result from the cleft or accompany it. Examples are low palatal vault (postoperative palate surgery) and narrow or foreshortened maxillary arch (also postoperative). No research data have been reported to indicate that there is a relationship between such structural deficits and compensatory articulation patterns but it seems likely that such a relationship may exist, particularly if there were more than one of these "marginal" kinds of structural malformations.

3. There is the matter of whether nasally-emitted consonant articulation can be learned behavior. As indicated above, the probabilities are very high that the nasal emission occurs because the patient is unable to effect velopharyngeal competence. There is one circumstance, however, when such nasal emission can be functional: when the velopharyngeal incompetence problem has been remedied by physical management yet the patient continues to produce speech as if it had not been. Examples of this are just after the cleft palate has been surgically repaired or just after a pharyngeal flap has been constructed, as secondary surgery. Usually, however, if such is the case, the patient will be able to demonstrate the newly acquired velopharyngeal competence during some speech task or nonspeech task. Further consideration of this matter will be provided in the section on diagnosis in this chapter.

4. Related to that question is the question of whether hypernasality can be considered as learned behavior. As indicated previously, the most likely etiological factor for hypernasality is

velopharyngeal incompetence. Certainly there are examples of nasality as an aspect of speech which is obviously learned: some French vowels, some American English dialects, etc. It seems pretty improbable, however, that a youngster would learn and retain over a period of time the hypernasal voice quality patterns of his mother who demonstrates so-called cleft palate speech. The odds seem higher that he would learn her articulation errors than her voice quality disorder. There may be examples of such a phenomenon but none seems to have been reported in the clinical literature.

In summary, then, inappropriate learning appears to be an important factor in considering etiology of the speech problems of cleft palate speakers. Some of these so-called functional errors appear unrelated to the cleft but the majority of them are probably adopted in an attempt to compensate for oral structure deficits.

There are a number of other factors which are of potential etiological significance to the communication problems of the cleft palate individual. Some of them have already been referred to. A hearing loss of moderate degree which is sustained for a period of time during the first six years of life is sure to have an effect on the development of speech and language. A moderately severe dental problem may result in deviant articulation although the individual may be able to compensate for that kind of deficit. The same holds true for other kinds of structural deficits.

The effect of psychosocial aspects of cleft palate on speech and language is more difficult to estimate. It seems very unlikely that the group finding of slightly depressed IQ score is of any significance since the difference from the normal is not great. Such factors as the adjustment of the parents, the possible lack of speech and language stimulation, and the effects of repeated hospitalization may be a different matter, however. Certainly all of these kinds of things may have an effect on the parent-child relationship and the type of communication model available to the child and, hence, on the development of his speech and language. Research to evaluate the possible effect of such factors is very difficult to design, however, and there are not many data upon which to base any conclusions.

In summary, the available evidence indicates that, for the cleft palate group, velopharyngeal incompetence and inappropriate learning are the two factors of major etiological significance to the communication problems of the cleft palate speaker. Other factors, such as hearing loss, dentition, and psychosocial aspects, appear not to be significant in the etiology of the communication problems of the cleft palate group but may well be of etiological significance for certain cleft palate individuals.

DIAGNOSIS

The diagnostic task, of course, is to describe the problem, to compare the patient's status with the expected status, and to make some decisions about what to do. Although it is simpler to consider each of these three steps singly in this discussion, there is in clinical practice a great overlap among the three kinds of activities that are involved.

As indicated above, the examiner needs to use appropriate procedures to describe the articulation, voice quality, and language of the cleft palate patient.

A. Articulation

In general, articulation tests should include word articulation tests, a sample of connected speech, and a stimulability test. The speech pathologist needs both the word and connected speech tasks because frequently the cleft palate patient performs differently on them. He needs to use a stimulability test because he will want to be able to estimate the extent to which the patient can improve his articulation with auditory and visual stimulation. The tests should be easy to administer, and attractive and interesting to the patient.

The tests must be designed to provide a sampling of the various kinds of articulation problems that a cleft palate patient can be expected to demonstrate. The test must include a variety of consonants to provide an index to general articulation ability. It must also include plosive, fricative, and affricative items because those are the consonants in English which require velopharyngeal competence. An example of such an articulation test is the Iowa

Pressure Articulation Test (Morris, Spriestersbach, and Darley, 1961; Templin and Darley, 1969).

If one objective is to compare the articulation proficiency of the cleft palate patient with the proficiency of normal speakers, then a test must be selected for which normative data are available. An example of such a test is the Templin-Darley Tests of Articulation (1969).

Considerable attention must be given to the technique to be used in evaluating and recording the responses of the patient to the items on the test. Many of the inferences to be made from the testing results will be drawn from information about the type of responses and not just whether the response was "right" or "wrong." One of the significant kinds of articulation error that a cleft palate speaker may demonstrate is distortion by nasal emission. Another is oral distortion. The use of glottal stops and pharyngeal fricatives must be noted. Other more commonly observed errors, such as substitutions and omissions, must be noted.

Many clinicians attempt to distinguish among varying degrees of distortion, whether nasal or oral, by rating the degree of distortion on, for example, a two-point or a three-point severity rating scale. While such a distinction may be meaningful to the individual clinician, there are indications that the reliability of such ratings between clinicians is not very high, and so comparisons of such results between clinicians should be made with care.

The connected speech sample can be used in several ways. A rating of general intelligibility or general articulation defectiveness can be made from the sample. Or the sample can be constructed in such a way that it constitutes a sentence articulation test in which performance on a specific speech sound in the sentence can be evaluated. An example is the test devised by Van Demark (1964).

If ratings of articulation defectiveness of connected speech are to be obtained, the clinician must decide whether clinical ratings will be adequate or whether psychological scale values will be needed. Clinical ratings are easier to make but are less reliable than are psychological scale values. The decision will probably depend on the purpose the values are to be used for. The reliability of clinical ratings can be increased by consistent use of a training tape which presents the extremes of the continuum to be considered or some examples of varying degrees of severity.

In a stimulation test, the clinician attempts to find out how much the patient can modify (improve) his articulation of a speech sound with auditory and visual stimulation. It is, in a sense, a one-shot therapy session. There are a number of approaches that can be used. The examiner can stimulate the speech sound in isolation, in a so-called nonsense syllable, in a phrase, etc. Formerly, many speech clinicians worked with what can be called a hierarchy of complexity. An isolated sound was considered to be "easier" than putting the sound in a syllable; using the sound in a syllable was considered to be easier than using it in a word, and so forth. Currently, however, the trend in thinking about such matters is that such a hierarchy is probably an oversimplification if, indeed, true at all. Maybe, then, the speech clinician will want to simply stimulate a speech sound in a variety of phonetic contexts, without trying to place those contexts on any kind of continuum of relative difficulty.

In reality, the business about stimulation is an attempt to make observations about a phenomenon which is vital to the speech clinician interested in articulation skill: consistency (or inconsistency) of production. In diagnosis, a crucial question is whether the patient has in his repertoire of speech sounds the speech sound under consideration. Another question, if the speech sound is in the patient's repertoire, is *How consistently does he use it in speech?* Information of both types is valuable in deciding about whether speech therapy should be provided and, if so, what kind of speech therapy should it be.

B. Voice

Describing voice quality disorders continues to be one of the most difficult tasks for the speech clinician. Usually, clinical judgments can be used to reliably indicate whether there is or is not a disorder but, as reported previously, such clinical judgments are not sufficiently reliable to assess degree of disorder.

Regarding hypernasality, there have been several attempts to design instrumentation which will yield reliable results about degree of severity. In every case, however, the standard by which the usefulness of the instrument is evaluated is judgment by listeners. If listeners' judgments are to provide the final word about degree of hypernasality, why bother at all with the instrument?

There are indeed problems in using listeners' judgments to assess degree of hypernasality or any other voice quality disorder. If the observation (or rating) is to be reliable, the method of psychological scaling must be used. Sherman (1954) has used psychological scaling extensively to assess degree of severity of voice quality disorder, and has described the method in detail several times. Usually the method requires the use of a number of listeners who are instructed to assign each of a number of speech samples along a multipoint scale (sometimes a seven-point scale, sometimes nine, and so forth). The speech samples are usually tape recorded and have been edited to a specific length, usually from five to ten seconds. The recordings must be of relatively high quality. Sometimes, if the examiner wishes the listeners to disregard articulation skill in making the judgments, the recorded speech samples are played backward to the listeners. The scale to be used is frequently defined as an equal-appearing intervals scale, so that the distance between points one and two is equal to the distance between points two and three, and so forth. (Other types of scales, such as direct magnitude estimation, may also be used). Many times, only the extremes of the scale are defined, least severe and most severe for example. The criterion measure is the median or mean scale value assigned to the speech sample by the group of judges. Reliability within judges and between judges has been reported to be high (above 0.90) by many researchers.

The speech pathologist will find it difficult to use the psychological scaling procedure in the clinical setting. He does not have access to a panel of listeners, the sample of connected speech which he elicits from the patient is not homogeneous in length or content, he has access to other information which may influence his judgment, and he needs the rating at the time the examination is completed. There are adjustments which he can make in his clinical rating procedure, however, that will make his ratings more reliable. The simplest adjustment is to use the same "yard-stick" for all his ratings. One way to do this is to adopt the use of a standard rating scale to be used for all clinical purposes. The clinician should construct a training tape for himself which is comprised of a number of speech samples representing the extremes of the continuum he wants to use. He should then "train" himself relatively often by listening to the tape. Another helpful procedure is to compare his standards with those of his colleagues. The procedure might be (a) training himself and his colleagues with a training tape, (b) rating a number of speech samples with his colleagues, and (c) comparing the judgments. If there are discrepancies, a second training session may be needed.

C. Language

In general, the language problems presented by cleft palate youngsters are not distinguishable from language problems demonstrated by youngsters without clefts. Therefore, there are no special diagnostic procedures to be used. For a discussion of language problems in general, the reader should refer to Chapter 3 in this text.

D. Physical Structures

Up until now, the discussion about diagnosis has pertained to communication skills. There is need, particularly with the cleft palate patient, to consider diagnostic procedures to be used in assessing the adequacy of structure of the mechanism, namely, velopharyngeal competence, the oral mechanism in general, and dentition.

1. Velopharyngeal Competence

There is no single satisfactory measure of velopharyngeal adequacy for speech, although there are a number of procedures which yield useful information. X-ray films have been used for a number of years to provide information about the relationship among the velopharyngeal structures. Typically, lateral cephalograms are made with the patient at rest and during a sustained production of /u/ or /s/. These x-ray films show the structural relationships in the midsagittal plane. Estimates can be made of how much difference there is in the structural relationships between the rest position and the speech task, how much palatal movement and pharyngeal wall movement seem to occur during speech (as opposed to rest), whether there is palatal-pharyngeal wall contact during speech, and, if there is not contact, how large the velopharyngeal opening is. Similar observations can be made from cinefluorographic (motion picture x-ray) films. The chief advantage of cinefluorographic films is that the sample of behavior observed is larger.

There are some rather obvious limitations to the use of x-ray films in making inferences about velopharyngeal competence. One is that only the midsagittal plane is observed and anything occurring in any plane lateral to midsagittal does not show on the film. Another is that sometimes the image of the mandible obscures the area of the velopharynx on the film and makes interpretation difficult. The third is indeed obvious, but needs to be commented about: the film shows only what the patient does and perhaps not what he is capable of doing. For example, a patient typically uses a nasally-emitted /s/ but can with stimulation produce an orally-emitted /s/. If an x-ray film is taken during the nasally-emitted /s/, he will show a velopharyngeal opening. If the film is taken during the orally-emitted /s/, he will not. Which one is true? Clearly, both are. The point is that information from the film can be interpreted only when the speech pathologist knows the kind of speech sample that was used. Because the speech sample is so important, it is usually wise to have the speech pathologist present when the films are taken, rather than simply discharging the procedure to an x-ray technician.

Another procedure or group of procedures which are useful in assessing velopharyngeal competence is the general technique for measuring air flow and air pressures. There are several such techniques: among them are the respirometer, the warm wire flowmeter, the dynagraph, and the pressure sensing tube. All are designed to asses oral or nasal air pressure or air flow during speech (or nonspeech) activities. From such information, inferences can be made about the physiological function of the velopharyngeal mechanism for directing the air stream orally. In general, these procedures have not been used clinically to any great extent, partly because of the complex instrumentation required and partly because of the data-reducing problem. They offer considerable promise, however, with further development.

A procedure which is useful clinically but which is a relatively gross tool for assessing velopharyngeal competence is the oral manometer.* A ratio or quotient is obtained by comparing the reading achieved by a nostrils-open trial with the reading achieved by a nostrils-occluded trial. If the two readings are the same, the ratio is 1.00 and the conclusion is that the patient can prevent nasal emission during blowing with the velopharyngeal mechanism as well as he can by mechanically blocking the nares. If the nostrils-open reading is less than the nostrils-occluded reading, the ratio is less than 1.00 and the conclusion is that the patient has a velopharyngeal opening during blowing. A constant escape of air pressure (sometimes referred to as "bleed") is needed in the manometer system to prevent the use of buccal pressure (created by tongue-palate valving) in performing the task.

There are several disadvantages to the use of the oral manometer. It is not very precise. There is intra- and intersubject variability that may be very significant in evaluating ratios obtained for an individual. The difference between a ratio of 0.40 and 0.85, for example, is not clearly related to size of the velopharyngeal opening. On the other hand, the instrument is small, simple to use and maintain, and inexpensive. The procedure provides the clinician with information about the ability of the patient to direct the air stream orally on a nonspeech task, which is often important, particularly with a relatively small child. In general, the advantages of the procedure seem to outweigh the disadvantages (Morris, 1966).

Probably the most valuable information which the speech clinician can use to decide about velopharyngeal competence comes from the articulation tests he uses. The usual question is, of course, whether the patient demonstrates errors on the articulation test which are characterized by nasal emission, whether he

---

*Hunter Manufacturing Company, Old Quarry Road, Coralville, Iowa 52240.

demonstrates nasally-emitted pressure consonants consistently or whether sometimes he produces those consonants orally, and whether he can be stimulated to produce those consonants orally. If the patient is able to make some of the pressure consonants orally, even inconsistently, the conclusion (actually, the working hypothesis) is that the patient is capable of velopharyngeal competence.

2. *The Oral Mechanism*

The speech clinician needs to examine the oral cavity of patients with cleft palate as a matter of course. Any standard examination of the oral mechanism, such as that one described by Johnson, Darley, and Spriestersbach (1963), will yield valuable information. There are in addition several other observations which need to be made for the cleft palate patient. For example, the palate should be examined relatively carefully for structural defects which are related to the patient's ability to direct the air stream orally. Examples of such defects may be an open cleft palate, congenital palatal insufficiency, an alveolar cleft which was left unrepaired in the palate surgery, or an oral-nasal fistula resulting from postoperative breakdown of palate surgery.

Clearly, an unmanaged cleft palate is significant in the patient's ability or inability to direct the air stream orally during speech. Mechanically, the patient is simply unable to separate the oral cavity from the nasal cavity. The situation is less clear in the case of either an alveolar cleft or an oral-nasal fistula. In many cases, the alveolar cleft (which results in a connection between the oral cavity and the labial sulcus) is frequently "closed" in the functional sense by the upper lip and consequently has no great impact on the patient's ability to direct the air stream orally. If the cleft seems to result in a leak of air significant in speech production, it can be occluded frequently by a prosthesis which many cleft palate patients need anyway to provide missing teeth.

The effect of an oral-nasal fistula on ability to direct the air flow orally is even more difficult to assess. If the fistula is very small, the effect is probably quite minimal. If it is larger, perhaps larger than one or two millimeters in diameter, it can play an important role in speech because of the escape of air through it from the oral cavity to the nasal cavity. If the fistula is at the juncture of the hard palate and the premaxilla, it can perhaps be occluded by a prosthesis which the patient may need anyway. If the fistula is in a more posterior location, perhaps at the juncture of the hard palate and the soft palate, additional surgery may be needed to repair the fistula.

The alveolar cleft and the postoperative fistula present some diagnostic problems to the speech clinician because it is difficult to tell whether the nasal emission results from the anterior palate "defect" or from velopharyngeal incompetence. In addition, one can speculate that a fair test of maximal velopharyngeal efficiency cannot be made so long as there is a possible avenue for nasal escape via some other opening, such as an anterior defect. For that reason, it seems best to delay decision about velopharyngeal adequacy until any alveolar cleft or oral-nasal fistula has ben physically managed.

A bifid uvula or submucuous cleft (which is associated frequently with bifid uvula) is not directly relevant to speech production. The relevancy comes about because a submucous cleft is frequently associated with a congenital palatal insufficiency which in turn results in velopharyngeal incompetence.

Notice that a decision about velopharyngeal competence cannot be made from an intraoral examination of an intact soft palate, whether the patient has a surgically repaired cleft palate or whether he is suspected of having congenital palatal insufficiency. Observations of length or mobility made from the intraoral view (the inferior aspect of the palate) are simply not reliable enough to estimate whether the patient achieves velopharyngeal closure. Other kinds of information, mostly relating to palatal *function,* are needed before such a decision can be made.

Several comments need to be made about tonsils and adenoids. In general, the tonsils are not oral structures which are relevant for speech unless they are so very large that they interfere with tongue movement, which is very unlikely, or unless they essentially occlude the oropharynx, which is also unlikely. They may of course be inflamed and show signs of infection which may relate to frequent upper respiratory infections and associated hearing loss.

The adenoids present some specific problems, however, related to speech production. For example, a large adenoid pad may provide a sufficiently large cushion in the nasopharynx that a palate which is in reality too short may make contact with the posterior pharyngeal wall-adenoidal pad structure. In such an event the patient may be able to effect velopharyngeal competence and show normal oral resonance and normal oral pressure consonant articulation. If the patient has an adenoidectomy for reasons of health the cushion is removed, and velopharyngeal incompetence may result. Typically, many patients experience a temporary velopharyngeal incompetence during the first twenty-four to forty-eight hours after adenoidectomy, but if the palate is of normal length and mobility, the patient is able to compensate for the enlarged nasopharynx relatively quickly. If the velopharyngeal problem persists for longer, however, the mechanism may be deficient and the patient may continue to demonstrate "cleft palate speech."

Unfortunately, there are no diagnostic tools currently available to be used in predicting which patients will have this kind of problem. For the patient without a history of cleft palate, one very gross screening device is to question the patient or preferably his parents about possible nasal emission of milk when he fed as a baby. Another screening device which may be helpful is to question whether the patient showed any kind of nasal speech during his early development. Either sign can be interpreted to mean that there may be trouble postadenoidectomy. Neither sign is very helpful for the patient with cleft palate because the nasal emission of milk and the hypernasal speech will probably be simply a result of the cleft palate! If the speech clinician considers postadenoidectomy velopharyngeal incompetence to be a possibility, the surgeon should be notified about such possible surgical sequelae. He may want to discuss the problem with the parents. If there are strong indications for the adenoidectomy, everyone involved may elect to proceed. If the procedure is considered elective in any sense, other alternatives may be considered preferable.

It is interesting to note that apparently velopharyngeal incompetence does not result from the normal process of atrophy of the adenoidal pad, even in the case of a short soft palate (at least, no documented case reports have been made in the literature of such an occurrence). The atrophy takes place over a considerable length of time and in very small gradations. Apparently the patient is able to compensate for such small decrements by equally small amounts of extension of palatal movement.

3. Dentition

Decisions about the relationships between dental structures and speech production are exactly the same for cleft palate patients as for patients without cleft palate. The major difference is that dental problems occur relatively frequently in the cleft palate patient, particularly those with clefts which extend through the alveolar ridge. In general, the need is for an adequate dental cutting edge across which to send the air stream for sibilants and for a functionally large enough oral cavity for the tongue to be used to manipulate the air stream.

The first requirement is sometimes not met in patients with gross dental problems in which there are several missing teeth and a large alveolar cleft. Sometimes there are problems meeting the second requirement in instances of severe Class II (overjet) or Class III (underjet) occlusions. Another problem frequently encountered in cleft palate patients is the effect of an orthodontic appliance on speech, primarily, again, the sibilants.

There are almost no generalizations to be made about the matter of dentition and speech. A large majority of speakers seem to be able to compensate to a remarkable extent for dental abnormalities. Sometimes of course the speech clinician needs to help a patient learn to compensate but, very often, by the time the individual is ten years or older he may have worked the matter out himself.

FORMULATING CLINICAL IMPRESSIONS AND PLANNING MANAGEMENT

Using the results of the various diagnostic procedures, the speech clinician arrives at one of several clinical impressions regarding the extent of the communication problem demonstrated by the cleft palate patient, the nature of the problem, and procedures of choice for management. Generally, the great difficulty for the clinician in doing cleft palate speech pathology is in deciding what component of the problem is velopharyngeal competence and what component is inappropriate learning. There are some guidelines to be used, however, from the various diagnostic tests results. The following groups seem pretty readily identifiable in the cleft palate or palatal problem population.

Group I, velopharyngeal competence, consists of patients who may have misarticulations but either the misarticulations are oral in nature (as opposed to characterized by nasal emission) or can be stimulated to be oral. Typically, they do not present hypernasal voice quality. Typically, there are no great differences between connected speech and speech on an articulation test, although sometimes patients with recently obtained velopharyngeal competence, such as immediately postoperative pharyngeal flap or palate surgery or obturator, may have poorer connected speech than shown on the articulation test. They do not show nares constriction (unless they have only recently become able to obtain velopharyngeal competence). Oral manometer ratios for the group are typically 1.00 or perhaps between 0.90 and 1.00. X-ray films show contact between the velum and the posterior pharyngeal wall.

For the speech pathologist, the key is the fact that the patient can demonstrate orally-produced pressure consonants, either on the articulation test in connected speech, or following auditory and visual stimulation. The inference to be made is that the patient is capable of oral speech and it is the speech pathologist's task to help him generalize the oral response to other speech tasks. Therapy, then, is essentially a process of generalization, like that used in other types of articulation therapy. No special procedures are needed, except, occasionally, with young children, some nonspeech tasks such as blowing may be used as a so-called nucleus task.

There may be other physical problems, of course, such as dentition or hearing loss, but essentially the problem is one of inappropriate learning and the procedure of choice for management is therapy.

Group III, velopharyngeal incompetence, is at the other end of the continuum. In Group III are patients who show no ability to direct the air stream orally in speech in any context. That is, on every speech task (word articulation test, connected speech, or stimulation test) and on nonspeech tasks, there is nasal emission of oral air pressure. The voice quality is clearly and consistently hypernasal. Oral manometer ratios are lower than 0.89, usually lower than 0.50. X-ray films show no contact between the velum and the posterior pharyngeal wall. The patient shows nares constriction in a highly consistent manner.

The important observation with this group is consistency. During no task does the patient evidence the ability to close the velopharyngeal port. There may be other components to the problem, such as inappropriate tongue placement or dental irregularities, but there is also a physical deficiency involving the velopharyngeal mechanism. The procedure of choice, if normally oral speech is the objective, is physical management: pharyngeal flap surgery, pharyngeal implant or injection surgery, obturation, or palatal lift.

Clearly, surgery for purposes of speech is not to be considered lightly. No specific guidelines can be given for use in deciding whether a specific patient should or should not have surgery. Each case must be decided individually. Prosthetic management is less risky since no general anesthetic is required but even so, construction, maintenance, and adjustment of the dental appliance require some special attention.

Speech therapy is indicated, of course, if there are speech errors related to inappropriate learning rather than the inability to direct the air stream orally, such as on the /r/ and /i/. Or language therapy may be indicated.

There is no research evidence at this time that velopharyngeal competence can be taught by behavioral methods. There have been recent suggestions about the use of electrical stimulation or mechanical exercise procedures to assist the patient in extending the range of palatal movement, but neither procedure has been shown to be effective by reported data. Blowing exercises have been used by some speech pathologists as a method for extending the range of palatal movement but, in the same way, the use of that procedure has not been supported by research data.

Sucking exercises have also been suggested as a useful procedure but clearly they are not. The sucking gesture involves the creation of negative pressure by valving between the tongue and the palate, not palate and pharyngeal wall. During sucking, then, the velopharyngeal mechanism is not even involved (Creating negative pressure on an oral manometer with bleed is a different case, since the presence of the bleed forces the individual to open the tongue-palate valve and to try to close the velopharyngeal valve).

If the decision is made against physical management of the velopharyngeal inadequacy, the speech pathologist may decide to provide speech therapy designed to help the patient compensate for the physical deficiency. Note that the goal here is not normally oral speech but rather the best speech the patient is capable of. Usually that is still somewhat defective speech.

In principle, compensatory therapy of this sort is directed at the goal of minimizing the effect of the nasal emission. One way to do this is to teach the patient to use very light contacts on pressure consonants. The pressure consonants should be articulated only enough to be perceived, but with not so much force that the nasal emission of air will be greatly evident. Another procedure used by many clinicians is to teach the patient to increase size of mouth opening. The theory is that in the presence of a velopharyngeal opening, the larger the mouth opening, the larger will be the oral pharynx, and the less great will be the hypernasal resonance.

In summary, in light of the available evidence it is not productive to use therapeutic procedures or exercises of some kind to try to teach the individual with an inadequate velopharyngeal mechanism how to extend the range of palatal or pharyngeal wall movement. Attempts to help such a patient achieve normally oral speech with behavioral therapy will be frustrating for both patient and speech pathologist. If normally oral speech is desired, physical management of some kind will be needed. Otherwise, about all the speech pathologist can do is help the patient accommodate to the physical deficiency as well as possible. The speech pathologist should keep informed about new developments in the field of behavior modification, however; perhaps one of the techniques which have been suggested may prove to be fruitful.

Group II, marginal or borderline velopharyngeal competence, constitutes a group of patients between Group I and Group III. These patients present the most difficulty to the speech pathologist in diagnosis and decision making. In general, the dilemma with the group is that certain of the diagnostic signs point to the capability of velopharyngeal competence yet that capability is not fully realized even after extended therapy.

There seem to be two subgroups in Group II. For the sake of convenience, they can be identified as the subgroup that almost-but-not-quite achieves closure, which can be referred to by the acronynm ABNQ, and the subgroup that sometimes-but-not-always achieves closure, SBNA.

The ABNQ subgroup is relatively consistent in performance. Throughout most speech tasks, there is a very small amount of nasal emission of oral air pressure (Sometimes the escape of air is slightly more noticeable during connected speech than on a word articulation test, but that usually is not the case.). Typically, the patient is not able to eliminate the slight amount of nasal escape upon auditory and visual stimulation. Oral manometer ratios are usually between 0.70 and 0.90. X-ray films show a small opening between the soft palate and posterior pharyngeal wall, if tissue definition on the film is very good. If it is not, the film may be difficult to read or it may be read as indicating no velopharyngeal opening.

With the ABNQ subgroup, the speech pathologist is apt to feel that if the patient could be induced somehow to extend the range of movement of either the palate or pharyngeal wall only a little bit, then competence could be achieved. And indeed, that is probably the case. The problem is that, very likely, the patient has "pushed" the mechanism as far as possible to achieve the extent of closure which he demonstrates and that going that last mile will be difficult indeed, if not impossible.

Considerations of using speech therapy or palatal exercises with the ABNQ subgroup are essentially the same as for Group III. In light of current information, it seems highly unlikely that such treatment will be effective. Nor is compensatory therapy apt to be very effective since the patient has probably made maximal compensation already, particularly if he is older than eight years of age. If he is to be helped further, physical management will be needed. Pharyngeal implants seem particularly suitable for this kind of problem because the gap to be filled by physical management is so small.

The SBNA (sometimes-but-not-always) subgroup is more difficult to manage. The problem is consistency of performance. Essentially, a patient with such a mechanism seems to be able to effect velopharyngeal closure on tasks which involve a relatively slow rate of movement or which do not require continued muscle action. For example, he may demonstrate relatively oral plosives, but nasal emission on fricatives. He may demonstrate oral pressure consonants on a word articulation test but nasal emission during connected speech. If he can manipulate oral structures somewhat, he can obtain an oral manometer ratio which is high (0.90 or above). If, on the other hand, the manometer mouthpiece is inserted relatively far into the oral cavity and he is told to blow quickly, the ratio may be considerably lower. Interpretation of x-ray films will vary according to the nature of the task he performed while the film was taken.

The general picture then is that the speech pathologist sees indications from the diagnostic tests that the patient is capable of velopharyngeal competence and that the task is essentially one of generalization of response. She hypothesizes that behavioral therapy will be effective and proceeds on that basis. The problem is that the patient is unable to generalize the response and continues to demonstrate the same inconsistency of behavior even after extended speech therapy.

Apparently, patients in this subgroup have velopharyngeal mechanisms which are neurologically impaired, at least in part.

The impairment is such that the patient is simply unable to manipulate the mechanism rapidly enough and with adequate timing to obtain velopharyngeal competence which is appropriate for normally oral speech. That being so, physical management is indicated, if normally oral speech is desired.

SOME COMMENTS

A. The Role of the Speech Pathologist in Cleft Palate Management

Frequently there is confusion about the role of the various professional people on the so-called cleft palate team. Clearly, there is a great deal of overlap among the members of the team, particularly with regard to such aspects of treatment as counseling. Furthermore, extensive interaction among the professions is required if an effective plan of treatment is to be devised to everyone's satisfaction.

One thing is certain, however. It is the responsibility of the speech pathologist to describe the communication problems of the patient, to decide about the etiological bases for the problems, and to decide whether speech therapy or physical management is indicated. The speech pathologist has appropriate tools available to her for that task (or has colleagues in speech pathology who have the appropriate tools) and she must not abdicate that responsibility to some other discipline. After all, she is the one trained in understanding the process of speech production and possible pathologies of the process.

Relative to that point, it is particularly important that the speech pathologist make very clear to the patient, his parents, the surgeon, the dentist, and to other members of the team the goals of her program of treatment. A lot of confusion can result from lack of clarity about those goals. For example, consider the instance in which the speech pathologist reports that a patient has velopharyngeal incompetence, that she cannot assist him to achieve velopharyngeal competence, and that physical management is needed before normally oral speech is possible. Yet she continues to schedule him for speech therapy for faulty productions of the speech sounds /r/ and /l/. Unless she points out very clearly that the /r/ and /l/ are not dependent on velopharyngeal competence and that even if he learns and uses the appropriate /r/ and /l/, the nasal emission and hypernasality in his speech will not change, the patient, the parents, and all concerned are apt to be confused about her recommendations for physical management and her continual speech therapy. The two decisions may seem contradictory and need to be fully explained.

She needs, then, to make her position very clear to all.

Sometimes the speech pathologist is asked by other members of the team to try speech therapy to improve the patient's speech even though she has predicted from her diagnostic tests that the problem is physical, not behavioral, in nature. Whenever possible she should be willing to test her hypotheses just as she expects the other members of the team to do. This kind of trial therapy is legitimate and certainly justifiable since no one wants to perform physical management for a problem which is in reality behavioral in nature. Consequently, she may agree to give trial therapy for a specified length of time and to achieve specified objectives. If, after that specified time, use of the criteria she specified indicates that therapy is not being beneficial and indeed perhaps harmful, she should not be reluctant to be firm in her decision to stop therapy and to indicate that her diagnosis of velopharyngeal incompetence is valid. If there is still opposition to her position from other quarters, she must be willing to stand by her decision to the extent of discharging the patient from her clinical practice if that seems indicated.

One thing must be remembered, however. The proof of the diagnostic pudding is the results of therapy. In a real sense, diagnosis involves a set of procedures designed to provide information which will give shortcuts in therapy. If the speech pathologist is not really sure whether the patient has an adequate physical mechanism or not, she can always give trial speech therapy. If the patient begins to show more skill at directing the air stream orally, then she can hypothesize that he has an adequate mechanism and proceed with therapy. If the patient does not demonstrate a change, then the odds are very high indeed that he does not have an adequate mechanism and will need physical management, if normally oral speech is the objective of treatment. The only real danger is that the speech pathologist will continue to expect normally oral speech in the presence of an inadequate mechanism, will continue to give therapy, and will continue to ask the patient to do things which he is physically unable to do. The end result is a patient who is highly frustrated with his lack of progress and highly distrustful of speech pathology in specific and cleft palate management in general. That kind of clinical practice is unproductive and unethical in the standards of clinical speech pathology.

Finally, the speech pathologist should realize that she has no corner on the market in regards to evaluating social adequacy of speech. There are certainly several standards by which such adequacy can be judged. One is in the sense of normal-abnormal, and that is probably the standard used by most speech pathologists. If the production of /s/ is slightly deviant, it is judged to be abnormal. The problem may be so slight, however, that the patient, the parents, or any of the other members of the cleft palate team considers it to be "insignificant." Occasionally, there is such a decision to make about a patient with slight nasal emission and slight hypernasality. The speech pathologist reports that articulation and voice quality deviate from the normal. Is the deviation enough to warrant physical management? Some members of the team may think so, others may not. Because there is discussion about that decision does not mean that the judgement of the speech pathologist is being questioned, but rather that there are in reality two different questions involved. It seems clear that, in the final analysis, the decision about management must be made by the patient and/or his parents. They are the ones who will take the consequences of the decision, good or bad.

B. Some Unanswered Questions

The material presented in this chapter is based on information currently available and it is important to point out that the body of knowledge in cleft palate management has expanded considerably during the last twenty years. However, there are still many unanswered questions and deficiencies in our understanding of the problem and procedures for management. Some of these un-answered questions are presented here to alert the speech pathol-ogist-in-training to issues which can be expected to receive con-siderable research attention during the next decade.

1. What are the requirements for velopharyngeal competence for normally oral speech?

The position presented in this chapter is that the speaker must be able to achieve complete velopharyngeal closure, and relatively easily so, to be able to use normally oral plosives and fricatives in connected speech. It may be that the normal speaker does not always demonstrate that competence during production of plosives and fricatives but he must be able to do so.

Clearly, additional research is needed. It may be that under certain circumstances a small velopharyngeal opening is permissi-ble. A better understanding of the normal mechanism will assist greatly in specifying the goals of management for the pathological palate.

2. What are the physical correlates of hypernasality?

Again, the position taken here is that the only way the phe-nomenon of hypernasality can occur is in the presence of coupling between the oral and nasal cavities (that is, velopharyngeal in-competence). Additional information is needed. The findings of Carney and Morris (in preparation) indicate that hypernasality may occur in the presence of velopharyngeal competence. If that is the case, the position taken here may represent an oversimplifica-tion. (Curtis, 1970, has provided a discussion of nasalized speech which will be helpful to the reader who is interested in this matter.)

3. Is it possible to assist an individual in extending the range of movement of the soft palate and/or posterior pharyngeal wall by therapeutic exercises or treatments of some sort?

As reported above, there is almost no information currently available which indicates that exercises or treatments are success-ful. There are several research programs either recently completed or now under way which provide additional information about the problem (Yules and Chase, 1969; Lubit and Larsen, 1969; Shelton,

Knox, Elbert, and Johnson, 1970; Shelton, Harris, Shales, and
Dooley, 1970; Tash, in press; and Peterson, in preparation).

*4. What is the procedure for physical management of cleft palate
which gives optimal results?*

This question is a very complex one, of course, and one that
will not be answered easily or quickly. There are currently a
number of options for physical management. One can choose
surgery or prosthetic management. If surgery is chosen, then there
are several surgical procedures from which the surgeon may select.
A part of the general question is not only what procedure works
best but what is the best time for the procedure to be used.

The speech pathologist can expect to get involved in the controversy. To begin with, the only reason that cleft palate is physically managed is for speech and so the criteria for deciding about
success of management will be speech proficiency. But, in addition, the speech pathologist has information from available research which is valuable in predicting success of various types of
management. She should be well informed about the status of information about the several aspects of the problem and be able to
make a contribution to the team in working out the general program of management for that center.

SOME CONCLUDING REMARKS

The last twenty years have been highly productive in improving the management procedures of cleft palate and associated
palate problems. The speech pathologist of today has a great deal
of information about the problem in general, diagnostic procedures to be used, and management techniques which have proved
beneficial. The speech pathology of cleft palate is complex and
involves aspects related to both physical deficits and problems of
inappropriate learning. The major task is to identify whether
there is a physical deficit, of either the velopharyngeal mechanism
or some other part of the oral mechanism. If there is, and if the
goals of treatment are normal speech, then physical management
by a plastic surgeon or a prosthodontist will be needed. Except in
certain instances, where experimental therapy is being tried, the

kind of speech therapy to be used for cleft palate patients is highly similar to that which is appropriate for other kinds of voice and articulation disorders.

With the combined efforts of the plastic surgeon, the prosthodontist, and the speech pathologist, there is a high probability that the majority of cleft palate patients can be habilitated to the level of good speech.

REFERENCES

Carney, P.J., and Morris, H.L.: Structural correlates of nasality. *Cleft Palate J*, in press.

Curtis, J.C.: The acoustics of nasalized speech. *Cleft Palate J, 7*:380-396, 1970.

Johnson, W.; Darley, F.L., and Spriestersbach, D.C.: *Diagnostic Methods in Speech Pathology.* New York, Harper, 1963.

Lubit, E.C., and Larsen, R.S.: The Lubit Palatal Exerciser: A preliminary report. *Cleft Palate J, 6*:120-133, 1969.

Morris, H.L.: The oral manometer as a diagnostic tool in clinical speech pathology. *J Speech Hearing Dis.,31*:362-369, 1966.

Morris, H.L.; Spriestersbach, D.C., and Darley, F.L.: An articulation test for assessing competency of velopharyngeal closure. *J Speech Hearing Res, 4*:48-55, 1961.

Peterson, Sally: Electrical stimulation of the soft palate. In preparation.

Pitzner, Joan H., and Morris, H.L.: Articulation skills and adequacy of breath pressure ratios of children with cleft palates. *J Speech Hearing Dis, 31*:26-40, 1966.

Sherman, Dorothy: The merits of backward playing of connected speech in the scaling of voice quality disorders. *J Speech Hearing Dis, 19*:312-321, 1954.

Shelton, R.L.; Harris, Katherine, S.; Sholes, G.N., and Dooley, Patricia, M.: Study of non-speech palate movement by scaling and electromyographic techniques. In Bosma, J.F. (Ed.) : *Second Symposium on Oral Sensation and Perception.* Springfield, Thomas, 1970, pp. 432-441.

Shelton, R.L.; Harris, Katherine, S.; Sholes, G.N., and Dooley, Patricia, M.: Study of non-speech palate movements by scaling and electromyographic techniques. In Bosma, J.F. (Ed.) : *Second Symposium on Oral Sensation and Perception.* Springfield, Thomas, 1970, pp. 416-431.

Spriestersbach, D.C., and Sherman, Dorothy (Eds.) : *Cleft Palate and Communication.* New York, Academic Press, 1968.

Tash, Earlene L.; Shelton, R.S.; Knox, A.W., and Michel, J.F.: Training voluntary pharyngeal wall movement in children with normal and inadequate velopharyngeal closure. *Cleft Palate J,* in press.

Templin, Mildred C., and Darley, F.L.: *The Templin-Darley Tests of Articulation*, 2nd ed. Iowa City, Bureau of Educational Research and Service, Division of Extension and University Services, The University of Iowa, 1969.

Van Demark, D.R.: Misarticulations and listener judgements of the speech of individuals with cleft palates. *Cleft Palate J, 1*:232-245, 1964.

CHAPTER SIX

ARTICULATION

JOHN V. IRWIN

with the assistance of

ALAN J. WESTON

P ROBLEMS OF ARTICULATION have typically constituted the bulk of the case load of the average practicing speech clinician. In particular, clinicians working in the schools have reported that articulatory problems constitute as much as 85 per cent of their total load (Johnson *et al.*, 1967). In consequence, a large body of literature on speech therapy with articulatory problems has developed. The traditional point of view has been well presented by such writers as Van Riper and Irwin (1958), Johnson *et al.*, (1967), and Eisenson and Ogilvie (1963).

Although this traditional body of literature has acquired considerable stature, it must not be assumed that a "standard" practice in articulatory therapy has ever been achieved. Tremendous variation exists with respect to implementation of the so-called traditional points of view. The present chapter, then, assumes some considerable familiarity with the conventional literature and in its turn will emphasize newer viewpoints. This deliberate omission of conventional materials in this chapter does not in any sense imply a rejection of the conventional viewpoints. Rather, this omission is simply a recognition that space does not permit a review of both the traditional and the new, that the traditional is already well represented in our literature, and that many of the newer viewpoints are not represented in our current, standard textbooks. A partial exception to this statement is, of course, *Articulatory Acquisition and Behavior* (Winitz, 1969), which presents many of the newer concepts with respect to articulation, but does not attempt to apply these concepts systematically to clinical programs.

THE PHONEME

Definition of Phoneme

The terms *phone* and *phoneme* need to be carefully differentiated. Phones are typically identified as families of sounds, families with sufficient perceptual and productive similarity to be regarded as being like each other and unlike other families. Phoneticians have studied these sound families in great detail and are able to transcribe them with considerable accuracy. In close phonetic transcription, the phonetician records with as much detail as possible those sounds that he hears. Here is an example of close phonetic transcription: (t' i m).

If such transcription is analyzed, it will be found that the phonetician frequently transcribes differences that are acoustically valid but semantically irrelevant. Thus, whether (t' i m) or (t i m) is said will not change the meaning of the utterance. That is, as the above example illustrates, some acoustic variations are relevant in a given language and some are irrelevant. Transcription at the level of the phone (that is, phonetic transcription) attempts to record all auditory deviations that can be reliably heard; transcription at the phoneme level (that is, phonemic transcription) seeks to record only those acoustic events that are significant in a particular language. In any one language, then, the phoneme is a grouping of sounds at a level that is significant. A phoneme family may include more than one phone.

The number of phonemes in different languages varies. Within any one language, disagreement may obtain as to the precise number of phonemes. Thus Irwin (1971), although explicitly recognizing the possibility of variation, suggests that American English may be regarded as having forty-one phonemes. These forty-one phonemes are listed in Table 6-I, the Phonemes of English. Note that this list excludes /hw/ as a phoneme of English on the grounds that the differences in the articulation of such words as *witch* and *which* are disappearing and that the /w/ is characteristically being employed in each instance.

TABLE 6-I
THE PHONEMES OF ENGLISH

Vowels and Dipthongs			Consonants		
Symbol		Example	Symbol		Example
1.	i	me	1.	p	*pep*
2.	ɪ	bid	2.	b	*baby*
3.	e	play	3.	t	*tot*
4.	ɛ	get	4.	d	*dad*
5.	æ	hat	5.	k	*kick*
6.	ɑ	rob	6.	g	*gig*
7.	ɔ	hall	7.	tʃ	*church*
8.	o	tone	8.	dʒ	*judge*
9.	ʊ	push	9.	f	*fife*
10.	u	pool	10.	v	*verve*
11.	ɝ-ɜ	bird	11.	θ	*ether*
12.	ɚ-ə	another	12.	ð	*either*
13.	ʌ	mud	13.	s	*sis*
14.	aɪ	smile	14.	z	*buzz*
15.	aʊ	ouch	15.	ʃ	*ship*
16.	ɔɪ	toil	16.	ʒ	*azure*
17.	ju	fuel	17.	h	*high*
			18.	m	*mom*
			19.	n	*nine*
			20.	ŋ	*sing*
			21.	l	*let*
			22.	w	*wit*
			23.	r	*run*
			24.	j	*yet*

Phoneme as Segmental Unit

In speech pathology, the phoneme has been the traditional unit of identifying defective articulation, of guiding modification, and of evaluating outcome. In recent years, the validity of the phoneme as a discrete unit in articulation has come under increasing attack. One type of attack has been based primarily on physiologic evidence. Data from a wide variety of sources (Daniloff and Moll, 1968; Malmberg, 1963; and Oehman, 1966) have tended to emphasize the importance of the coarticulation concept, to emphasize that in connected speech the speaker does not produce a string of individual phonemes, but rather executes complex interrelated movements of the articulatory apparatus. Little physiological evidence can be found to support the existence of the isolated phoneme in connected speech. Similar evidence has come from acoustical data. If acoustic spectrographs based on continuous speech are examined, it is essentially impossible to delineate either the boundaries between phonemes or even the unmodifed central position of phonemes. Indeed, Deese (1970) has emphasized that no single acoustic stimulus can be uniquely associated with a given phoneme. Obviously, this combination of physiological and acoustical evidence has cast doubt upon the validity of the phoneme as the unit of articulatory therapy.

In general, the traditional defense of the speech pathologist for his continued use of the phoneme has been somewhat intuitive. First, he has argued that he is able to make judgments concerning phonemes in connected speech. That is, despite the evidence that the phoneme has neither acoustical nor physiological discreteness, the practicing clinician has demonstrated his ability not only to isolate such phenomena in connected speech and to make judgments of the appropriateness or inappropriateness of individual phonemes, but to teach children to do the same. Second, the speech pathologist has argued that the technique has worked; he has cited observed changes in articulatory behavior subsequent to such application. Finally, on occasion, the more sophisticated (or desperate) clinician has occasionally had the courage to ask the scientist, "If I don't work with phoneme, what unit do I use?" Perhaps because the clinician has not pressed this question, the scientist has not clearly answered it.

Recently, some support for the validity of the phonemic concept has come from psycholinguistics. Langacker (1968), for example, although admitting the validity of both physiological and acoustical arguments aginst discreteness, insists upon the discreteness at a competence level. Deese (1970), who recognizes that the acoustical stimulus of speech is not segmented, emphasizes that we perceive speech as being segmented into discrete and separate sounds. And, Tikovsky, in a forthcoming manuscript (Tikovsky, in press), describes phonemes as the smallest segmental units of the language and notes that it is generally easy to teach native speakers of the language to write and to read with an alphabet that is based on phonemes.

If one grants that, despite the evidence that no acoustical and no physiological discreteness exists, but that discreteness does exist at a competence level, one finds not only a possible resolution of this specific dilemma but also strong data to support the view that communicative difficulties may be viewed either from a competence or a performance aspect. In any event, the validity of the phoneme as a discrete unit has found renewed support and will need further examination.

Classifications of Phonemes

It is customary to classify phonemes in two major groupings: Vowels and Consonants. Each type is, of course, produced by the articulatory mechanism. That is, both the vowels and consonants of English are typically produced on an expired air/sound stream that is modified in its passage through the larynx, the pharyngeal cavities, and/or the oral and nasal cavities. The essence of the modification is the (a) degree, (b) mode, and (c) locus of constriction. Thus, /z/ and /i/ represent differences in degree of constriction; /b/ and /m/ in mode; and /b/and /k/ in locus. With this recognition that the two types of phonemes, i.e. vowels and consonants, share both a productive apparatus and a productive technique, each will now be described separately.

Unfortunately, as of this moment, agreement does not exist as to the most appropriate way to describe the essential characteristics of phonemes. Recent literature (Chomsky and Halle, 1968; Jakobson *et al.*, 1963, and Winitz, 1969), has emphasized the importance of the distinctive feature approach. Most distinctive matrices are binary, that is, a feature is either present or absent. In general, any distinctive feature serves to differentiate at least one phoneme from one other phoneme or one class of phonemes from another class. Thus voice, as a distinctive feature, serves to differentiate between /b/ and /p/ or between those pairs of English consonants known as cognates.

The clinical applications of distinctive feature approach are just being recognized (Fisher, 1970; and McReynolds and Huston, 1970). This chapter, because of its clinical orientation, will recognize the increasing importance of the distinctive feature approach, but will emphasize established descriptive techniques because of their demonstrated clinical utility.

Vowel and Vowel-like Sounds

Table 6-II, Physiological Characteristics of the Vowels of English, which is based on the work of Wise (1957) and of Thomas

TABLE 6-II
PHYSIOLOGICAL CHARACTERISTICS OF THE VOWELS OF ENGLISH

	Front		Central		Back			
					Unrounded		Rounded	
	Tense	Lax	Tense	Lax	Lax	Tense	Lax	Tense
High	i	ɪ					u	ʊ
Mid	e	ɛ	ɝ-ɜ	ɚ-ə ʌ			o	
Low		æ				ɑ	ɔ	

(1958), summarizes the major productive features of English vowels. Three variables are indicated: (a) position within the oral cavity of the highest arched portion of the tongue, (b) tenseness and laxness of tongue, and (c) degree of lip rounding. Neither orality-nasality nor voicing-unvoicing has been indicated; in English, each vowel is normally oral and normally voiced. Note that in English, as indicated in Table 6-III, lip rounding is important only for the back vowels.

TABLE 6-III
STRESS PATTERN IN THE PHONEMIC DIPHTHONGS OF ENGLISH

Diphthongs*	Key Words
↓ /aɪ/	ice
↓ /aʊ/	now
↓ /ɔɪ/	toy
↓ /ju/	feud

* ↓ = Stressed Member

The difference between vowel and vowel-like sounds now needs to be emphasized. At a phonemic level the basic class of vowel-like sounds is the diphthong. The conventional phonemic diphthong of English consists of two vowels, produced sequentially without interruption, but with a major difference in the stress or relative intensity of the two vowels. In most phonemic diphthongs of English, the stress is on the first of the two vowels. Table 6-III, Stress Relationships in the Phonemic Diphthongs of English, presents three phonemic diphthongs in which the first of the two vowels is emphasized. But in the final diphthong, that symbolized by /ju/ as in *feud,* the stress is on the second or final of the two members.

You should also note that many nonphonemic diphthongs are characteristic of English. Thus, in using the word *boat* as the subject of an oral sentence, most speakers of English pronounce the word as [boUt] rather than as [bot]. But, because English has no pair of words that is differentiated semantically by the articulation of [boUt] or [bot], distinction is not recognized at phonemic levels and the word *boat* is typically rendered as /bot/ irrespective of phonetic differences in the production of the vowel element. Ordinarily, vowels or vowel-like elements constitute the intensity peak of a syllable in multisyllabic words or of the word itself in a single syllable word. Thus, deviant vowels can be very conspicuous auditorily. Perhaps fortunately, most functional articulatory deviations seem to involve consonants rather than vowels. Nevertheless, with speakers in whom organic factors (such as hearing loss or paralysis or integrity of the palatal structures) are important, or with speakers whose linguistic orientation is different (as in either foreign accent or ghetto variations) vowel differences can become crucial.

Consonants

Table 6-IV, Physiological Characteristics of the Consonants of English, specifies these factors: (a) variation in the locus of constriction, as bilabial or glottal; (b) variation in the mode of articulation, as a glide or a plosive; and (c) variation in voicing.

Place of Constriction. So far as the phonemic consonants of

TABLE 6-IV
CLASSIFICATION OF ENGLISH CONSONANTS

MODE OF ARTICULATION	Area of Constriction													
	Bilabial		Labio-Dental		Lingua-Dental		Lingua-Alveolar		Lingua-Palatal		Lingua-Velar		Glottal	
	u*	v*	u	v	u	v	u	v	u	v	u	v	u	v
Glide		w						r		j				
Lateral								l						
Nasal		m						n				ŋ		
Fricative			f	v	θ	ð	s	z	ʃ	ʒ			h	
Affricative							tʃ	dʒ						
Plosive	p	b					t	d			k	g		

*u = Unvoiced
*v = Voiced

English are concerned, the essential points of constriction are from front to back through the oral cavity: lips, lips-teeth, tongue-teeth, tongue-gum ridge, tongue-hard palate, tongue-soft palate, and the vocal bands.

Note that all possible physiological points of constriction are not used. For example, in English no constriction is normally present between the tongue and either upper or lower lip, although such constriction is physiologically possible. This principle is true of other languages as well. That is, no language uses either (a) all possible points of physiological constriction or (b) all modes of release at any one point of constriction.

So far as consonants are concerned, the place of constriction is so important that it is usually specified first in naming a phoneme physiologically. Terms derived from anatomy are usually employed. Thus, as indicated in Table 6-IV, the consonants of English are first classified as bilabials, labial-dentals, and so forth.

Mode of Production. The basic variations in mode of production refer to the handling of the pressure component in the production of the sound.

Glide. Certain consonants of English, classified here as glides but sometimes classified as semivowels, are characterized by both (a) relatively open constriction and (b) movement of the articulators during the production of the sound. You should probably remember that the nature of a glide is somewhat changed by whether the movement is from a vowel to the glide or, perhaps more characteristic, from the glide to the vowel. Thus the glides symbolized by /w/, /r/, /j/, and /l/, to a vowel are typically regarded as consonants; on the other hand, the glides from a vowel to /r/, /j/, and /l/ are frequently transcribed as vowels rather than as consonant glides. The glide to /w/ is not usually recognized in English; that is, final /w/ does not appear in English words.

Lateral. In English, the only lateral is /l/. That is, in producing /l/ the air-sound stream must go laterally around the tongue while it is in the target position. /l/ also has glide characteristics.

Nasal. At the present writing, neither the precise acoustic characteristics of nasalization nor the precise productive mechanisms that result in nasalization can be specified. Nevertheless, speakers of English are able to recognize with considerable reliability that which they characterize as acceptable nasality and that which they characterize as unacceptable. Moreover, the degree of openness of the velo-pharyngeal valve correlates significantly with this distinction. Indeed, data available to use from many sources now suggest that perhaps 85 per cent of what we construe as nasality can be related to the degree of closure of the velopharyngeal valve.

With these restrictions in mind, it is now possible to suggest that only three of the phonemes of English, /m/, /n/, and /ɔ/ are produced with the oral cavity essentially closed and the nasal cavity essentially open. These three phonemes, because of their transmission route, are specified as nasals. As used in this sense, the term nasal has no interpretation of either abnormality or of undesirability. Indeed, so acceptable is nasality in these contexts that the *denasal* is applied clinically to describe /m/, /n/, or /ŋ/ that is not produced with sufficient opening of the nasal transmission cavity. On the other hand, the production of other consonants (or vowels) of English is significantly affected if the nasal passageway is open. Clinically this is particularly likely to be true in children with congenital cleft palate.

Fricative. In English fricatives, although the degree of constriction is acute, the closure is not complete. These sounds, like vowels and nasals, can be produced continuously but, unlike vowels and nasals, are produced with considerable frictional noise.

Affricative. In English, two affricatives are recognized. Affricatives, as is indicated in the symbolization, begin with a plosive and end with a fricative.

Plosive. The plosives of English are characterized by three pressure stages. After the constriction is complete at the point specified, (a) flow of the air or air-sound stream is impounded (implosion), (b) the intra-oral pressure builds (plosion), and (c) finally the constriction is released quickly and the pressure escapes (explosion).

Voicing-Unvoicing. In English eight pairs of consonants are differentiated primarily by the way the sound is produced with or without voicing. Three of these pairs are plosives; one of these pairs, affricative; and four of these pairs, fricatives.

PHONEMIC ACQUISITION

The phonological development of a child has been widely studied. Underlying such studies has been the tacit assumption that the knowledge of phonological development would be helpful to the field both in (a) understanding the relevant variables in such development and (b) making critical decisions more meaningful. As a result of such interest, some general knowledge of the relevant variables, particularly for the Western European languages, now exists.

Discussion

The literature on phonological development is, unfortunately, influenced by the assumptions, the techniques, and the designs employed by the various investigators. Thus, despite the relatively large body of literature that exists, and despite the relative consistency of much of this literature, the basic limitations on our knowledge must be carefully kept in mind. Some of the more obvious and important problems will now be considered.

Learning Versus Biological Theories

Children possess an amazing capacity to learn language; they do not seem to need to be taught in any conventional sense; they seem only to need to participate in language situations.

The standard body of learning theory has maintained, sometimes implicitly and sometimes explicitly, that human language behavior is like all other behavior. In particular, the view has frequently been advanced that language is a set of verbal habits, that it is explainable by a stimulus-response model, and that the basic mechanisms are classical and instrumental conditioning with appropriate reinforcement. Representative paradigms of this approach are those of Skinner (1957), Mowrer (1954), Staats (1968), and Osgood (1968).

Recently, however, this basic interpretation has been seriously challenged. Beginning primarily with the writings of Chomsky (1957), but supported also by the work of other individuals such as Lenneberg (1967) and McNeil (1968), the importance of a biological predisposition for language has been urged. Supporting arguments range from the uniformity of language acquisition throughout the human race, the fantastic rapidity with which language is acquired by the child, to the language behavior of handicapped children. It is now possible to interpret human communication as a species specific form of behavior.

One cannot predict now the ultimate resolution of these conflicting points of view. But, in the meantime, one should note that most of the normative data available to us are based—at least implicitly—on a learning based explanation of language acquisition. Thus, such research tends to emphasize isolated performance as opposed to generalized competence.

Sample Limitations

It has not been generally recognized that the major norms now existing for phonemic development such as those of Templin (1957), Wellman *et al.* (1931), and Irwin (1947) have all been based on studies of white, middle-class, English speaking children. As of this writing, similar norms are not available for other groups such as inner-core blacks.

It is imperative, first, that this fact be recognized. It is also imperative that the implications of this fact be recognized. For, if the assumption previously noted is true, that is, that normative data enable the clinician to put the articulatory deviations of the individual into meaningful perspective, then the speech pathologist is indeed handicapped in his attempts to evaluate the child from the black ghetto. Furthermore, although it may seem intuitively reasonable to assume that the predictors noted apply to ghetto children as well as to white middle-class children, the degree of agreement has not been demonstrated. For example, it is possible that sex differences will be more important in the development of the articulation of the black ghetto child or of the Spanish-American child than in the development of the articulation of the middle-class white. Unfortunately, until we have actually collected comparative data, such speculation can remain only speculation.

Production Versus Reception

In general, investigators of phonological acquisition have emphasized productive rather than receptive skills. Hence data with respect to relationships—either at the performance or competence level—between reception and production are not well understood.

Methodological Problems

Much of the basic literature on phonological development—as for example the splendid series of studies by Orvis C. Irwin (1947) —reflects the phonemic concepts of listeners with one language standard. Data in process should broaden our understanding of the effect of this limitation.

PREDICTORS

As our sophistication with respect to the acquisition of oral language increases, speech pathologists have become more and more loath to speak in terms of cause and effect. Perkins and

Curlee (1969) have discussed relevant issues. But, although correlational relationship of one factor with another factor does not necessarily imply cause and effect, the relationship may still be of clinical utility. In this section, then, following the previous analysis of Irwin (in preparation), the terms *predictors* and *outcomes* will be used. These terms have the advantage of recognizing possibly useful relationships without any assumption as to the nature of the relationship.

A brief discussion of some of the more obvious predictors now follows.

Language Spoken

Although the importance of biological predispositions for language is conceded, it must be emphasized that learning factors too play an important role. Thus, although the infant during the first few weeks of life may produce a pattern of sounds that is independent of the language used about him, the phonemes that he ultimately uses purposefully will reflect the phonemic structure of the language (or languages) that he hears. Unfortunately, as has been previously suggested, although phonological variations within such major language groups as English, German, and French have been recognized, variations within the varieties of American English, for example, have not been given specific attention.

Age

In all known languages, children master the necessary phonemic structure in a pattern that is roughly correlated with time. That is, during a critical period the articulation of children improves with age. In English, purposeful use of phonemes begins at about age one; complete mastery of the phonemic structure is ordinarily achieved at about age eight. The progression is relatively orderly for large groups of children. Certain age norms are presented later in this chapter. For the moment, however, it is sufficient to recognize that early sounds such as /m/ and late sounds such as /r/ can be recognized. But, the phonemic development of any one child may and usually does vary widely from the statistical or group norm. Nevertheless, the concept of phoneme age has been of considerable utility to the clinician.

Socioeconomic Factors

Various studies, as, for example, Templin (1957), have established that the pattern of phonemic development is related to socioeconomic background. Although the precise impact of the factors within different socioeconomic backgrounds has not truly been pinned down, the assumption has been freely made that phonemic development is favorably influenced by the amount and variety of speech, the reinforcement of speech, and other educational and social factors. Presumably, the higher the socioeconomic status, the greater the impact of these features. Assuming that TV either has or will penetrate the American home irrespective of socioeconomic status, the future impact of the socio-economic variable may be reduced. It is not likely to be eliminated entirely.

Intelligence

Inasmuch as articulation is at least partly learned, phonemic development would seem to be related to intelligence. In fact, despite obvious operational difficulties in defining intelligence, such a relationship does seem to exist. Perhaps the most useful concept is to regard intelligence not so much as a variable that correlates highly with articulatory development but rather as a variable that serves as a prerequisite to articulatory development. Thus, if one assumes low normal or higher intelligence, the correlation between articulation and intelligence, although positive, is very slight. Thus, low normal or higher intelligence can be viewed as a prerequisite to articulatory development. On the other hand, assuming intelligence of below normal down to and including institutional levels, a relatively higher correlation exists. That is, the severely retarded will ordinarily demonstrate greater deviation in and reduction of articulatory development than will the moderately retarded or the normals.

Sex

Historically, the articulatory development of females has been shown to be somewhat advanced relative to that of males. More recent studies, however, have tended to minimize this difference.

Indeed, although a review of the world literature would certainly fail to support the contention that boys develop more rapidly than do girls, the traditional notion that the articulation of girls is the more highly advanced is also not supported. On the basis of present data, the best judgment seems to be that the patterns of phonemic development for girls may be somewhat different but not necessarily superior to that for boys. Data to be presented later in this chapter will clarify this point.

Organic Deviations

Sensory Deficits. The major sensory deficits recognized in our culture are blindness and deafness. As might be anticipated, inasmuch as speaking is essentially auditory, vision is not closely related to phonemic development. On the other hand, as has been reviewed in Johnson, *et al.* (1967), Van Riper and Irwin (1958), and Winitz (1969), an impressive array of studies supports the conclusion that auditory deficits up to and including deafness not only delay articulatory development but, in some instances, actually change the nature of the development. Thus, the child who is deaf from birth may not—at least without instruction—acquire purposeful use of such phonemes as /k/ and /s/. On the other hand, children with acquired losses restricted to the highest frequencies may acquire phonemes such as /s/ and /k/ but not make them well.

More recently, investigators such as Bosma (1967) and Ringel (1970) have been concerned with the effect of tactile-kinesthetic-proprioceptive deficits on articulatory ability. Data from experimental and pathological sources are not conclusive, but in general the assumption seems warranted that oral sensory deficits of the type indicated do interfere with the development of articulatory skills.

Motor Deficits. Articulation is, of course, one of the most highly skilled acts performed by humans. It follows, then, that paralyses—whether of neural or muscular origin—will reduce the efficiency of articulatory performance. The nature and extent of the interference will vary both with the production requirements of particular phonemes and with the type of paralysis. Although motor defects will be treated more specifically in other chapters of this text, it is appropriate here to note that because of such defects a particular organ, as the tongue, may not be able to move, may not be able to relax, or may not be able to resist extra movements. The nature of the articulatory deviation will tend to reflect the nature of the paralysis.

Structural Deficits. Inasmuch as articulation involves the basic structures of the oral, nasal, and pharyngeal cavities, it would seem to follow that deviations in the structure of these areas would result in articulatory deviations. This assumption is basically true. But, because of the extreme flexibility of the mechanism, particularly in the oral region, repeated studies as those by Fairbanks and Green (1950) ; Fairbanks and Lintner (1951), and Bloomer (1957), have shown that structural deviations must indeed be severe if the effect on articulation is to be clearly measurable.

So far as actual effect on articulation is concerned, the clinical defect of major importance is cleft of the hard and/or soft palate. Such clefts, either if unrepaired or if repaired unsuccessfully, may make it difficult or impossible for the speaker to close mechanically the nasal passage from the oral passage and thus to direct the air-sound stream through the oral passage. As described in the chapter in this text on "Cleft Palate" by Morris, such structural deviations have a marked effect on the phonemes of English generally and particularly on those consonants requiring a buildup of pressure such as the plosives and fricatives.

If the normal relationship between the upper and lower jaws is not maintained, that is, if the lower jaw (mandible) extends forward of the upper jaw (maxilla), or if conversely the lower jaw is retracted excessivly, articulatory deviations may result. West (1957) has stated that prognathic mandible (bull dog or excessively undershot jaw) is difficult to compensate for, because the lower jaw, although capable of sliding forward, cannot be easily retracted.

Finally, many studies such as that of Bankson and Byrne (1962) have shown that missing teeth, particularly missing front teeth, may affect the articulation of certain consonants.

Currently, speech pathologists are reluctant to attribute articulatory deviations to structural variations in the mouth and nose, unless (a) deviation is extreme, (b) compensatory movements are not possible, and (c) the nature of the articulatory deviation can be precisely related to the nature of the structural defect.

Clinical Retardation. The relationship of articulatory development and intelligence has been previously discussed. The present author explicitly recognizes that experiential as well as biological factors may be important in retardation. Nevertheless, in extreme instances of organic retardation such as those associated with hydrocephaly, cretinism, and Mongolism, a considerable degree of articulatory retardation can be predicted.

Emotional Disturbances

As presented on this occasion, emotional disturbances are treated as functional rather than organic. This separation is for convenience and for clarity; it does not seek to imply that all emotional disturbances are nonorganic. Indeed, present data would suggest that the emotional involvement of children may stem both from functional and organic factors.

Precise data are lacking as to the exact relationship between phonological development and emotional problems. Rousey and Moriarty (1965) has formulated the most explicit statement of this relationship. But, irrespective of whether the degree of relationship attributed by Rousey does or does not exist, both psychologists and speech pathologists recognize that the articulation of the emotionally involved child may deviate from normative patterns.

OUTCOMES

General Considerations

On the basis of our present data, it is usual to recognize two major divisions in the sound development process. The first division, which is concentrated in the first weeks of life, is concerned with the nonpurposive use of sounds. The second division, which begins during the latter months of the first year, is concerned with the purposive use of sounds in a language structure. Irwin's studies (1947) overlap these two periods; the studies of Wellman

(1931), Poole (1934), Templin (1957), Hall (1962), and Healey (1963) emphasize the second period.

Bearing in mind the limitations stated earlier in this section, the following generalizations about speech and sound production can be made:

1. The number of different sounds—whether viewed phonetically or phonemically—increases with age.

2. The total number of sounds produced per unit of time increases with age.

3. Although vowels are more common than consonants initially, the proportion gradually reverses until an approximation of the adult vowel-consonant ratio is reached.

4. Infants begin with a heavy production of front vowels and back consonants; the relative consonant-vowel back-front proportion reverses itself with age.

5. Phonemic development is essentially complete by age seven or eight.

Specific Normative Data

Normative data for the purposive use of English phonemes in language context are presented in two tables. Table 6-V, Age Level for Selected English Vowels and Consonants, is based on the general literature and does not attempt to specify differences between boys and girls. Table 6-VI, Age Norms for the Consonants of English by Sex is based on the doctoral dissertations of William Healey and William Hall. The data in both tables are relatively compatible.

ARTICULATORY ERRORS
Definitions

It is difficult if not impossible to frame a completely satisfactory verbal definition of an articulatory error. Basically, such a definition should recognize that an articulatory error must constitute a difference that makes a difference either to the listener or to the speaker or to both. Definitions to date have tended to emphasize listener effects rather than speaker effects; furthermore, previous definitions have tended to emphasize acoustical and phy-

TABLE 6-V
COMPOSITE AGE NORM FOR SELECTED VOWELS AND
CONSONANTS OF ENGLISH*

Representative Vowels		Representative Consonants	
Phoneme	Age	Phoneme	Age
i	3	w	3
ɪ	3	m	3
e	3	n	3
ɛ	3	ŋ	3
æ	3	f	3
ɑ	3	r	4
ɔ	3	b	4
o	3	d	4
ʊ	3	k	4
u	3	s	4.5
ʌ	3	ʃ	4.5
ə	3	tʃ	4.5
ɝ	3	v	6
		t	6
		ɵ	6
		z	7

*Possible ages below 3 not shown.

sical deviation in contradistinction to perceived handicap. In fact, however, if the articulation of a given individual, whether validly

TABLE 6-VI
AGE NORMS FOR THE CONSONANTS OF ENGLISH*

Phoneme	Sex		Phoneme	Sex	
	M	F		M	F
w	3	3	l	7	4
m	3	3	f	7	6
n	3	3	j	5	5
h	3	3	dʒ	6	5
p	3	3	r	7	6
b	3	3	ʃ	7	6
d	3	3	tʃ	7	6
ŋ	4	3	v	7	7
ʍ	6	6	ð	7	7
g	3,5	3	s	7	7
k	3	3	z	7	7
ʒ	6	6	θ	7	7
t	3	4			

*Based on the Hall-Healey studies, using 90% achievement as age criterion.

or only as a perceptual artifact, is interpreted as handicapping either by his listeners or by himself, the speaker may be legitimately held to have an articulatory problem. This present concept of articulatory deficit places its emphasis, as is appropriate, upon the presumed handicapping effect of the deviation, whether auditory, visual, or motor-contact. In practice, however, it must be recognized that speech pathology does not have available any standardized measure of either the inter- or intra-handicapping nature of articulatory deviations.

In actual practice, then, articulatory deviations tend to be identified not in terms of handicapping effect, but rather in terms of (a) degree of variation from acoustic (and to some extent visible) norms or, and less often, (b) presumed effect upon the oro-facial structures. The assumption is then made that the greater the degree and kind of deviation, the greater the handicap. In day-to-day clinical practice, articulatory errors are defined as the inability to produce in an easy, automatic perceptually acceptable manner (a) each of the phonemes of a given language in (b) each of the usual combinations in which the phoneme appears. Clinicians, in applying such a definition, make allowance for such characteristics of the subject as age, linguistic background, and role. For example, a three-year-old inner-core black who cannot produce /s/ in all of its usual phonetic combinations would not ordinarily be regarded as having an articulatory problem. Yet a nine-year-old child of white, middle-class parents in good health and from a happy home would, with the same articulatory deficit, be regarded as having a problem. By the same token, a nine-year-old English speaking child who cannot produce /x/ would not be regarded as having articulatory problems; a German speaking child of the same age would be so regarded.

Finally, it should be noted that verbal description of the type offered here can never be adequate. Ultimately, whatever the principle may be, the concept must be taught in actual auditory and visual discrimination sessions.

CLASSIFICATION OF ARTICULATORY ERRORS

Traditional Categories

The traditional classification of articulatory errors has been (a) fourfold and (b) based on a combination of auditory and phonemic factors. The usual categories are as follows:

Omission. If the speaker fails to produce a phoneme at a position in a word in which a phoneme is expected, the error may be classified as an omission. Thus, if the word *coat* is articulated as /ko/, that is, if the final /t/ is not articulated, the articulatory deviation is an omission.

Substitution. If the speaker articulates the word *soup* as /oup/, that is, with /ө/ instead of /s/ in the initial position, the deviation may be classified as a substitution. Stated more generally, an error of substitution is one in which as accepted phoneme of a given language is substituted for another accepted or standard phoneme.

Distortion. If the speaker articulates the word *tip* as [t'ip], that is, with [t̪] rather than /t/, the error may be classified as a distortion. A distortion is the substitute of a nonstandard sound for a standard phoneme.

Addition. Finally, if the speaker articulates the word *soup* as [psup], that is, with the phoneme /p/ at the beginning of the word, the error may be classified as an addition. In errors of addition, as the name suggests, an extra sound—standard or nonstandard—is added. Ordinarily, addition—or insertion, as it is sometimes called—is the least common of the errors.

Other Classifications

Van Riper and Irwin (1958) have noted that both the error of substitution and the error of distortion are, in fact, actually substitutions. The only difference is that in one instance a standard phoneme is substituted and in the other a distorted phoneme is substituted. In fact, these authors state: "There seems to be some justification for the thesis that all articultory errors belong in the category of substitutions." But, in a bow to established clinical reality, the authors employed the standard classification in the balance of the book. Other bases of classification have had some viability. For example, the distinction is sometimes made between functional and organic articulatory deviations. More specifically, West, Ansberry, and Carr (1957) extend the etiological basis of classification as follows: (a) Dysarthrias are recognized as disorders of articulation resulting from lesions of those portions of the cerebrospinal nervous system directly involved in the control of the organs of articulation; (b) Dyslalias are recognized as disorders of articulation due to structural anomalies of the organs of articulation or to impaired auditory control; and (c) Dysphemias are recognized as including articulatory involvements of primary emotional or intellectual deficits and diseases.

More recently, articulatory disorders are being tentatively classified as phonetic or phonemic. As used here, the term *phonetic* implies that the individual is unable to make the sound in question because of biosocial, psychobiological, or reinforcement factors. As so classified, an ariculatory deviation is, indeed, a deficit in performance. The term *phonemic,* on the other hand, implies that both the sounds used and the sounds not used are parts of a different but not deficient linguistic structure. In the *phonetic* type of explanation, then, articulatory deviations represent an inability on the part of the subject to measure up to a standard. The *phonemic* explanation, on the other hand, interprets articulatory deviations as normal manifestations of a different standard. Obviously, a given child might exemplify both types of error. For example, he might produce a somewhat mushy /s/ because of a high frequency hearing loss but fail to make the /θ/ in *toothbrush* because, in his linguistic structure, /f/ is uniformly articulated for the medial /θ/ of toothbrush.

This last category, which seeks to explain rather than describe deviations, has potential significance to the speech clinician. Undoubtedly, this last concept will affect the clinical procedures of the future.

EVALUATING ARTICULATION
Purposes

Irwin (in preparation) has defined the following steps in the clinical process:

(1) Identification is the process by which the clinical team selects low and high risk individuals. (2) Management includes the systematic (a) observation and/or (b) intervention. (3) Termination refers to removal from the program by (a) clinical decision or (b) default. (4) Validation is the process by which the communicative behavior of the individual is realistically assessed and rigorously related to data and procedures.

The purposes of testing articulation vary with each of the above steps. In identification, the purpose is to establish the present status of articulatory behavior against individualized norms of the subject concerned. In the management phase, the purpose is to assess changes in articulatory behavior over time. In dismissal phases, the purpose is to predict future articulatory behavior in naturalistic situations. In the constantly ongoing validation process, the purpose is to verify the soundness of decisions and procedures.

Techniques

To date, two basic types of techniques for the evaluation of articulation have evolved in the field of speech pathology: (a) scaling techniques and (b) phoneme-centered techniques. As of the present writing, the phoneme-centered approach has been the most widely used clinically. But, because the scaling technique is demonstrating increased potentiality, it will also be described.

Scaling Techniques

In the evaluation of articulation by scaling, a listener is instructed to react to an overall impression of a speech sample rather than to individual phonemes. In the literature of speech pathology, the equal appearing interval scale, using five, seven, or nine points, has been most widely used. Recently, however, increased attention has been given to the possibility of using direct magnitude observation scales.

Despite the fact that scalar measures correlate closely with phonemic measures, can be done quickly, and can have high reliability, the scaler technique has not been basically employed in evaluating articulation. Why? At least two reasons can be given. First, research has shown that scaling is done most accurately by a panel rather than by an individual judge. Most therapists have not been in a position to use a panel for their judgments, and hence the scale has been deemed clinically impractical. Second, and perhaps more fundamentally, the scale—by the very nature of its function—does not provide specific information with respect to the phonemic behavior of the individual. Most therapists today, whether they employ the traditional medical model or the newer behavioral model, build their therapy around specific phonemes and hence must have knowledge of these phonemes. Scaling techniques simply do not provide this type of information.

Phoneme-centered Tests

Many methods have been evolved for testing the capacity of an individual to articulate each of the phonemes of his language in each of the usual phonetic contexts of that language. Traditionally, practicing clinicians have tended to categorize articulation tests primarily on the basis of the method of eliciting the speech sample (Table 6-VII). Comparison of Five Modes of Eliciting Speech Samples in Evaluating Articulation, which is reproduced with permission from *Introdutcion to Communicative Disorders* (Irwin, in preparation), summarizes the essential effects as they vary with method of stimulation.

In this text, however, a somewhat different system of organization will be emphasized. Here, tests will be categorized under the following headings: (a) isolated word unit; (b) tests in depth; and (c) conversational tests. Each of these categories will now be analyzed in turn (Table 6-VIII). Comparison of Representative Articulation Tests on Selected Factors, also reproduced with permission from *Introduction to Communicative Disorders,* facilitates this description.

The Isolated Word Test. The isolated word test has been the most widely used in this country. Among the more common examples of this type of test available commercially are the Templin-Darley, the Photo-Articulation Test, and the Goldman-Fristoe Articulation Test, although this test has in addition a narrative section.

Basically, all of these tests are similar in that they provide

TABLE 6-VII
COMPARISON OF FIVE MODES OF ELICITING SPEECH SAMPLES IN EVALUATING ARTICULATION

Key Characteristic	Say-After-Me	Reading	Mode of Stimulation Picture-Object Recognition	Narrative Stimuli	Conversation Simi	Veri
Usual Response Unit	Word or Phrase	Word, Phrase, or Sentence	Word	Word, Phrase, or Sentence	Word, Phrase, or Sentence	
Phonetically Systematic	Yes	Yes	Yes	Difficult	Difficult	
Validity	Relatively Low	Doubtful	Relatively Good	Relatively High	Very Good	Best
Interestingness	No	No	Yes	Yes	Varies	

TABLE 6-VIII
COMPARISON OF REPRESENTATIVE ARTICULATION TESTS ON SELECTED FACTORS

TEST CLASSIFICATION	Specific Test	Phonemes Tested	Phonemically Systematic	Consistency Effect — Right or Wrong	Consistency Effect — % Right	Stimuli Type — Picture	Stimuli Type — Repetition	Stimuli Type — Speech	Stimuli Type — Word	Context — Word Units	Context — Sentence	Judgment Task — Specific	Judgment Task — General
ISOLATED WORD	Templin Darley	Consonants, vowles, & blends	Yes	X		X			X			X	
ISOLATED WORD	Photo-Artic. Test	Consonants, vowels, & blends	Yes	X		X			X			X	
ISOLATED WORD	Goldman-Fristoe (Part I)	Consonants & blends	Yes	X		X			X			X	
REPEATED SAMPLE	McDonald (Deep & Screening)	Selected Consonants	Yes		X	X				X		X	
REPEATED SAMPLE	Shelton 30 Item	Selected Consonants	Yes		X		X				X	X	
FREE SPEECH	Picture Narration	Any (in large samples)	No (Improves with sample size)		X	X					X		X
FREE SPEECH	Simi-Conversation	Any (in large samples)	No (Improves with sample size)		X			X			X		X
FREE SPEECH	Veri-Conversation	Any (in large samples)	No (Improves with sample size)		X			X			X		X

picture stimuli for the purpose of eliciting isolated words. The test words are so arranged that a representative selection of the common phonemes of English appears in each of the possible word position, that is, initially, medially, and finally. This statement does not hold, of course, for those few phonemes of English that do not appear in each of these three positions. For example, /ŋ/ does not appear initially in English; /w/ does not appear in final position. Although practice varies, these tests also sample some of the more common blends, that is, combinations in which two or more consonants appear in a "blended" position. The word *sprint* is an example of an /spr/ blend. Blends are tested because certain data (Spriestersbach and Curtis, 1951) suggest that consonants may appear either in blends or in simple positions somewhat independently of each other.

Ordinarily, this type of test is evaluated by indicating whether a phoneme is articulated acceptably or unacceptably in a particular position. For example, in the Templin-Darley, /f/ might be scored as wrong in initial and medial positions but as correct in the final position. Ordinarily, each phoneme is tested only once in each position. In addition to recording correctness and incorrectness, some testers may seek to record (a) the type of error and (b) the degree of error.

In addition, this type of test may include a stimulability section. If stimulability is employed, the clinician calls the error phoneme to the attention of the subject, makes the error phoneme clearly and distinctly either in isolation or in a test word, and then specifically asks the subject to imitate him. The degree of stimulability is measured by any change in the articulation following stimulation from the articulation as recorded during simple elicitation from the picture stimuli. The form reproduced as Table 6-IX, from the Triota Articulation Analysis, provides for these discriminations.

The Isolated Word Test makes certain assumptions. First, the assumption is made that each of the phonemes should be tested in each of the positions in which it ordinarily occurs. As a consequence, although information is collected uniformly, the data are not always appropriate to the interests of the clinician. Second, the

TABLE 6-IX
SAMPLE ARTICULATION TEST FORM

Item No.	Phoneme	Judgment c | d | s | o | a	Severity 1 | 2 | 3 | 4	Stimulability Yes | No
		| | | |	| | |	|
		| | | |	| | |	|
		| | | |	| | |	|
1. saw	S—	| | | |	| | |	|
		| | | |	| | |	|
2. glasses	—S—	| | | |	| | |	|
		| | | |	| | |	|
3. kites	—S	| | | |	| | |	|
		| | | |	| | |	|
		| | | |	| | |	|

assumption is made that the isolated word is said as it would be said in a nontest situation. That is, this type of test assumes that eliciting the test word by picture approximates true spontaneous conversational articulation. This assumption is actually double-barreled: (a) it assumes that articulation in an isolated word is representative of larger phonetic contexts, and (b) it assumes that the test situation is not sufficiently artificial to put the subject on guard so far as articulation is concerned. Both of these assumptions are, of course, open to serious question. Finally, the assumption is made, as least implicitly, that if a phoneme is right initially in the one test word in which it is tested, then it is right initially in all words used by the individual. That is, the basic judgment is made that a particular phoneme in a particular position is either always right or always wrong. Contrast this conception of rightness and wrongness with the conception to be described in the next section.

Tests in Depth. Two typical representatives of this type of test procedure are the McDonald Deep Tests and Shelton Thirty Item Tests. The McDonald, which uses picture stimuli as generally administered, repeatedly samples the consonants of English in varied (but very brief) context. The Shelton, as the name implies, samples a particular consonant phoneme thirty times in a brief sentence. The Shelton ordinarily uses the repetition technique.

Both of these tests have the advantage of obtaining the sample in a situation that more nearly approximates normal phonetic context than does the isolated word. In the McDonald, the context is brief but the stimulation is reasonably spontaneous and the combinations are varied. In the Shelton, stimulation is less spontaneous but the context is longer and the sample is more varied.

But, in both of these tests it is important to note that the phoneme is not reported as right or wrong per position but rather as right or wrong in a stipulated percentage of occurrences. Thus, by utilizing multiple presentation, this type of test is better equipped to represent the inconsistency of articulation than is the conventional isolated word test.

Free Speech Tests (Conversational Tests.) In the storytelling tests, as represented in the Memphis State Communication Kit,* a picture stimulus is employed not for the purpose of asking the child to name a specific object but rather for the purpose of eliciting a spontaneous story or narrative based on the picture. Such a story, if told with either no or minimal interruption by the clinician, provides a sample not only of the articulatory ability of the child but also of the complexity and range of his communicative behavior.

(Conversational Tests) Irwin (in preparation) has defined two types of conversational tests. This is an important distinction and will be cited here:

> As speech pathologists begin to make increasing use of conversation as a measure of communicative ability, it is important that distinctions be drawn with respect to these conversational situations. At least two types need to be recognized. (1) the simi-conversation is a situation in which the therapist or a therapist designatee carries on a conversation or series of conversations with the subject usually in the therapy room or in an environment provided by the school or clinic. Unless unusual precautions are taken, these conversations tend to lose their spontaneity. The simi-conversation is worth doing; its limitations, however, must be recognized. (2) The veri-conversation, on the other hand, is a conversation held under completely naturalistic conditions. Participants must be real life members of the subject's environment; the physical environment must be one frequented norm-

---

*In press.

ally by the subject; and the observation-recording process must be completely concealed.

Both the simi- and veri-conversation share many characteristics. Both can result in lengthy contextual units, and both are difficult to make phonetically systematic. The big difference, of course, is that the veri-conversation represents the stronger validation of the therapeutic process.

At the moment, we do not have data with respect to the degree of difference in these two techniques. It is probable that (a) the degree of difference will ultimately be shown to be slight and that (b) it may be possible to predict from the simi-conversation the behavior in the veri-conversation. But, at least until such data are available, the field must be careful to recognize this distinction.

Special Applications

Screening Procedures

In situations in which large numbers of presumably normal children are seen, as in the schools, it may be efficient to administer a brief screening test of articulation rather than one of the more complete measures described previously. Many practicing clinicians, for example, use a brief screening test such as counting to ten, saying the days of the week, or identifying selected pictures from the Standard Articulation Test, usually, in each instance, following this portion of the test by a brief conversation. On the basis of these data, the clinician is usually able to identify children with some degree of articulatory deviation.

Considerable variation exists as to the next procedure. Many therapists will now give a complete isolated word type test such as the Templin-Darley. Others will proceed to a test in depth such as the McDonald Deep Screening or the Shelton Thirty Item. Again, still other therapists will, in addition, employ stimulability tests. Although present practices are not uniform, identification as to low or high risk can be made on the basis of such factors as number, type, and percentage of errors; stimulability; chronological age versus phonemic age; existence of related organic or emotional conditions; evaluation of cultural backgrounds.

Referral Situations

If the child is referred specifically for an articulation problem, or if background conditions leading to the referral are such that the probability of articulatory involvement is high, the clinician is likely to begin with a complete isolated word type test, follow this with stimulation and deep testing, and then make decisions with respect to management.

INTERVENTION

As cited earlier, after *Identification* the next basic step in the therapeutic process is *Management*. In articulatory therapy two types of management are possible: (a) systematic observation with emphasis on rate and direction of change in articulatory behavior, and (b) systematic intervention with emphasis on controlled acceleration of change in articulatory behavior. This section will deal with intervention.

Goals in Intervention

The primary goal in articulatory intervention is to modify articulatory behavior as it occurs in naturalistic circumstances. It is important that this goal be stated forthrightly and openly, for if one watches articulatory therapy and seeks to derive a goal from such observation, one might conclude that the goal in articulatory intervention is to develop "correct" articulatory behavior for use in small rooms in game situations with adult speech clinicians.

In all instances, socially acceptable articulatory behavior in naturalistic circumstances is not always achievable. In such instances, additional goals become (a) acceptance by the subject of the articulatory competence possible for him and/or (b) in extreme instances the development of substitute forms of communication.

Traditional Viewpoints

Although it is common practice in our literature to refer to "traditional articulatory therapy," no valid consensus as to the precise nature of traditional therapy can be held to exist. It is impossible to reconcile completely the viewpoints of West, Ansberry, and Carr (1957), Backus and Beasley (1951), Barbara (1960), and Van Riper and Irwin (1958). Yet, after recognition of the fact that no true uniformity has existed, certain very general core practices can be recognized.

Traditional Theory

In our conventional textbooks and courses, if not in our actual clinical practice, the assumption is that deviant articulatory behavior is a symptom of an underlying cause. Although the typical underlying causes have been named and described variously, ordinarily they can be grouped under some such headings as the following: (a) physical, including hearing loss, cleft palate, cerebral palsy, etc.; (b) emotional, including autism, childhood schizophrenia, negativism, and other problems; and (c) environmental including the home situation with its child rearing practices, the school and/or other institutional environments, and the general cultural background in which the individual lives.

In the traditional viewpoint, the total articulatory symptom picture of the child, the case history, and other relevant physical, emotional, and environmental data are, through a process known as diagnosis, related to each other. If a relevant-remedial cause can be conceptualized, that is, if a cause can be diagnosed that can both reasonably account for the symptoms and at the same time be corrected, treatment is instituted against the cause. With certain types of causes, the treatment procedures—usually instituted by related professional disciplines—have been quite successful. For example, surgical and dental intervention has been successful in minimizing the consequences of cleft palate; certain types of conductive hearing loss can be relieved by medical or surgical treatment; certain emotional problems have been reduced by psychotherapeutic intervention; and some behavioral problems have been minimized by drug treatment. Limited success has also been obtained in treating familial environments; to date we have probably been less successful in manipulating total cultural environments.

Etiological therapy, if done early enough and done well enough, sometimes proves sufficient. But if it cannot be done well, if it cannot be done soon enough, or if it cannot be done at all as in certain incurable conditions, direct teaching—symptomatic therapy—becomes necessary.

In articulatory therapy, particularly in mass situations such as the schools, the tendency of the field has been—except in obvious instances of gross causal deviations—to attempt direct teaching first and to reserve systematic, differential diagnosis for those instances in which direct intervention is unsuccessful. Although logically somewhat unsatisfying, this approach has much to recommend itself in practical instances.

Practice

As already noted, no truly standard traditional practice can be described. Yet, based both on the literature and on considerable observation, traditional therapy seems to involve such factors as auditory training (with correct and incorrect phonemic stimuli), production techniques (which conventionally move from producing the error phoneme in isolation to practice syllables, to words, and to larger contextual units but which may be initiated in larger contextual units), and carryover techniques in which the new articulatory behaviors achieved in the clinic situation are, hopefully, developed for use in naturalistic circumstances. Typically, this therapy is done in game or drill situations, although it may be done in conversational situations. But, even if this general pattern is accepted as descriptive, one must immediately recognize the many variations that do exist. For example, attitudes toward using the traditional method in group and in individual therapy vary and, if in group, vary as to the size and the composition of the group. Ordinarily, traditional therapy seems to advocate working on one phoneme at a time with a particular child, but the precise principles for selecting a particular phoneme sequence and for timing the introduction of the phonemes in the sequence are not clear. Finally, tremendous variation exists in the length and frequency of training periods, the time over which training periods are maintained, the methods of reinforcement, and the degree of supporting services.

It is easier to make negative statements about traditional articulatory therapy than positive statements. Thus one can say that identification procedures have not been uniform, that reinforcement procedures in direct teaching have varied widely, and that in a large scale sense precise data have not been kept. All in all, it is probably more accurate to say that a sharply defined traditional therapy does not exist than to seek to describe such therapy.

CURRENT VIEWPOINTS

Theory

Increasingly, in the field of articulatory intervention, the so-called behavioral model has become increasingly prominent. In the behavioral model, the articulatory difficulty—whether substitution, distortion, or omission—is seen as the problem rather than as the symptom. Advocates of this behavioral model, then, do not attempt diagnosis with its thoughtful seeking for causal relationships. Rather, in this model the goal is immediate modification of the deviant articulatory behavior.

Two basic types of conditioning—classical and instrumental—are emphasized in behavioral intervention.

Figure 6-1, Classical and Instrumental Conditioning, diagrams both types. Classical or Pavlovian conditioning has been most successfully used in attitude and concept modification. By presenting the attitude or concept that is to be learned in conjunction with an established concept or attitude, the desired response can be achieved.

Instrumental conditioning has had wide application in changing motor behavior and thus relates easily to articulatory modification. The Three-step Skinner Paradigm is shown in Figure 6-1. This Paradigm is best understood by beginning with the central R. This formula says that a response R that is systematically followed by a reinforcing stimulus SR, will have a high probability of future occurrence. The first part of the formula, SD, says that if the reinforcement typically occurs only in the presence of a particular stimulus, usually known as the discriminatory stimulus, the response will ultimately be brought under the control of that stimulus. This relationship of course is subject to many of the elements of classical conditioning.

The basic difference, then, between traditional practices—

Classical   Instrumental

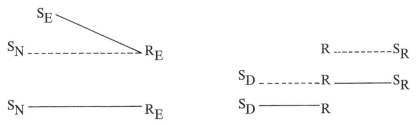

Figure 6-1. Classical and instrumental conditioning. Classical: If a new stimulaus (S_N) is presented systematically in advance of an established stimulus (S_E), the established response (R_E) can be conditioned to the new stimulus (S_N). Instrumental: 1. If a desired response (R) is systematically followed by a reinforcing stimulus (S_R), the probability of the occurrence of the desired response will be increased. 2. If systematic reinforcement occurs to a desired response (R) subsequent to the presentation of a discriminatory stimulus (S_D), the desired response is said to come under the control of the discriminatory stimulus.

whether orientated physically or emotionally—and some current thinking is the relative importance of causal factors. The traditional therapy emphasized causal change; much current thinking emphasizes behavior change.

Practice

To date, except for relatively limited demonstrations as reported in the writings of such individuals as Mowrer (1968), McLean (1970), and McReynolds (1970), rigidly controlled operant techniques have not had wide application. Recently, Weston and Irwin (1971) have described the Paired-Stimuli Technique. But, in general, one must concede that broad scale clinical evidence of the effectiveness of the new techniques has not been achieved.

Dismissal Criteria

As of the present writing, dismissal criteria in articulatory therapy have not been well established. In the first place, each of the

problems described in connection with the definition of an articulatory defect becomes relevant if one seeks to define successful
intervention. Thus, just as articulation is defective if it constitutes
a real or a perceived handicap to either the listener or the speaker,
so is intervention successful when the articulation ceases to be a
handicap either real or perceived to speaker or to listener. Unfortunately, the central problem of evaluating the extent of this
handicap is still present. Lacking such a measure, the field has
tended to define successful intervention as a program that enables
the subject to use easily and automatically each of the phonemes
of his language in all of the usual combinations in which that
phoneme appears. Performance as opposed to handicap becomes
the criterion. Unfortunately, even if one grants the validity of the
performance criterion, technical problems in the measurement of
articulation in naturalistic circumstances have resulted in a general failure to develop criteria either for (a) the prediction of
adequate carryover or (b) the measurement of carryover. Until
these goals are achieved, dismissal will remain more art than
science.

REFERENCES

Backus, O., and Beasley, J.: *Speech Therapy with Children*. Boston, Houghton Mifflin, 1951.

Bankson, N., and Byrne, M. C.: The relationship between missing teeth
and selected consonant sounds. *JSHD, 27:*341-348, 1962.

Barbara, D. (Ed.): *Psychological and Psychiatric Aspects of Speech and
Hearing*. Springfield, Thomas, 1960.

Bloomer, H.: Speech defects associated with dental abnormalities and
malocclusions. In Travis, L.E. (Ed.): *Handbook of Speech Pathology*.
New York, Appleton-Century-Crofts, 1957.

Bosma, J. F.: A syndrome of impairment in oral perception. In Bosma, J. F.
(Ed.): *Symposium on Oral Sensation and Perception*. Springfield,
Thomas, 1967.

Chomsky, N.: *Syntactic Structures*. Mouton, The Hague, 1957.

Chomsky, N., and Halle, M.: *The Sound Pattern of English*. New York,
Harper and Row, 1968.

Daniloff, R., and Moll, K.: Coarticulation of lip rounding. *J Speech Hearing Res, 11:*707-721, 1968.

Deese, J.: *Psycholinguistics*. Boston, Allyn and Bacon, 1970.

Eisenson, Jon, and Ogilvie, Mardel: *Speech Correction in the Schools*. New
York, Macmillan, 1963.

Fairbanks, G., and Green, E.: A study of minor organic deviations in 'functional' disorders of articulation: Dimensions and relationships of the lips." *JSHD, 15:*165-168, 1950.

Fairbanks, G., and Lintner, M.V.H.: A study of minor organic deviations in 'functional' disorders of articulation: The teeth and hard palate." *JSHD, 16:*273-279, 1951.

Fisher, H.: Distinctive feature analysis in testing articulation competence. Paper presented at the Annual Convention of the American Speech and Hearing Association, New York, 1970.

Hall, W.: A study of the articulatory skills of children from three to six years of age. Ph.D. Dissertation. The University of Missouri, Columbia, Missouri, 1962.

Healey, W.: A study of the articulatory skills of children from six to nine years of age. Ph.D. Dissertation. The University of Missouri, Columbia, Missouri, 1963.

Irwin, J.V.: Disorders of articulation. Indianapolis, Bobbs-Merrill, (in press, 1971).

Irwin, J. V.: *Introduction to Communicative Disorders.* Boston, Allyn and Bacon (in preparation).

Irwin, O. C.: Development of speech during infancy: Curve of phonemic frequencies." *J Ex Psychol, 37:*187-193, 1947.

Jakobson, R.; Fant, G., and Halle, M.: *Preliminaries to Speech Analysis.* Cambridge, M.I.T. Press, 1963.

Johnson, W.; Brown, Spencer, F.; Curtis, James F.; Edney, Clarence W., and Keaster, Jacqueline. *Speech Handicapped School Children.* New York, Harper and Row, 1967.

Langacker, R. W.: *Language and Its Structure.* New York, Harcourt, Brace, and World, 1968.

Lenneberg, E.: *The Biological Foundations of Language.* New York, Wiley, 1967.

McLean, J.: Shifting stimulus control of articulation responses by operant conditioning. *ASHA Monographs, 93-*153, 1970.

McNeill, D.: On theories of language acquisition. In Dixon, T.R., and Horton, D.L. (Eds.): *Verbal Behavior Theory.* Englewood Cliffs, Prentice-Hall, 1968.

McReynolds, L.: Contingencies and consequences in speech therapy. *JSHD, 35:*12-24, 1970.

McReynolds, L., and Huston, K.: A distinctive feature analysis of children's misarticulations. Paper presented at the Annual Convention of the American Speech and Hearing Association, New York, 1970.

Malmberg, B.: *Phonetics.* New York, Dover, 1963.

Mowrer, D.; Baker, R., and Schutz, R.: Operant procedures in the control of speech articulation. In Sloane, H., and MacAuley, B. (Eds.): *Operant*

Procedures in Remedial Speech and Language Training. Boston, Houghton-Mifflin, 1968.

Mowrer, O. H.: The phychologist looks at language. *Amer Psychol, 9:*660-694, 1954.

Oehman, S. E.: Coarticulation in VCV utterances: Spectographic measurements. *J Acoust Soc Amer, 39:*151-168, 1966.

Osgood, C.: Toward a wedding of insufficiencies. In Dixon, T.R., and Horton, D.L. (Eds.) : *Verbal Behavior and General Behavior Therapy.* Englewood Cliffs, Prentice-Hall, 1968.

Perkins, W., and Curlee, R.: *Causality in Speech Pathology. JSHD, 34:*231-238, 1969.

Poole, I.: Genetic development of articulation of consonant sounds in speech. Elem Eng Rev, *11:*159-161, 1934.

Ringel, R. L.: Oral sensation and perception: A selective review. *Speech and the Dentofacial Complex: The State of the Art.* ASHA REPORTS NO. 5. American Speech and Hearing Association, Washington, 1970.

Rousey, C. L., and Moriarty, A. E.: *Diagnostic Implications of Speech Sounds.* Springfield, Thomas, 1965.

Skinner, B. F.: *Verbal Behavior.* New York, Appleton-Century-Crofts, 1957.

Spriestersback, D., and Curtis, J.: Misarticulation and discrimination of speech sounds." *QJS, 37,* 483-491, 1951.

Staats, A.: *Learning, Language, and Cognition.* New York, Holt, Rinehart and Winston, 1968.

Templin, M.: *Certain Language Skills in Children.* Minneapolis, U. of Minnesota Press, Minneapolis, 1957.

Thomas, C. K.: *An Introduction to the Phonetics of American English.* New York, Ronald, 1958.

Tikovsky, R.: The structure of language. In Irwin, J. V., and Marge, M. (Ed.) : *Language Disorders of Children.* New York, Appleton-Century-Crofts, (in press).

Van Riper, C., and Irwin, J. V.: Voice and articulation. Englewood Cliffs, N. J., Prentice-Hall, 1958.

Wellman, B. L.; Case, I. M.; Mengert, I. G., and Bradbury, D. E.: Speech sounds of young children. *University of Iowa Studies in Child Welfare, 5(2):* 1931.

West, R. Ansberry, M., and Carr, A.: *The Rehabilitation of Speech.* New York, Harper and Brothers, 1957.

Weston, A. J., and Irwin, J. V.: The use of paired stimuli in the modification of articulation. *J Percept Motor Skills, 32:*947-957, 1971.

Winitz, Harris: *Articulatory Acquisition and Behavior.* New York, Appleton-Century-Crofts, 1969.

Wise, C.: *Applied Phonetics,* Englewood Cliffs, Prentice-Hall, 1957.

CHAPTER SEVEN

THE MANAGEMENT OF DISFLUENCY IN ITS EARLIEST DEVELOPMENTAL STAGES

ROBERT L. MULDER

THE LITERATURE concerning the treatment of the advanced stages of stuttering is considerable (Murphy and Fitzsimons, 1960; Van Riper, 1963; Johnson et al., 1967). Although increasing attention is being paid to management of the elementary school-age child (Chapman, 1959; Williams and Roe, 1960; Luper and Mulder, 1964; Fraser, 1964; Emerick, 1970), the emphasis on therapy for the child in the preschool period, roughly between the ages of two and six years, has been on preventative measures. This indirect approach to the child has evolved because most of the investigations of the preschool child have described the onset of stuttering as related to the child's parents.

The main focus of this chapter will be concerned with an examination of the rationale that has led to indirect therapy for the incipient stutterer and an exploration of a modified rationale which allows for the development of direct, child-centered interventional procedures. This approach is not viewed as a replacement for traditional procedures, but rather as an alternate strategy appropriate for some young children who stutter. Although an attempt is made to discuss therapy for stuttering in its earliest developmental stages, this is not always possible. Therapy only rarely, if ever, coincides with onset and subsequent identification. The child under consideration is young and has been stuttering for a relatively short time. He may be a preschooler, but he also may be found enrolled in elementary school.

THE DEVELOPMENTAL PHASES OF STUTTERING

An easily documented observation is that symptoms change as stuttering develops to its most advanced form. In order to differentiate between the symptoms commonly displayed by people when they begin to stutter with the symptoms when their stuttering is in its advanced form, Bluemel (1932) introduced the terms *primary* and *secondary* stuttering. Primary stuttering was defined as ". . . a simple disturbance of speech in which a delay ensues between the commencement and completion of a word." Secondary stuttering was defined as "consciousness of the defect and attempts to control and conceal it, employing starters, synonyms, etc." Van Riper (1954) introduced the term *transitional stuttering* to describe the behaviors that occur as the child experiences increasing awareness of his disfluency as it shifts from primary to secondary stuttering.

Bloodstein (1960), after carefully pointing out that the development of stuttering is actually a continual process to which any sharp definition into phases does some violence, concluded, for convenience in classification, that stuttering could be regarded as passing through four major phases in its development.

Bloodstein (1969) described the four phases as follows:

> *Phase One.* The preschool period, roughly between the ages of two and six years, is one in which a large number of stutterers are to be seen. During this early period there are some six characteristics that may be said to typify most stuttering cases.
>
> 1. *The difficulty has a distinct tendency to be episodic.* One of the best indications that stuttering is still in its most rudimentary form is that it appears for periods of weeks or months between long interludes of normal speech. During this phase there is apparently a high percentage of spontaneous recoveries from stuttering that consist essentially of cases in which episodes of stuttering have failed to recur. How high this percentage is would be very difficult to determine. It is not improbable that single episodes of stuttering so mild and brief that they are overlooked or soon forgotten, are exceedingly common during these years.
>
> 2. *The child stutters most when excited or upset, when he seems to have a great deal to say, or under other conditions of communicative pressure.*
>
> 3. *The dominant symptom is repetition.* This must be hastily qualified. Practically any of the integral or associated symptoms of stuttering may be seen in some of the youngest stutterers, and in some cases there seems to be little or no repetition. For

the most part, however, the more severe symptoms appear briefly and intermittently in these children, and relatively simple repetition is far more common. In some cases repetition is practically the only symptom to be observed. While much of it consists of repetition of initial syllables, as it does in older stutterers, there is also usually a marked tendency to repeat whole words of one syllable.

4. *The tendency for stutterings to occur at the beginning of the sentence is exceptionally marked in many cases during this phase.* In some of the youngest children stuttering seems to be limited almost entirely to the first word of the sentence.

5. *In contrast to more advanced stuttering, the interruptions frequently occur on the "small" parts of speech—the pronouns, conjunctions, and prepositions.* Stuttering on such words tends to consist of whole-word repetitions. In short, there is frequent repetition of such words as "like," "but," "and," "so," "he," "I," and "with."

6. *Most of the time children in the first phase of stuttering show little evidence of concern about the interruptions in their speech.* This is not to say that they are completely unconscious of them. It is commonplace for children as young as two or three to show acute frustration when they stutter by refusing to speak, crying, beating the wall with their hands, or saying, "Why can't I talk?" Such reactions are usually brief and sporadic, however, in contrast to the chronic fear and embarrassment of many older stutterers. Furthermore, the characteristic reaction of the Phase I stutterer may be epitomized by saying that when he reacts at all it is usually in response to the immediate experience of being thwarted in his efforts to communicate rather than to the ramified implications of the knowledge that he "is a stutterer."

Phase Two. The second phase in the development of stuttering is marked by the following:

1. *The disorder is essentially chronic.* There are few if any intervals of normal speech.

2. *The child regards himself as a stutterer.*

3. *The stutterings occur chiefly on the major parts of speech—nouns, verbs, adjectives, and adverbs.* There is much less tendency to stutter only on the initial words of sentences and phrases, and whole-word repetitions are no longer common.

4. *Despite his self-concept as a stutterer, the child usually evinces little or no concern about his speech difficulty.* There is an absence of such features of more advanced stuttering as conscious anticipations of stuttering, substitution, circumlocution, avoidance of speaking, and word, sound, and situation fears.

5. *The stuttering is said to increase chiefly under conditions of excitement or when the child is speaking rapidly.*

Phase Three. The third phase of stuttering has these typical features.

1. *The stuttering comes and goes largely in response to specific situations.* Among the situations that the person often reports to be especially difficult are classroom recitation, speaking to strangers, making purchases in stores, and using the telephone.
2. *Certain words or sounds are regarded as more difficult than others.*
3. *In varying degrees, use is made of word substitutions and circumlocutions.* This tends to be done only occasionally and more often as a reaction to frustration, or its imminence, than in actual fear of stuttering.
4. *There is essentially no avoidance of speech situations, and little* evidence of fear or embarrassment.

Phase Four. At the apex of its development stuttering is marked by:
1. *Vivid, fearful anticipations of stuttering.*
2. *Feared words, sounds, and situations.*
3. *Very frequent word substitution and circumlocution.*

The Preventative Approach. In the first developmental stage of stuttering, the therapy of choice that has evolved is environmental or indirect. No attempt is made to work directly with the child or his speech or language symptoms. In the traditional indirect approach considerable reliance is placed on the following: (a) preventing the child from thinking of himself and what he is doing as stuttering, (b) modifying his speech symptoms through attempts to eliminate or alter pressures in the child's environment felt to be adversely affecting fluency, mainly via parental counseling.

There are a number of reasons for an indirect approach to the management of the incipient stutterer. One of the principal reasons is related to a point of view concerning the onset of stuttering as expressed by Johnson's (1944) *diagnosogenic* theory.

1. Practically every case of stuttering was originally diagnosed as such, not by a speech expert, but by a layman—usually one, or both, of the child's parents.
2. What these laymen had diagnosed as stuttering was, by and large, undistinguishable from the hesitations and repetitions known to be characteristic of the normal speech of young children.

3. Stuttering . . . as a definite disorder was found to occur, not before being diagnosed, but after being diagnosed.

Later in a widely read textbook (Johnson, 1956) on speech disorders he succinctly stated this point of view as follows:

> No child should be diagnosed or classified as a stutterer by the classroom teacher, or by his parents or anyone else merely because he seems to speak hesitantly and with repetitions. So long as the child shows no anxiety-tension with respect to his speech nonfluencies, certainly nothing is to be gained by placing him under a cloud by calling him a stutterer, and it is clear that doing this can have seriously harmful consequences.

This point of view coupled with the belief that stuttering is an emotional disorder of childhood has gained wide acceptance among some professional workers. Typical of this point of view is one by Bloodstein (1961) who states that the most important goal of therapy for the Phase One stutterer is "to prevent the child from gaining the dangerous image of himself as a stutterer which underlies the disorder in its more chronic forms, and once acquired, is so difficult to erase."

Studies of quondam stutterers attribute their improvement to a variety of factors including some management practices contrary to traditional speech therapy approaches (Ellis, 1968). Salient features of these studies related to speech therapy for incipient stuttering give rise to questions regarding the significance of the admonishment of early stuttering, which lead to questions concerning whether therapy for the beginning stutterer should be limited to indirect therapy.*

The Importance of Labeling Per Se. The evaluation of stuttering *per se* does not appear to have a universal effect on the remission of stuttering symptoms. For example, Bryngelson's records (1938, 1943) indicate that approximately 40 per cent of young children who had been identified as stutterers stopped stuttering by the time they were seven or eight years of age. In a study by Glasner and Rosenthal (1957), almost half of 153 children who

---

*Part of this section is based on a paper delivered by the author at the 1968 meeting of the Council for Exceptional Children, New York City, "Investigations of the quondam stutterer: The effects on early stuttering therapy."

were evaluated by their parents as having stuttered before beginning school had stopped stuttering. An additional 14 per cent
was reported as stuttering only occasionally at the time of the
study. Dickson (1965) requested parents of children in grades
kindergarten through nine to check twenty-three items pertaining
to incipient stuttering. Approximately 10 per cent of the parents
in each grade reported incipient stuttering symptoms. There were
196 or 55 per cent of the subjects who were reported to have
experienced spontaneous remission of these symptoms.

Shearer and Williams (1965) in their study of recovery from
stuttering point out that since most quondam stutterers were
aware of their early stuttering difficulty and were able to recover,
it would seem that self-awareness or self-labeling *per se* need not
be a negative factor in recovery.

Wingate (1962) in his evaluation and stuttering series concerning identification of stuttering and the use of a label, states:
"Research findings yield no tangible basis for the belief that the
presence, and use, of a term for stuttering has etiological significance in the disorder."

Admonishment of Stuttering Behavior. Traditionally, at the
onset of stuttering, it is advocated that management efforts should
avoid drawing a child's attention to his way of talking. Approaches
directed at doing something about the speech symptoms do not
necessarily have a negative effect on stuttering. Milisen and Johnson (1936), reporting a study of differences between young stutterers and young quondam stutterers, indicated that the parents of
twelve of the thirty-two recovered cases had made the child stop
and repeat. In another case, recovery was claimed to be effected
by spanking the child every time he stuttered. In the study reported by Glasner and Rosenthal (1957) of parental diagnosis of
stuttering, almost half of the children who were actively corrected
by their parents were reported to have stopped stuttering. It is
interesting to note that the approaches used by the parents, i.e.
telling the child to repeat or stop and start over, talk more slowly,
etc., are in contradiction to those usually advocated by some
speech pathologists.

Consciousness of the act of stuttering *per se* does not seem to be a negative factor in recovery. Wingate (1964) reported that half of the fifty quondam stutterers he investigated described the change as determination to change or overcome the problem. Shearer and Williams (1965) reported that of fifty-eight quondam stutterers, 96 per cent felt that speaking more slowly helped in recovery from stuttering.

Wingate (1962) in the first of his evaluation series found that 18 per cent of the fifty-five older recovered stutterers reported that the only help they had concerning what to do to stop stuttering was from receiving 'lay' advice and suggestions from parents and others. Wingate goes on to say ". . . there is no direct evidence to support the contention that expressing concern about speech fluency or the use of a 'label' is etiologically significant in stuttering. On the contrary, there is evidence that such factors either have been immaterial or have had a salutary effect."

There is little question but that the term *stuttering* can be loaded with emotional significance. In the best interest of the child, it is sound practice to prevent the child from thinking of himself as a stutterer. When this can be accomplished the effort is well spent. Unfortunately, the prevention of awareness is not always possible.

Our society has a name for this kind of behavior. Right or wrong they call it stuttering. One of the things that can be overlooked is that parents are not the only people in the world capable of calling this particular behavior stuttering. All of the youngsters on the block can do this, the check-out girl at the supermarket can do this, his Sunday School teacher can, anyone can—and often will. But when a child first begins to call what he is doing stuttering, all we really know at that point is that the youngster is sophisticated enough to know that there is a word that classifies his behavior and that he has made a connection between his behavior and the word. We don't really know about the child's reaction to the word at that time. All we know is that he has been intelligent enough to pick it up and use it. At this point, it doesn't mean that his self-labeling has necessarily harmed him one iota, nor that he has acquired a so-called self-concept as a stutterer.

The Watch and Wait Approach. An unfortunate and unin-

tended outcome of the indirect speech therapy approach to incipient stuttering based on evaluational theories is that some young
children who stutter do not receive speech help until their symptoms worsen dramatically.

Emerick (1965) says it this way: "In their fear lest they do
something harmful and create stuttering, some therapists do nothing at all." He points up three undesirable approaches common
in the public schools: (a) pretending that stuttering doesn't exist,
(b) waiting until the child outgrows it or grows older, or (c) placing him with an articulation case.

According to Sanders (1959), the child who requires systematic help may not receive the kind of help he needs when he needs
it, because "some therapists never get beyond the *don't-label-him-a-
stutterer* type of counseling." As Sanders points out it is not
sufficient simply to tell parents that the child will "out-grow" the
problem or that they have "nothing to worry about."

It goes without saying that a speech clinician is a responsible
person who does not want to set things into motion which may
have harmful consequences. One interpretation of the evaluational theory of stuttering is that an unusual show of interest in
youngster's symptoms could be construed as a diagnosis of stuttering. The speech clinician feels constrained to display much interest in the child's manifestations of stuttering because his interest
may increase rather than decrease concern. Thus, his cautions
have focused around injunctions to parents and teachers to refrain
from exaggerations of the significance of the observed behavior.
But, sometimes, even when the child's parents heed the injunctions to refrain from dealing with or acting as if the child's stutterings are symptoms of the onset of stuttering, the results are not
always as expected—the child's symptoms may worsen. The result
is time lost. Unnecessarily long delays may result before more
appropriate management procedures are instigated. In the interim
there may be a significant deterioration of the child's fluency, and
growing confusion or anxiety on the part of the child's parents—
and perhaps the child himself.

When it is recommended to parents to watch and wait to see
if there is something significant to be concerned about, the

criterion used by the clinician for justifying the wait is to see, hopefully, if the speech behavior changes for the better. Care must be taken to assure that parents do not suspect the clinician of being less than candid. There is good reason for this caution. A clinician may protest that parents should not fear that what their child is doing is something to be anxious about and yet be so concerned himself that his efforts at reassurance reveal overtones of anxiety (Mulder, 1961). Efforts to minimize the problem must also include an acknowledgement of the possibility that the child's symptoms may get worse. Because constant surveillance is required to find out if the symptoms worsen, this can work against the clinician's efforts to keep the parent's anxiety under control.

When speech clinicians feel constrained to avoid open reference to a child's stutterings they may also avoid covert probing. As a consequence a child may be aware that society calls his behavior "stuttering" and may have been thinking of his behavior as stuttering long before his parents or clinician discover his level of awareness. If no one says anything about it to him, the child may come to believe his condition is partly or even completely undesirable, unmentionable or that no one knows how to help him.

There is an interesting argument that can be raised for earlier attempts at direct therapy that is based on the kinds of results that are now obtained in therapy. Although we do not have complete assurance that a child will recover from his stuttering if he receives early direct speech therapy, it may be that the recovery rate could be raised if direct systematic therapy were started earlier. Sheehan and Martyn (1966) in their study of spontaneous recovery from stuttering make an intriguing point. They observed that the more severe a young stutterer is, the more likely he is to receive speech therapy, but, the more severe a young stutterer is, the less likely he is to recover. Further emphasizing this point, they point out that speech therapy is thus most likely to be directed at those who have the poorest prognosis, using severity as the predictor. Their data do not indicate the age level when therapy work was attempted nor the nature of the therapy, but it seems reasonable to hypothesize that if the therapy were begun sooner when the symptoms were less severe, the prognosis would be better.

THE APPROPRIATENESS OF THE SPEECH CLINICIAN'S TRAINING

Sheehan and Martyn (1966) point out that even if a child is admitted to early therapy, he may not receive the kind of help necessary to mitigate his symptoms. They noted that both quondam and active stutterers:

> reflected a feeling of vague uneasiness and confusion as to the goals of therapy, and as to their relationship (if any) to the methods. For example, 'we read stories,' or 'we played speech games,' or 'we just talked.' The sheer irrelevance of speech techniques served chiefly to heighten the stutterer's apprehension that there was something unmentionably wrong with him that could not be dealt with directly (p. 129).

At stake here is the type of training provided by our college and university programs in speech pathology. Williams (1970) estimates that approximately 75 per cent to 85 per cent of all the elementary school-age children in the country who receive help with stuttering receive that help from the school clinician. These clinicians are trained in university programs in speech pathology and audiology where their practicum experience concerning stuttering is mainly with adults who stutter and with counseling parents about prevention of the problem. According to an unpublished study (Williams, Melrose, Silverman, and Cox, 1969) of eighty-nine Iowa school clinicians trained at thirty-three different institutions, 72 per cent had less than ten hours of supervised experience with elementary-age stutterers. In certain instances, the "supervised experience" consisted solely of observing another clinician work with a child of this age. Williams (1970) assumes that comparable data would be obtained from other states, and this author concurs. He goes on to say that "in many instances the school clinician is asked to work with a stuttering child of an age with which the clinician has had little experience, and concerning whose stuttering problem and therapy procedures little has been written." Although he is talking about the child from seven to twelve years of age, comparisons can be made concerning the training background of speech clinicians working with the preschool child who is beginning to stutter.

WHO SHOULD RECEIVE DIRECT HELP?

The case has been presented that theoretical biases have miti-gated against a child-centered approach to the preschool disfluent child. Procedures which indirectly involve the child in face-to-face therapy do not contraindicate the significance of preventative approaches.

These approaches should be followed insofar as possible. What we need to know is how to differentiate between the child who should be treated indirectly and the one who should receive systematic direct help. Because this is not an easy task, many clinicians employ the "watch and wait" approach. They wait to see if the symptoms get severe enough to warrant direct interven-tion. This is not so much a problem if a child is under the observa-tion of a speech clinician because his parents are bringing him to a speech clinic. When the parents are motivated to help, counsel-ing and careful observation can be systematically planned.

Many children who are beginning to stutter have entered school before therapy is made available. In these instances some of the parents of these children are not available for or amenable to clinical guidance. In those instances where the child is already in school and his parents desire help, the time available to the school clinicians for parental counseling may be severely restricted for a number of reasons: size of case load, available time, administrative policy restricting reimbursement to actual child-centered therapy, and others. One of the very real problems facing the clinician is that in the early developmental stages the stuttering symptoms come and go. Clinicians whose philosophies of therapy hold that stuttering is an emotional disorder of childhood sometimes resolve these conflicts by not listing the beginning child who stutters on their active case rolls.

The question of whether to employ direct or indirect therapy is probably ill-phrased. Perhaps it is more appropriate to ask, "How directive should the therapy program for this child be at this time?" (Luper and Mulder, 1964). They discuss major levels of directness with the degree of directness reading down the list.

1. No direct involvement with the child.

2. Direct contact between child and therapist but with no attention being focused on speech production.
3. Direct contact with attention focused on speech improvement but not directly on stuttering.
4. Direct therapy with the child's attention focused on reducing stuttering but with labeling and complexity of techniques held to a minimum.
5. Direct therapy with emphasis upon stuttering and with considerable attention being directed at the attitudes connected with stuttering and at the maladaptive speech behaviors associated with the stuttering (p. 64-65).

Age. Traditionally, therapists were enjoined that the younger the child the better it was to concentrate on environmental approaches and to be less directive. It was felt that the younger the child, the more likely it was that he would "forget" unfavorable speech experiences.

Awareness. Bloodstein (1969) points out that even though children in the first developmental phase of stuttering show little evidence of concern about the interruptions in their speech, this is not to say that they are completely unconscious of them. He goes on to point out that it is commonplace for children as young as two or three to show acute frustrations when they stutter by refusing to speak, crying, beating the wall with their hands, or saying, "Why can't I talk?" (Bloodstein, 1969, p. 23). Traditional therapy has handled the child's frustration by attempting to reduce or eliminate the frequency of these occurrences through restructuring the child's environment to reduce the pressures that brought on these behaviors. Since some of these pressures come from the child's ability to handle his language, some of them from attitudes unknown to his parents and/or therapists, indirect therapy was only partially successful in helping the child maintain fluent patterns of speech.

Severity. According to Bloodstein (1960), "The concept of a primary stage of stuttering has fastened the assumption that the stuttering of early childhood is simple and innocuous. While this is true in many instances, there are actually hardly any more severe cases than some of those to be found in the first phase of stuttering" (p. 370). Significant here is the fact that diagnosis and planning for therapy is not clean-cut. Only little research has been conducted concerning the process of development of stuttering. Bloodstein (1969) maintains that the outline of stuttering phases he has developed appears to be typical, not universal. His phases are descriptions of reference points along a continuum. Many of the young stutterers who are under discussion here are in transition between phase one and phase two.

Along with severity, the characteristic type of speech symptoms the child is employing should be considered. Glasner and Vermilyea (1953) who investigated how the term "primary stuttering" was defined and used by professional pathologists found that 87 per cent of the workers felt that there is definitely something in the speech of some young children that compels both parents and therapists to do something about it. Parents also are a reliable source. Stromsta (1965) in a study designed to describe the characteristics of disfluencies displayed by certain young children and labeled as abnormal by their parents found that thirty-eight cases so identified were described as stuttering ten years later.

This "something" mentioned above consists predominantly of sound and syllable repetitions and prolongations. Thus, when a child of four or younger is stuttering quite severely with sound and syllable repetitions and prolongations, the clinician should consider direct face-to-face therapy as part of this therapy.

Language Skills. Many children who stutter frequently tend to be slow in developing language skills. (Berry, 1938; Morley, 1957; Bloodstein, 1958). Stutterers are more likely than nonstutterers to have other speech defects, chiefly defects of articulation, or have histories of such defects (Berry, 1938; Bloodstein, 1960; Darley, 1955; Schindler, 1955; Morley, 1957; Johnson *et al.,* 1959; Andrews and Harris, 1964).

Traditional speech therapy approaches have been aimed at manipulation of factors in his environment to reduce pressures affecting his fluency without involving the child himself directly. Because of the very nature of indirect therapy, due consideration is not always given to improving language ability. Although clinicians have little compunction about working with a very young child who is delayed in speech or who has troublesome articulation errors, some of them tend to regard children beginning to stutter differently, as if they do not need direct help in learning the mechanics of speech and language. Part of the trouble encountered by a child who is disfluent stems from the fact that he is a novice just starting to learn to talk. His vocabulary is restricted and the intricacies of grammar as well as articulation affect the prosodic aspects of his speech.

An unpublished study of Rutherford and Telser (1969) aimed at studying word retrieval abilities in young children has generated normative information to verify the existence of word-finding problems of minimal nature in some children who stutter. The technique employed was based upon the response latency in naming pictures of common objects shown to the child one at a time on cards. During trial one, the child is presented each card unhurriedly and asked to name what he sees to familiarize the child with the cards. Any cards not recognized or which seem unfamiliar to the child are removed. During trial two, the card is flipped in front of the child with a snap.

Responses which produce stuttering, undue latencies (longer than two seconds) , or misnaming are noted.

In clinical use, the diagnosis of a word finding problem is a matter of the qualitative analysis of abnormally long latencies.

A characteristic of the dysnomic individual is that his symbol-retrieval skills will fatigue rapidly, so that he encounters more frequent and severe word lapses on later trials than on the first two trials. Conversely, normals (including nondysnomic stutterers) adapt to the materials and are more fluent on later trials than on initial runs.

The diagnosis of a symbol retrieval problem is made on the basis of clear evidence that pictures named on previous trials cannot now be correctly named, or are named only after obvious groping for the word. The use of synonyms *(Canine* for *dog),* associated responses *(fork* for *spoon),* or function words *(cutting thing* for *saw)* should be carefully explored, for they often are signs of word lapses which have been circumvented.

It is rare that the examiner cannot distinguish a word lapse from a stuttering block. Usually the word lapse is not accompanied by struggle behavior or an articulatory attempt. Not infrequently, however, he may partially produce the initial sound or syllable, only to discover that he does not know the word he is attempting to say. Rutherford and Telser suggest that the programming of the motor sequences for syllable and word production precedes any conscious awareness of the word which is to be uttered. When there is doubt in the examiner's mind, careful questioning usually will indicate whether the word was in mind but could not be spoken (a stuttering block) or not yet in mind (a word lapse).

As to the question about the examiner's ability to distinguish a stuttering block and a word lapse, Rutherford and Telser comment thus: "Occasionally it is not possible, but in most instances the word lapse is marked by complete absence of struggle or starter behavior, and upon questioning the child can tell you whether the word was in his mind or not."

They point out two characteristics noted with great consistency in stutterers who have word-finding problems. Stutterers who do not have a word-finding problem adapt to the test materials rapidly. They may have severe blocks on the initial trial, fewer on the second, and may be completely fluent on the third. The stutterer who also has a word-finding problem seems not to adapt; he either remains the same, showing approximately the same number of word lapses on subsequent trials as on the first, or he gets worse (Rutherford and Telser, 1969).

A comment is due here concerning a re-examination of the traditional injunction about helping a child to say his troublesome words. In those instances where a word-finding problem is discovered, these children may profit from concentrated help aimed at establishing better word-recall.

Not only do we find that children are delayed in speech development but we will find that some speech failure is due, as Weiss (1964) contends, to the child's efforts to avoid cluttering. Oral reading difficulty in the classroom may be a contributor, particularly when the constant threat of failure present in such a situation is intensified by a teacher's impatience or the child's emotional insecurity (Bloodstein, 1969, p. 226).

Clinicians should work at mutually profitable cooperative efforts so that parents and preprimary and kindergarten teachers of these children can become acquainted with available language learning approaches and encouraged in their use. This should take the form of helping the child to learn to use speech and language so that he may hear himself speak smoothly in an integrated fashion. Certainly, not to be overlooked is that special attention should be provided for specific problems of articulation, vocabulary building, etc. unique to individual children.

The child should have at least one person to serve as a speech model to imitate. This should be a person who consistently speaks in short, simple sentences. If a model is not readily available, the clinician should train himself, or one of the child's parents or a teacher, to talk this way. This way of talking should provide him with uncomplicated ways of saying things automatically, reducing the necessity for fumbling as he manufactures sentences.

Various means for hearing himself speak without breakdown have been advocated. Not to be overlooked is the desensitization approach advocated by Van Riper (1963). Once a basal level of fluency is established efforts should be aimed at toughening the child to interruption and disturbances.

He should learn to experiment with more flexible use of his vocal mechanism. Methods such as those described by Van Riper and Butler (1955) in their book *Speech In The Elementary Schools* can be adapted to the specific needs of these children.

New development in linguistics and the study of language development certainly must be adapted in order to help the child through his early attempts at language acquisition more gracefully. More definitive tests of language functions are needed so that language deficits can be discovered early. Thus can the efficacy of early language training for the young child who stutters be determined.

Interaction. It is difficult to demonstrate that self-awareness (Shearer and Williams, 1965) and labeling (Wingate, 1962) as such are causative or maintaining factors in stuttering. What is easier to demonstrate is that the significance attached to awareness and labeling are important considerations. Although prevention of stuttering via these means is desirable, the evaluations themselves should be made accessible and amenable to therapy. Because awareness and labels can materialize rapidly, it behooves the clinician to insure that the child's (and the child's parents) concepts of stuttering be guided so as not to be acquired willy-nilly and possibly injuriously. Therapy should aim to assure that possible adverse effects of the self-evaluations are offset by objective, reassuring appraisal.

The clinician must take into account such factors as age, awareness of disprosody, severity of the disfluency on display, and deficits of other language skills before deciding the level of directness of therapy. Brutton and Shoemaker (1967) pointing up the significance that classical conditioning has for stuttering, base their theory on the observations that stress may produce in normal speakers autonomic reactions capable of disrupting speech fluency.

In incipient stuttering, if a child regularly encounters stress in a situation, the negative emotion aroused may become a conditioned response to neutral stimuli in the situation. Each time the situational cues are present, the child now experiences emotional arousal and its consequent fluency failure. The assumption that stuttering is a problem that is learned (Williams, 1970), points out that in this learning there is a disruption in interaction between the child and his listening environment. Williams (1970) bases his therapy program on the nature of the stuttering problem as expressed by Johnson (1961). Williams interaction hypothesis assumes that the child, at approximately three or four years of age, is repeating or prolonging sounds to a degree that bothers the important listeners in his environment. Because they react adversely to him as a speaker, he in turn reacts to their reactions, prompting a feeling and a belief on his part that the way he talks —and possibly he as a person—are not acceptable to them.

As a result, he begins to develop a cautious, hesitant way of talking that is highlighted by increasing tensing behavior with undue efforts to "talk right." "Talking right" is often construed to mean "not talking wrong." It is the wrongness that receives attention. The child begins to do things behaviorally to "not talk wrong." He begins to develop belief about the reasons that he talks the way he does—and begins to associate his internal feelings with the occurrence of "talking wrong." Therefore, with increasing frequency, when he is called upon to talk he attends to his internal feelings for "cues" as to whether he can or cannot say acceptably what he wants to say—and then acts accordingly.

This author feels strongly that in too many instances the unresolved barrier to successful stuttering therapy turns out to be the clinician himself. As Williams points out, these ways of talking are reinforced in inappropriate ways by the important listeners because of their own beliefs about the nature of the problem. Essentially these beliefs carry assumptions: that he "has trouble getting certain words out." and that he needs to do something special to help himself (by this it is meant things that other people don't have to do) to 'get the word out.' According to Williams the more he tenses, struggles, and does "special things to help him talk," the more that people (and he) evaluate this as "talking wrong," and therefore seemingly the only thing left to do is "try harder."

This author encourages the interested clinician to give careful attention to Williams' (1970) therapy program which emphasizes a positive approach to learning: (a) by examining the child's basic assumptions about stuttering and what, as he thinks, causes it, (b) by providing considerable information about talking (not only about stuttering—but primarily about the total process of talking), (c) by helping him understand and accept his feelings, (d) by helping him to become more aware of the purpose of talking, that is, of verbal communication, (e) by helping him to experiment with and to explore the versatility of his behavior that we call talking, and (f) by demonstrating and then reinforcing the kinds of things he can do to talk easily and spontaneously in any situation where he is called upon to speak.

SUMMARY

Acceptance of direct interventional procedures for the child who is beginning to stutter is dependent on the validity of the rationale intended to support this approach. The design of this chapter is an attempt to support such a position. It is too early to know whether a child or even which child will recover from his stuttering if he receives early direct child-clinician oriented therapy. The concern here is with providing ways to increase the recovery rate.

It seems fair to view the paucity of available interventional techniques as being due in part to the existence of considerable well-established, reasonable approaches advocating top priority to prevention. This traditional approach has provided considerable relief to numerous children and their rightfully concerned parents. But, because disfluency is not always smoothed out by removing disturbing influences or even by keeping the child from being disturbed by his disfluencies, the need for alternative strategies is brought home. Hopefully, this point of view will be tested by thoughtful speech clinicians. New approaches and modifications of existing approaches should suggest themselves. Certainly constructive caution is necessary when new concepts are attempted. Watching and waiting to see whether the disfluency will increase in frequency or be accompanied by tension and struggle, however, is seen as a poor measure of the effectiveness of preventative techniques.

REFERENCES

Andrews, G., and Harris, M.: *The Syndrome of Stuttering.* Clinics in Developmental Med., No. 17. London, Spastics Society Medical Education and Information Unit in association with Wm. Heinemann Medical Books, 1964.

Berry, M.F.: Developmental history of stuttering children. *J Pediat, 12:*209-17, 1938.

Bloodstein, O.: The development of stuttering: II Developmental phases. *J Speech Hearing Dis, 25:*336-376, 1960.

Bloodstein, O.: The development of stuttering: III Theoretical and clinical implications. *J Speech Hearing Dis, 26:*67-82, 1961.

Bloodstein, O.: *A Handbook on Stuttering.* Chicago, National Easter Seal Society for Crippled Children and Adults, 1969.

Bluemel, C.S.: Primary and secondary stammering. *Quart J Speech,* XVIII, 1932.

Brutton, E.J., and Shoemaker, D.J.: *The Modification of Stuttering.* Englewood Cliffs, Prentice Hall, 1967.

Bryngelson, B.: Prognosis of stuttering. *J Speech Hearing Dis, 3:*121-123, 1938.

Bryngelson, B.: Stuttering and personality development. *Nervous Child, 2:*162-166, 1943.

Chapman, Myfanwy: *Self-Inventory: Group Therapy for Those Who Stutter*, 3rd ed. Minneapolis, Burgess, 1959.

Darley, F.L.: The relationship of parental attitudes and adjustments to the development of stuttering. In Johnson, W., and Leutenegger, R.R. (Eds.): *Stuttering in Children and Adults*. Minneapolis, U. of Minneapolis Press, 1955.

Dickson, Stanley: Incipient stuttering symptoms and spontaneous remission of non-stuttered speech. Unpublished paper presented at ASHA meeting, Chicago, 1965.

Ellis, P.: Critical incidence relevant to the remission of stuttering symptoms by quondam stutterers. Unpublished M.S. Thesis, Oregon College of Education, 1968.

Emerick, L.: Therapy for young stutterers. *Exceptional Child, 398-402*, 1965.

Emerick, L.: *Therapy for Young Stutterers*. Danville, Ill., Interstate, 1970.

Frazer, M.: *Treatment of the Young Stutterer in the School*. Memphis, Speech Foundation of America, 1964.

Glasner, P.J., and Vermilyea, F.D.: An investigation of the definition and use of the diagnosis, "primary stuttering." *J Speech Hearing Dis, 18:*161-168 (1953).

Glasner, P.J., and Rosenthal, D.: Parental diagnosis of stuttering in young children. *J Speech Hearing Dis, 22*, 288-95, 1957.

Johnson, W.: The Indians have no word for it. I. Stuttering in children. *Quart J Speech, 30:*330-37, 1944.

Johnson, W.: *Stuttering and What You Can Do About It*. Minneapolis, U of Minn. Press, 1961.

Johnson, W. et al.: *Speech Handicapped School Children*, rev. ed. New York, Harper and Bros., 1965.

Johnson, W. et al.: *Speech Handicapped School Children*, 3rd ed. New York, Harper and Row, 1967.

Johnson, W. et al.: *The Onset of Stuttering*. Minneapolis, U of Minneapolis Press, 1959.

Luper, H. L., and Mulder, R.L.: *Stuttering: Therapy for Children*. Englewood Cliffs, Prentice-Hall, 1964.

Milisen, R., and Johnson, W.: A comparative study of stutterers, former stutterers and normal speakers whose handedness has been changed. *Speech, 1:*61-86, 1936.

Morley, M.E.: *The Development and Disorders of Speech in Childhood*. Edinburgh, Livingstone, 1957.

Mulder, R.L.: The student of stuttering as a stutterer. *J Speech Hearing Dis, 26:*168-179, 1961.

Murphy, A.T., and Fitzsimons, R.M.: *Stuttering and Personality Dynamics*. New York, Ronald, 1960.

Rutherford, David, and Telser, Elsa: Word-finding abilities of kindergarten and first grade children. Northwestern University, Presented at Convention of the *American Speech and Hearing Association,* November, 1969.

Sander, E.K.: Counseling parents of stuttering children. *J Speech Hearing Dis, 24*:262-271, 1959.

Schlinder, M.D.: A study of educational adjustments of stuttering and non-stuttering children. In Johnson, W., and Leutenegger, R.R. (Eds.): *Stuttering in Children and Adults.* Minneapolis, U of Minn. Press, 1955.

Shearer, W.W., and Williams, J.D.: Self-recovery from stuttering. *J Speech Hearing Dis, 30*:288-290, 1965.

Sheehan, J.G., and Martyn, M.M.: Spontaneous recovery from stuttering. *J Speech Hearing Res, 9*:121-135, 1966.

Stromstra, C.: A Spectographic study of dysfluencies labeled as stuttering by parents. *De Therapia Vocis et Loquelae,* Volume 1, Societat Internationalis Logopaediae at Phoniatric XII Congressus Vindobonate Anno MCMLXV, Acta, August, 1965.

Van Riper, C., and Butler, K.G.: *Speech in Elementary Classroom.* New York, Harper and Row, 1955.

Van Riper, C.: *Speech Correction: Principles and Methods,* (3rd ed.). Englewood Cliffs, Prentice-Hall, 1954.

Van Riper, C.: *Speech Correction: Principles and Methods,* (4th ed.). Englewood Cliffs, Prentice-Hall, 1963.

Weiss, D.A.: *Cluttering.* Englewood Cliffs, Prentice-Hall, 1964.

Williams, E.D.: Chapter entitled "Stuttering therapy for children." In Travis, L.E.: *A Handbook of Speech Pathology* (in Press). New York, Appleton-Century-Crofts, 1970.

Williams, E.D.: A point of view about stuttering. *J Speech Hearing Dis, 22*:390-397, 1957.

Williams, E.D., and Roe, A.: Teachers, parents, and stutterers. *Education, 80*:471-475, 1960.

Wingate, M.E.: Evaluation and stuttering. Part I. Speech characteristics of young children. *J Speech Hearing Dis, 27*:106-116, 1962.

Wingate, M.E.: Evaluation and stuttering. Part III. Identification of stuttering and the use of a label. *J Speech Hearing Dis, 27*:368-377, 1962.

Wingate, M.E.: Recovery from stuttering. *J Speech Hearing Dis, 29*:312-321, 1964.

CHAPTER EIGHT

APHASIA IN ADULTS

ROBERT J. DUFFY

Aphasia is the name applied to a broad range of disturbances of communication caused by damage to the brain and characterized by difficulty using language symbols. This chapter is concerned with aphasia in adults as a clinical communication problem and how it is treated by the speech pathologist. Other aspects of aphasia are also discussed in order to provide background necessary to understanding communication problems and their treatment.

Aphasiology is an extensive field of study which is of interest to many disciplines other than speech pathology. Psychologists have long been interested in aphasia because of its relationship to problems in memory, thinking, imagery and other behaviors. Neurologists view aphasia as a clinical symptom of brain damage which may be helpful in locating sites of lesions. Psychoneurologists study aphasia because it contributes to our knowledge of the relationship between structure and behavior. Linguists have contributed much theory and technique to the analysis of aphasic language behavior.

INCIDENCE AND PREVALENCE OF APHASIA

Despite the fact that aphasia has been under investigation for over a hundred years, reliable figures on the incidence and prevalence of aphasia are lacking. One estimate places the prevalence at one million aphasics for the entire population of the United States. Increased high speed transportation can be expected to increase the number of accident victims with head injuries. Also as life span increases there is an increase in the size of our older population which is prone to heart and circulatory disorders resulting in brain damage. Thus, the increases in the number of persons sustaining cerebral injuries combined with medical advances in the ability to preserve life will result in greater numbers of persons surviving cerebral trauma with residual aphasia. The prevalence of aphasia will continue to increase until preventive measures can reduce the incidence of cerebral trauma.

DEFINITION OF APHASIA

It is difficult to understand aphasic behavior without some direct exposure to at least a few aphasics representing different degrees of severity or types of communication difficulties. If possible the student should have the opportunity for case presentations, films, videotapes or recordings throughout his study of the problem. Case histories and personal accounts of experiences with aphasia are also helpful (Buck, 1957; McBride, 1969; Ritchie, 1961; Sies and Butler, 1963).

A mild but dramatic occurrence of aphasia was that of Dwight Eisenhower while he was president of the United States. He described his experience in his autobiography (Eisenhower, 1965):

> Following a light lunch I walked to my office to resume work. At my desk I found papers waiting for signature. As I picked up a pen, I experience a strange, although not alarming feeling of dizziness. Since the sensation lasted only a moment, I reached for another paper. Suddenly I became frustrated. It was difficult for me to take hold of the first paper on the pile. This finally accomplished, I found that the words on it seemed to run off the top of the page. Now more than a little bewildered, I dropped the pen. Failing in two or three attempts to pick it up, I decided to get to my feet, and at once found I had to catch hold of my chair. . .
>
> I sat down quickly and rang for my secretary. As Mrs. Whitman came to my desk I tried to explain and then came another puzzling experience: I could not express what I wanted to say. Words—but not the ones I wanted—came to my tongue. It was impossible for me to express any coherent thought whatsoever. I began to feel truly helpless.
>
> Actually my performance must have been worse than I suspected, for Mrs. Whitman, unable to make any sense out of my words—which I was fully aware were nothing but gibberish—called for General Goodpaster.

Andy Goodpaster wasted no time asking questions. He concentrated on getting me to my room in the Mansion. Though I was not yet convinced that I was the victim of anything more than a temporary dizzy spell, I was so puzzled by my futile efforts to communicate that I responded without protest to Goodpaster's grasp of my arm and his urgent 'Mr. President, I think we should get you to bed.'

I had no difficulty in walking and felt no pain. In my room, Goodpaster helped me to undress and lie down. The doctor soon arrived. Having resigned myself to bed I spent no time worrying about the source of my trouble; I just turned over to take a nap.

Sometime later there arrived the inevitable medical consultants, two very gifted neurological surgeons. By this time I could communicate a little, but only a little. The doctors, following a lengthy examination, arrived at a tentative conclusion.

I had suffered, they said, a minor 'spasm'—and I am not sure whether of a nerve or a small blood vessel. In any event the result was temporary interruption in communication between my mental 'dictionary' and the thought I wished to express. So far as vocabulary was concerned I had a loss of memory. The doctors said I had improved even during the period of their visit, and predicted a full recovery in a matter of days, possibly of hours.

Gradually, memory of words returned: the doctors pronounced 95 per cent recovered and said that before long I should be completely cured.

They were not wholly accurate. From that time onward I have frequently experienced difficulty in prompt utterance of the word I seek. Even today, I reverse syllables in a long word and at times am compelled to speak slowly and cautiously if I am to enunciate correctly.

This particular illness was of a kind that could, if it became severe, create a situation in which the patient might be incapable of analyzing difficult problems and making reasonable decisions. Possibly he could become unable to express his thoughts—in the case of the President, be unable to express a decision to resign.

Eisenhower's description of his episode provides an intuitive definition of aphasia. A formal definition which would readily be acceptable to all disciplines concerned with the problem would be difficult to give. One must be prepared to encounter a number of definitions of aphasia as he begins to read more widely and especially as he crosses boundaries into other disciplines. However, most speech pathologists would probably agree that the term aphasia* *refers to an impairment in the ability to communicate due to disorders of symbolic language processes caused by lesions of those cerebral mechanisms which normally underly language processing.*

An aphasic is similar to a person who suddenly finds himself in a strange country where everyone is using a language which he does not know. Although he can hear and see, he cannot comprehend what is being said or read because he does not know the language code. He does not know what "meaning" the auditory or visual patterns (words) stand for (symbolize). Even though he can accurately repeat the words which he hears or can copy the words that he sees, he does not understand their meaning; there is no association between the word and its referent. Similarly he cannot speak or write a meaningful message because he does not know the phonological, semantic or grammatical system of the language. Both the aphasic and the stranger have difficulty communicating because of deficiencies in the knowledge and/or use of the symbolic language code.*

Further specification of the definition indicates what aphasia is *not*. It is an impairment of the language process itself and not an impairment in the *use* of language because of (a) mental dysfunction, or (b) sensory loss of motor dysfunction. These two conditions may also be produced by cerebral damage and can result in communication disturbances but they are clinically distinguishable from aphasic communication disorders.

---

*The prefix *a* means *without;* and *dys-* means *impairment of*. Since aphasics are rarely completely without speech, the term *dysphasia* is a descriptively more accurate clinical term for most cases. However, tradition and common practice favor the use of the term *aphasia* regardless of the degree of impairment. The term aphasia will be used in this chapter to refer to all degrees of severity of language disturbance. Similarly, the terms *agnosia, apraxia* and *dysarthria* will be used without implication concerning the degree of severity of impairment.

*The analogy between the foreigner who does not *know* a language and the aphasic might not be quite accurate. Unlike the foreigner the aphasic perhaps does retain his *knowledge* of the linguistic code but his deficiency may be in the activation or utilization of this knowledge for communicative purposes. The question whether aphasia is an impairment of linguistic competence (knowledge) or performance (use) is currently under discussion (Schuell, 1969, p. 119).

COMMUNICATION DISTURBANCES DUE TO MENTAL DYSFUNCTION

Brain damage may produce nonaphasic disturbances in communication as a result of impaired mental functioning. Verbal behavior reflects cognitive and affective states. Therefore, verbal behavior will show disturbances due to disorders of memory, attention, retention, orientation, thinking, ability to function abstractly, and emotional states. These persons may be "dull," passive and withdrawn with little expressive behavior of any kind. However, when they are required to use verbal abilities they can usually do so; unlike the aphasic, they can name, read, write, and understand single words and short phrases and sentences quickly, easily and accurately. They can communicate adequately concerning immediate concrete needs but have difficulty with the understanding or expression of long, complex or abstract ideas such as defining words, explaining proverbs, etc. In formal testing and spontaneous conversation they exhibit adequate phonological, semantic and grammatical performance. In contrast to the aphasic it is the *content* of their message which is disturbed rather than its form or construction.

Darley (1964) gives examples of disturbed verbalization due to impaired mental functioning:

> Productions such as the following suggest that the patient is confused rather than aphasic since the response is uttered fluently and is grammatical but is completely irrelevant to the situation. A hospitalized patient in response to a request to tell three things he did today said, 'I watered the roses in the cemetery, talked to you guys on the edge of the stream, and brought some dirt for your roses.' Another patient explaining the proverb 'Don't put all your eggs in one basket,' said, 'Means something to do with old Farrington and stuff that you have; something new the people used for old sewing machines.' Another patient listing three things he did today said, 'I don't know if I tried any desserts. I suppose I did. You'd have to figure them out. Gave friends new models of things to go by, I suppose.'

Geschwind (1964) has described other types of nonaphasic language disturbances due to mental dysfunction.

TRANSMISSIVE DISTURBANCES OF COMMUNICATION: AGNOSIA, APRAXIA, DYSARTHRIA

In addition to aphasia (symbolic language dysfunction) and mental dysfunction, communication can be disturbed by impairment of cerebral systems used in the transmission of speech signals. Visual, auditory and other sensory channels carry the coded message to the cerebral language processing mechanisms involved in the decoding and encoding of messages. Coded messages must be transmitted and transduced into muscle activity for their expression. Thus, impairment in the transmission of visual or auditory stimuli or impaired motor function of the hands or speech mechanism can produce nonaphasic comprehension, reading, writing, gestural or speech disorders. Wepman, Jones, Bock and Van Pelt (1960) have presented an operational diagram of language functions which distinguish aphasia, a problem in symbolic formulation and recall, from transmissive impairments of communication due to central nervous system dysfunction (see Fig. 8-1).

In describing their diagram they state:

> The model presented in Figure 1 (is) meant to suggest not a duality of language function within the central nervous system, but at least a triad of functions: input transmission leading to integration leading to output transmission. Input and output (are) seen as being modality-bound, while integration itself (has) modality-linkage to some degree, but is not bound by it. This permit(s) the concept of agnosia and apraxia as transmissive, non-symbolic processes of disruption . . . . Aphasia (is) seen as a disruption of integration with little specific modality relationship, and neither a sensory nor a motor problem.

*Agnosia** is a failure in the recognition of sensory stimuli. Even though the sensory receptors such as the eye or the ear are intact, the pattern of received stimuli is misperceived, i.e. distorted in some way, so that recognition of the stimulus is interfered with. Since stimuli must be recognized (perceived) before they can be comprehended (i.e. associated with their "meaning"), agnosic difficulties will interfere with language comprehension.

---

*Sigmund Freud first used the term "agnosia" in 1891.

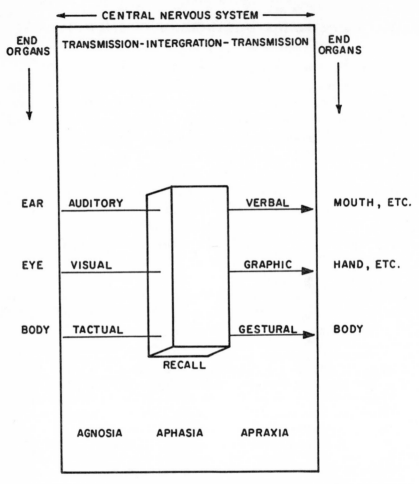

Figure 8-1. An operational diagram of language functions in man. (Wepman, Jones, Bock and Van Pelt, 1960).

Auditory verbal agnosia has been compared to listening to "double talk"—speech which sounds familiar but does not make any sense. Visual perceptual distortions can result in interference with reading and writing. The agnosias are subsymbolic nonaphasic communication disorders.

Output transmissive impairments will affect the motor acts of speaking, writing and gesturing. *Apraxia* is a disturbance in the execution of deliberate purposeful organized motor acts in the absence of any paralysis, weakness or incoordination of the muscles themselves. The apractic may have difficulty in initiating or controlling the direction and extent of motor acts when he is attempting them consciously and deliberately. He may have no difficulty when he performs the same act spontaneously or reflexively. For example, when asked to puff his cheeks and blow a column of air the apractic will not be able to do so, but when a lighted match is held before him, he can blow it out easily and effortlessly. Often he does the opposite of what he is asked to do. He locks his mouth tight when asked to open it; he retracts his tongue when asked to protrude it. Hughlings Jackson (Brain, 1961) first described this phenomenon in the 1860's.

Apractic involvement of the oral structures can affect speech. Similar involvement of the extremities may result in difficulty in writing or copying forms; the apractic may not be able to guide his pencil in the correct direction to form letters even when he "knows" how he is supposed to do it. Apraxia is difficult to understand until it is actually observed. Films, case demonstrations, tape recordings are particularly helpful in developing an understanding of apraxia. Apraxia, like agnosia, is a subsymbolic nonaphasic communication disorder.

Dysarthria is also an impairment in the motor production of speech, but it is due to a specific neuromuscular dysfunction. The lesion may be in the central or peripheral nervous system. Damage to the brain or spinal cord may produce muscular weakness, paralysis or incoordination. If the affected muscles are part of the speech production mechanism, phonation and/or articulation of speech sounds may be impaired resulting in speech problems ranging from slight slurring to complete unintelligibility or absence of speech.

In summary, damage to the brain can produce aphasia as well as the nonaphasic communication disturbances of agnosia, apraxia, dysarthria and those disturbances resulting from mental dysfunction. Nonaphasic problems can exist independently or can combine with each other and with aphasic disorders.

APHASIC DISTURBANCES

Schuell (1965) has reported that there are recurring combinations of various aphasic and nonaphasic disturbances which can form the basis for clinical classifications and which have diagnostic and prognostic implications. The nonaphasic disturbances have been described above. The various types of aphasic language disturbances will now be described. The range of severity and types of aphasic behavior are great and only the most common characteristics will be described.

The essential problem in aphasia is the disturbance of vocabulary and the rules of the language by which words are strung together to convey meaning. This basic impairment in langauge processing will reflect itself across all language modalities—speech, verbal comprehension, reading and writing. Therefore, although each langauge modality will be discussed separately, it should not be inferred that disturbances will be found in only one modality.

Speech

The hallmark of the aphasic is his expression, "I know what it is but I can't think of the name." He has most difficulty when attempting to use words propositionally, i.e. to use words to convey specific propositions or messages. When attempting to name an object or express some concept, the aphasic will be slow and hesitant as he searches for the word; he may circumlocute, or say a wrong but associated word. Errors are not usually random but may be "in class" errors, that is, belonging to the same class or category of events, e.g. "girl" for "boy," "table" for "chair," etc. Other errors may be due to acoustic ("feet" for "eat") or phonetic ("by" or "pie" for "my") similarity.

Some aphasics may produce a stream of unintelligible sounds when they attempt to speak *(jargon)*. Others may produce a flow of comprehensible speech with sounds or words reversed or substituted *(paraphasia)*.

Some authors have suggested that word recall difficulty (anomia) can exist without concomitant syntactic disturbance, and that syntactic disturbances (syntactic aphasia) can exist without word recall problems. Schuell, Jenkins and Jimenez (1964), however, state that both systems—semantic and syntactic—are disturbed concurrently.

Except for the very severely impaired, most aphasics can produce certain automatic types of speech even when they are unable to use words propositionally. Words used automatically are not used as language symbols; they are "empty" words inasmuch as they have only form but no specific meaning. Automatic level speech consists of emotional expressions, profanity, series speech (e.g. counting, reciting the alphabet, days of the week), strong rhythmic speech (e.g. singing, rhymes, poems) and other over-learned or memorized words (e.g. prayers, greetings).

Verbal Comprehension

The aphasic's basic disability in integrating and associating words with their meanings is also observed in his attempts to comprehend what is said to him. He can hear a word, perceive it correctly as evidenced by his ability to repeat it, but cannot associate it with its correct meaning. When asked to point to "chair," the aphasic may repeat the word several times, look around the room searchingly and give up or may point to the table. Such confusions as "table" for "chair" are similar to the "in class" errors of speech.

Reduction of verbal retention span is also a frequent aspect of aphasia. Some aphasics can comprehend single words but not longer units of speech such as phrases, sentences, or stories of various lengths. By the time the speaker has gotten to the end of his utterance, the aphasic may have failed to retain the beginning and therefore loses the message.

Impairment of verbal retention span can also affect the aphasic's speech production. If the aphasic is making a statement and does not retain its beginning, he cannot complete it accurately. He may "forget what he started to say" and simply give up or he may meander through the expression of a number of disconnected ideas.

Reading and Writing

The difficulty that the aphasic has in integrating word with meaning and with verbal retention span will also reflect itself in reading and writing. When he looks at the printed word *C-H-A-I-R* he may not be able to match it with the object *chair*. He can copy the word (or even read aloud) showing that he is seeing and perceiving it but he cannot connect the visual symbol with its meaning.

It is important to realize that reading and writing are not simply visual symbol systems. The visual and visuomotor symbols of reading and writing are learned years after children have learned the primary receptive-expressive auditory language system. The visual symbol system is superimposed on the auditory language system; the visual is a symbol system of a symbol system. Therefore, when the primary symbol system is impaired reading and writing behaviors will reflect that impairment.

The aphasic may be able to read aloud, copy printed words and write them to dictation quite accurately showing that the basic visual and visuomotor systems subserving reading and written language are intact. However, he may have difficulty understanding or expressing meaning through these systems as a reflection of the basic symbolic language disturbance of aphasia.

Verbal retention span can affect reading and writing in a manner similar to that described for speech and verbal comprehension.

All Language Modalities Affected

Since aphasia is basically an impairment of the integration of meaning and langauge symbols, it is reasonable to expect that all of the modalities used in language coding and decoding—speech, verbal comprehension, reading and writing—would reflect this impairment equally. Clinical observation, however, indicates that there is a hierarchy of difficulty with verbal comprehension and reading easier than speech and writing. The passive language activities of reading and listening are usually more functional than the active tasks of speaking and writing. Written langauge is generally the most impaired modality, perhaps because it is the last learned and involves the integration of more systems—auditory-language, visual and motor.

The unity of the language impairment across all language modalities is, however, demonstrated by the observation that similar kinds of errors occur in each modality. And even though some modalities of language may be somewhat more functional than others, the overall degree of functional impairment is about the same across modalities. Thus a moderate problem in verbal comprehension would be accompanied by moderate problems in speaking, reading and writing, but within this level of impairment speaking and writing show more disturbance than reading and verbal comprehension.

A number of clinicians, both within and outside of the field of speech pathology, do not accept the concept of a unitary breakdown of language functioning across all modalities. They believe that each language modality can be impaired independently or that receptive and expressive processes can be independently disrupted in aphasia. Specific diagnostic terms used to describe language impairments such as *expressive aphasia, receptive aphasia, motor aphasia, sensory asphasia, anomia, agraphia, alexia,* may be found in clinical reports with the implication that only certain specific aspects of the language process are independently impaired. The bases of the belief in independent language systems and disorders can best be understood from a review of the history of aphasia which is presented in a following section.

Nonlanguage Disturbances of Aphasia

The term "language" is loosely used to indicate any organized system of symbols or signs. These systems may be verbal, that is using *words* in either their spoken or written form, or nonverbal, such as gesture and pantomime. Although the central problem in aphasia is generally considered to be the disturbance of the verbal symbolic communication process, it has often been noted that some aphasics also show disturbances in nonverbal communication. These aphasics cannot substitute for their impaired verbal communication the use of gestures, pantomime, drawing, picture boards, pointing to indicate a desired object, or even simply nodding the head for "yes" or "no." Similarly, deaf aphasics may be impaired in their ability to use sign language and finger spelling. Such observations have led some investigators to broaden their definition of aphasia beyond that of a verbal symbolic disturbance to include impairments in the use of any kind of sign or symbol (asymbolia). For example, Henry Head's (1926) studies of the verbal and nonverbal aspects of aphasia led to his classic definition of aphasia as an impairment in "symbolic formulation and expression." He states:

> By symbolic formulation and expression I understand a mode of behavior in which some verbal or other symbol plays a part between the initiation and execution of the act. This comprises many procedures, not usually included under the heading of the use of language. If clinical experience shows that some particular aspect of behavior is affected in association with these speech defects, it must be included. . . in the purely descriptive term, 'symbolic formulation and expression' (p. 211).

Other investigators consider aphasia to be a reflection of a general cognitive disturbance resulting from cerebral damage. Piere Marie (Brain, 1961) concluded that aphasia is the effect of a general diminishment of intellect. E. Bay (1964) states that "aphasia is a disorder of conceptual thinking rather than of speech."

Between 1929 and 1934 Weisenburg and McBride (1964) conducted an intensive investigation to "study the actual nature of the psychological changes occurring in aphasic conditions." While there still remain considerable differences in points of view regarding the basic nature of aphasia, their conclusion probably reflects the current opinion of most clinicians:

> Aphasia is first and foremost a disorder of language. That is the primary conclusion which the analyses of these cases indicate. But it is not limited to the language processes. In practically every case it clearly involves some deterioration in so-called non-language performances and it also involves changes in the patient's reactions to practical, everyday problems and to matters of social response and relationship. Thus the extent of the disorder varies from one case to another; sometimes there are comparatively limited changes in

mental functioning and sometimes widespread changes, but in clear-cut cases of aphasia, there is never a general deterioration (p. 429).

In contrast to the veiws that some nonverbal communication disturbances may be due to a general symbolic disturbance or a general cognitive impairment is the conclusion of Goodglass and Kaplan (1963) that impairment in gesture and pantomime is the result of a specific movement disorder, an apraxia for manual activities.

HISTORY OF APHASIA

Familiarity with the history of aphasia is necessary to an understanding of many of the present-day beliefs and practices regarding aphasic and nonaphasic language disturbances. This is particularly true regarding the beliefs in the independence of the various language modalities and their disorders, cerebral localization of language disorders and clinical classification systems which have been developed.

Although impairment of speech and language due to cerebral damage had been described for centuries (Benton and Joynt, 1960), it was not until the mid-nineteenth century that a concentrated study of aphasia began. The initial interest in speech disorders resulting from cerebral damage was a by-product of the more general problem of discovering how the brain functioned and how clinical symptoms were correlated with sites of brain lesions. In the early 1800's Franz Joseph Gall challenged the prevailing medical theory that the brain was a uniform mass which functioned as a single organ. Gall suggested that the brain was made up of separate centers which subserved the various "vital, intellectual and moral faculties of man." By 1825, Bouillaud, a young physician who later was to become a powerful figure in the medical circles of Paris during the time of Paul Broca, had several publications defending the localization of various functions in different areas of the brain. Head's description of Bouillaud's activities shows that the early interest in speech disturbances was only one aspect of the broader question of cerebral localization.

(Bouillaud) narrates a series of cases of cerebral disease, attempting to show that the symptoms differ according to the site of the lesion. He devotes his attention to disorders of motion, of sensation, and of the intellectual functions, particularly speech. . . (Head, 1926).

It was amidst this continuing controversy as to whether the brain functioned as a single organ or consisted of separate functional areas that Paul Broca presented the case of "Tan" in support of the cerebral localizationist point of view. In 1861, he described a man whose only problem was inability to speak but who was essentially normal in other respects.

> He was perfectly well oriented and intelligent and did not differ from a healthy man except in his ability to speak. He walked about the hospital where he was known as 'Tan.' He understood everything said to him; even his hearing was excellent; but no matter what question was addressed to him, he always answered: 'tan, tan' accompanied by various gestures designed to make himself understood. . . . 'Tan' was regarded as egotistical, vindicative, mean and his comrades, who hated him, accused him of being a thief. These traits may have been due to his cerebral lesion, anyhow, they were not pronounced enough to be called pathological . . . He was regarded as a man who was perfectly responsible for his acts (Kann, 1950).

After "Tan's" death, Broca examined his brain and concluded that damage to the third frontal convolution of the cortex had produced the loss of speech. Broca added other case studies in support of his theory that the third frontal convolution was specifically related to the faculty of "articulated speech."* This cortical area is popularly known as *Broca's area* (see Fig. 8-2) and the type of speech disturbance assumed to result from damage to it is called *Broca's aphasia* (also, *motor aphasia*).

Following Broca a number of investigators postulated "centers" in the brain for various activities such as verbal understanding, reading and writing (see Fig. 8-2). These centers were presumed to be interconnected by neural pathways. A popular practice of the time was for each investigator to illustrate his theories of brain functioning by using diagrams of the brain showing different centers and connecting pathways and demonstrating how each of various sites of lesions could result in different and specific

---

*Broca originally used the term *aphemia* to describe the speech disturbance he observed but later used the term *aphasia*.

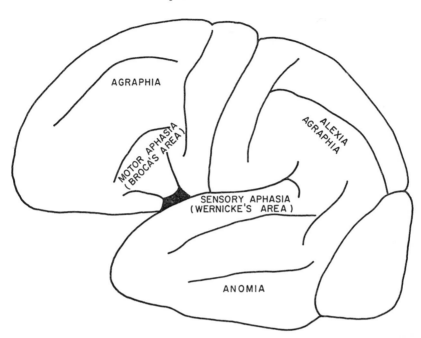

Figure 8-2. Historical cortical localization of specific disturbances. Agraphia has been localized in both the frontal lobe and the angular gyrus by different investigators.

disturbances of communication. Clinical disorders were formed and classified on the basis of these theoretical schemata rather than upon careful descriptive observations of clinical symptoms. This unscientific approach to the study of aphasia reached its peak in the 1870's and is the period referred to by Head as the era of the "diagram makers." The more dynamic and psychological theories of aphasic disturbances such as those of John Hughlings Jackson, an English physician, were not as popular and had little influence until over fifty years later.

The initial studies of the clinical problems of aphasia were strongly influenced by the "structuralists" (also, known as "localizationists"). The clinical terminology and classification of aphasic disorders reflected the view of a direct relationship between physical structure and clinical behavior, e.g. *motor aphasia, sensory aphasia, conduction aphasia, transcortical aphasia.* The orientation to and influence on the study of aphasia by the structuralists is historically understandable. It is difficult, however, to understand the extent to which these ideas have persisted and influenced the present day clinical study of aphasia.

One of the most durable and persisting beliefs of the early investigators is that of independent impairment of separate language modalities. This belief remains today and influences clinical observations despite the fact that it is not supported by experimental data nor daily clinical observation of aphasics. Wherever careful observations and testing have been used in the examination of substantial numbers of aphasics (Head, 1926; Weisenburg and McBride, 1964; Wepman, 1951; Schuell, Jenkins, Jimenez, 1964), no investigators confirm the presence of isolated impairment of single modalities (Schuell, 1969).

Neither does the routine clinical evaluation of aphasic disturbances support the belief in separate language dysfunctions. Yet this belief persists. An example of the biasing effect that such a belief can have on clinical observation is the frequent report found in medical charts and other reports that "the patient has expressive aphasia, but understands everything said to him." However, when these patients are carefully and systematically examined they do, indeed, show impairment in verbal comprehension, many with rather gross deficiencies. Commenting on the tendency for observers to find what they are looking for, Schuell, Jenkins, Jimenez (1964) state:

> Historical case material is invaluable for extending one's own frame of reference in regard to aphasia. It is, however, necessary to view reported judgments with considerable skepticism. . . The report, 'He understood everything that was said,' occurred again and again in the protocols of early investigators. Somehow or other, that is something people always say about aphasic patients, particularly when they have no speech. It is said, again and again, about patients who cannot follow directions as simple as "Put the spoon in the cup." Patients with little or no speech are usually highly motivated to communicate and to perform well. They frequently respond appropriately by making maximal use of visual cues, situational cues, and occasional words they grasp. They observe the social amenities, smile, and appear responsive when spoken to. Since they have little or no speech they tend not to give themselves away when they misunder-

stand, as hard-of-hearing individuals frequently do. Sometimes when the patient makes an obvious error, the speaking person ascribes it to his own difficulty communicating with the aphasic patient. This is a very curious phenomenon (p. 21).

In view of the preceding discussion, the clinician should be wary when he encounters a patient who is reported to have language disorders confined to only one or two language modalities. Examination procedures must be careful and thorough to determine whether the problem is truly aphasia, or one of the nonaphasic visual, auditory, or motor transmissive problems described above.

A familiarity with the history of aphasia is essential to anyone who wishes to understand present-day concepts about the nature of aphasia and the bases for its clinical treatment. A number of reviews are available (Head, 1926; Weisenburg and McBride, 1964; Schuell *et al.*, 1964).

CAUSES OF APHASIA AND ASSOCIATED IMPAIRMENTS

By definition aphasia is a language disorder due to brain injury. Destruction or dysfunction of the brain tissue may result from a variety of causes. The most common cause is disruption of the blood supply due to some type of cerebral vascular accident (CVA), commonly called a *stroke*. When the blood supply to some portion of the brain is diminished by hemorrhaging or blockage of an artery (due to a thrombus or embolus), the brain cells are deprived of oxygen and die within a very short period of time. The damaged part of the brain may become edematous resulting in generalized and temporary dysfunction of large portion of brain area. The results will be an initially severe symptom pattern which will show gradual improvement as the edema subsides and the initial effects of trauma wear off. The severity and number of symptoms which remain depend upon the location and extent of the permanent tissue damage.

In addition to cerebral vascular accidents brain damage may be caused by infections, toxins, direct trauma (e.g. bullet wound) or brain tumors. There appears to be little difference in the types of aphasic behavior produced by the different causal agents.

In addition to the aphasic and nonaphasic transmissive communicative impairments already discussed, injury to the brain can result in physical, mental and behavioral impairments. It is important for the student to recognize that aphasia may be only part of a more extensive constellation of disorders in order to gain a proper perspective of the role of the speech pathologist in the total rehabilitation program. The aphasia clinician must become familiar with related problems in order to participate effectively in the evaluation and treatment of the aphasic's needs. A comprehensive review of the process of rehabilitation may be found in Rusk (1964) and Hirschberg, Lewis and Thomas (1964).

Physical Symptoms

The brain is separated into two cerebral hemispheres each of which is responsible for the innervation of the motor and sensory activity to the opposite side of the body. Thus the left hemisphere contains the motor and sensory tracts to the right side of the body due to the crossing over (decussation) of these tracts in the brain stem, or spinal cord. Since aphasia is usually found to result from damage to the left cerebral hemisphere, it will be associated with physical disturbances on the right half of the body. Some of the common physical impairments resulting from brain damage associated with aphasia are the following:

1. Hemiplegia—paralysis or paresis (weakness) of the extremities on the right side of the body.
2. Facial or oral muscular weakness on the right side.
3. Visual disturbances
   a. homonymous hemianopsia—blindness in one half of the visual field in each eye.
   b. blurring of vision; diplopia—double vision.
4. Loss of general body sensations on the right half of the body, e.g. touch.

Hearing acuity is usually not affected by unilateral cerebral damage because each ear has neural connections with both cerebral hemispheres. Thus damage to the auditory area of the left hemisphere will not result in loss of hearing acuity in the right ear because the right ear still maintains connections with the undamaged right cerebral hemisphere.

Behavioral and Personality Symptoms

Damage to the brain also may result in a variety of behavioral and personality alterations. Wepman (1951) lists the following:

Loss of attention and concentration
Loss of memory
Reduced association of ideas
Abstract-concrete imbalance (loss of ability to abstract; concrete concept formulation)
Poor organizing ability
Poor judgment
Perseveration
Constriction of thought and interest
Reduced ability to generalize, categorize, group, or plan action
Reduced general level of intelligence
Reduced ability to inhibit internal emotional forces which disturb the action of the intellect
Inability to shift
Psychomotor retardation
Feelings of inadequacy
Egocentricity
Increased irritability and fatigability
Euphoria
Social withdrawal and seclusiveness
Reduced ability to adjust to new situations
Catastrophic reactions
Reduced initiative
Disinterest in the environment; both physical and human
Externalization of behavior; a lack of introspection or self-criticism
Reduced spontaneity
Perplexity (a distrust in one's own ability)
Automatic verbalization
Impulsive behavior
Regressive, infantile behavior

Impotence (the inability to correct behavior one knows is wrong)

Posttraumatic psychotic behavior showing illusions, hallucinations, delusions and extravagant behavior.

Anxiety and tension

Changing personality profile, the emergence and submergence of characteristics

The aphasia clinician must take these aberrations into account in the course of his evaluation and treatment of the patient.

EVALUATION OF APHASIA

The clinical evaluation of the aphasic's communication problems is primarily the responsibility of the speech pathologist. Many factors will be reflected in the patient's communicative behavior—his medical and physical condition, mental status, educational background, family and social situation. Although this type of information is generally provided by other professional personnel such as the physician, social worker and psychologist, the speech pathologist must take these factors into account in his evaluation. His specific function is to obtain a description of the patient's current speech and language abilities and limitations, the identification of the particular factors (e.g. auditory recall, verbal retention span, visual discrimination, visuomotor, etc.) underlying the disordered communication, and the planning and execution of an appropriate treatment program.

The formal tests of aphasic language behavior used by the speech pathologist should meet the requirements of any good psychological test instrument: standardized administration and scoring, quantification, reliability and validity. For the clinician the test should also yield results which have implications for treatment planning and prognosis. Many of the aphasia "tests" which have been developed over the years reflect the subjective experience of their originators in regard to the choice of specific behaviors to be tested, selection of test items and the interpretation of the results. Few tests of aphasia can meet the rigorous requirements of an acceptable phychological test instrument.

Minnesota Test for Differential Diagnosis of Aphasia (MTDDA)

One of the most thoroughly developed and clinically useful tests of aphasia is the *Minnesota Test for Differential Diagnosis of Aphasia* by Hildred Schuell (1965). Although not published until 1965, test development began in 1948 at the VA Hospital in Minneapolis and underwent periodic refinement and revision based on its clinical use and statistical analysis. The first step was to assemble and administer a large number of language and language related tests to aphasic patients. Continued analyses of the results of this testing program resulted in the elimination of tests which did not contribute information on language disturbance, were difficult to administer or to interpret or duplicated information on other tests. As hundreds of patients were tested and retested it was noted that symptoms began to group themselves in a number of recurring patterns. These patterns were stable and patients continued to demonstrate the same types of errors throughout their recovery period even though the number of errors had decreased.

Certain groups of symptom patterns were indicative of good potential for recovery of communication abilities and others were associated with poor potential. A variety of therapy procedures were used with the patients. Some error patterns showed no response to treatment and communication remained below functional levels. Some therapy procedures were effective with some groups but not with others. Thus it became possible to use the empirically obtained classification of aphasics by error pattern to indicate prognosis. The seven groups of symptom patterns and their prognoses for recovery described by Schuell (1964b) are the following:

> Group I. Simple Aphasia—characterized by reduction of available language in all modalities with no specific perceptual or sensorimotor impairment and no dysarthria. Prognosis—excellent recovery of all language skills. Treatment is usually required for maximal return of language and successful vocational adjustment.
>
> Group II. Aphasia with Visual Involvement—characterized by reduction of available language in all modalities, with coexisting impairment of discrimination, recognition, and recall of learned visual symbols. Prognosis—excellent recovery of langauge as in Group I.

Reading and writing improve more slowly than speech. Rate of performance tends to remain retarded, and occasional inconsistent visual errors tend to persist. Former reading and writing levels are approximated, however.

Group III. Aphasia with Sensorimotor Involvement—characterized by severe reduction of language in all modalities accompanied by difficulty in discriminating, producing, and sequencing phonemes. Prognosis—recovery of limited but functional language skills. Patients are able to communicate needs through intelligible speech, although responses are often slow and labored and reflect severe disruption of language processes. Reading and writing remain limited, also.

Group IV. Aphasia with Scattered Findings Compatible with Generalized Brain Damage—characterized by reduction of available language, with scattered findings that usually include both visual involvement, and some degree of dysarthria. The patient is able to communicate voluntarily in either speech or writing, though both processes are usually defective to some extent. Prognosis—limited by the general neurophysiological status of the patient. Group IV patients often work well with the clinician, and make gains in auditory comprehension, word finding, and intelligibility. They are usually incapable of persistent self-directed effort.

Group V. Irreversible Aphasic Syndrome—characterized by almost complete loss of functional language skills in all modalities. Prognosis—auditory comprehension may show functional improvement, and reactive responses increase, but langauge does not become functional or voluntary in any modality.

Minor Syndrome A. Aphasia with Partial Auditory Imperception—characterized by severe impairment of auditory perception, with some functional speech retained or recovered early. Prognosis—limited but functional recovery. Auditory comprehension usually improves to a functionally significant degree, although residual difficulty tends to persist and to be reflected in all language modalities.

Minor Syndrome B. Mild Aphasia with Perisisting Dysarthria—this syndrome resembles Group I, except for the accompaniment of persisting dysarthria. Prognosis—excellent recovery of language as in Group I. Normal articulation patterns can be acquired, but disintegrate when conscious control is not exerted. Automaticity and fluency are not regained.

In addition to assessing the aphasic's level of functioning in each language modality and indicating prognosis for recovery, the MTDDA is diagnostic. It is diagnostic in that a number of test items attempt to identify the specific cause of the patient's impairment. For example, in addition to testing whether the aphasic can copy or write single words, phrases, sentences or paragraphs, the test procedures attempt to determine whether an impairment in writing is due to problems in visual discrimination, spatial disorientation, visual recall of letter forms, visuomotor disability, auditory recall of spelling, word recall or verbal retention span. By identifying the particular impairment underlying the "writing" problem the clinician can direct his therapy activities at that specific cause.

In summary, the MTDDA was constructed as a descriptive, diagnostic and prognostic instrument which has direct implication for clinical management. The standardized administration and scoring of the test items permits the reevaluation of patients from time to time, and by different examiners, in order to determine amount of improvement. Its empirical foundations are impressive and it is a valuable instrument in the hands of an experienced clinician.

Porch Index of Communicative Abilities (PICA)

The PICA (Porch, 1967) was published after a number of years of development and use with a large number of aphasic patients. Careful attention was paid to the development of the scoring system. A unique sixteen point binary choice scale was developed which permits the examiner to score each response on a continuum from an "accurate, responsive, complex, immediate, elaborative response" (a score of "16") to "no awareness of the test item" (a score of "1"). Such a scale is sensitive to slight differences in performance and provides a more accurate numerical index of behavior than does a "plus-minus" (correct-incorrect) scoring system. For example, using the "plus-minus" scoring, if a patient names a picture correctly after considerable delay and hesitation, he receives the same "plus" score as the patient who names the picture immediately. On the PICA scoring the patient would receive a "16" for an accurate and immediate response but only a "13" for an accurate but delayed response.

The PICA scoring also distinguishes among types of errors. There are many types of aphasic errors, some of which are better than others. The aphasic who tries to name "chair" and says "table" is giving an in-class associated response which is a "good" error. If he gives no response, an unrelated response, or an unintelligible response, these are poorer errors than the in-class error. The qualitative differences in types of errors are not reflected in "plus-minus" scoring. On the PICA test a "table" for "chair" response receives a score of "7," an unrelated response is a "6," unintelligible is "4," and no response is a "1."

The test samples performance on a range of language, gestural and matching tasks from simple to moderately difficult. The PICA is particularly useful with severely impaired aphasics because it samples tasks from the easier end of the language continuum. It is sensitive to subtle changes which will appear on the easier tasks before the more difficult ones.

PICA test results may be plotted in graphic form and comparisons made with a large number of aphasic patients. The shape of the profile indicates which tasks are most responsive to treatment and where to begin therapy. At the present time data are being prepared which will permit the prediction of the eventual level of recovery from early test performance.

In addition to the MTDDA and the PICA, two other tests in current use are the Language Modalities Test for Aphasia (Wepman and Jones, 1961) and Examining for Aphasia (Eisenson, 1954). Many clinicians have developed and use their own test procedures and materials based on their clinical experience.

APHASIA THERAPY

Aphasia therapy is more than speech therapy for the aphasic. It is more than administering therapeutic activities designed to improve isolated linguistic deficiencies, such as naming or spelling or speech production. The goal of aphasia therapy is to assist the aphasic to achieve the highest level of communication possible and to develop a person capable of interacting and relating effectively with the society in which he lives. Wepman (1951) describes the goals of aphasia therapy:

> . . . recovery of the ability to speak, to read, or to write while the patient is still unable to adjust to society is a wasted resource.

A resumption of social intercourse in a manner mutually acceptable to the patient and to society, a controlled reduction of the effects of the personality aberrations which follow brain injury, stability of psyche, and insight into the physical limitations imposed by the brain insult seem to be the important goals. Language should be considered as the means of interpersonal relations, not the end result of recovery (p. 4).

The aphasia clinician can improve the communication of the aphasic in two ways, by improving his speech and language skills and by improving the ability of others to communicate with the aphasic. The important "others" are the family and the professional staff who care for the patient. An essential foundation for successful communication and adjustment for the aphasic is a thorough understanding of the nature of aphasia by the family and others, and by the patient himself. Often the first reaction of the patient and the family is bewilderment by the loss or strangeness of the language behavior. Has he lost his mind? Can he speak but won't? Can it be cured? How long will he be like this? What causes it? Why can words burst out at times but then he can't or won't repeat them again? The patient and family are embarrassed and perplexed when he tries to speak and cannot think of the word, or produces jargon, or says a wrong word (sometimes socially unacceptable words). The aphasia clinician can provide the answer to the many questions which naturally arise. He can replace fear and bewilderment with information and help achieve a climate of understanding, encouragement and support in which the aphasic can be free to attempt communication. There are a number of pamphlets available which would serve as a good basis for counselling the layman concerning aphasia (Boone, 1965; Buck, 1968; Horowitz, 1962; Wepman, 1965). Counselling is not something that is done only in the initial phase of treatment, but it is a continual on-going process as new problems, questions and needs arise.

In addition to setting an optimal climate for the aphasic, the clinician can demonstrate ways of helping him communicate by showing listeners how to take a more active role in the communication process. A speaker and a listener are required for communication to take place. Normally, the listener is the passive participant while the speaker actively constructs and transmits his message. When the aphasic speaker is impaired in his ability to send the message it is possible for the listener to take a more active role in order to facilitate communication. For example, it was mentioned that the aphasic can often comprehend somewhat better than he can speak messages. It is, therefore, possible for the listener to formulate probable messages which the aphasic can verify or reject with a nod or simple "yes" or "no." The listener can narrow down the range of possible messages with questions like, "Do you want to tell me about something in this room?," "It it about someone in the family?" The process can be continued until the topic is identified and the appropriate message formulated by the "listener." "You want me to bring you your pipe and tobacco from home?" When the aphasic finally indicates "yes" —usually with a sign of relief and satisfaction—he has transmitted his message even though the "listener" had done all of the talking. The essence of communication is that messages be exchanged; how they are exchanged is secondary. It may be possible for the "listener" to facilitate communication with the aphasic through the use of word or picture boards, writing or drawing when shown how by the aphasia clinician.

Recovery from Aphasia

Knowledge about the course of recovery from aphasia is based primarily on clinical experience rather than well-controlled longitudinal studies. Clinical experience suggests that there are three phases of recovery in which the needs of the aphasic and his family change and for which the clinician must vary his treatment as appropriate.

Phase I

The first, or acute phase, of recovery takes place in the first four to six weeks after the onset. In the very early days the family and the patient are stunned by the severity and suddenness of a multitude of problems. The paralysis of the arm and leg, the disrupted speech, and the question of life and death prevail. In this phase of recovery the speech pathologist mainly provides psychological support to the aphasic and his family in various ways. Early contact with, and evaluation of, the aphasic not only provides a baseline against which future improvement can be measured but it gives the clinician the opportunity to inform and counsel the family (and patient, if possible) at a crucial time. This first phase of recovery usually takes place in a hospital or rehabilitation setting. The patient and the family are reassured in knowing that there is an "expert" available to assume responsibility for the management of the problem. These early contacts provide needed psychological support for the aphasic and family and allow the speech pathologist to keep other professional persons concerned with patient's rehabilitation informed of his status.

The first phase of recovery is not generally the time for the initiation of direct intensive speech therapy activities. The aphasic may be still medically unstable, physically weak, euphoric, emotionally unstable or unable to focus his interest and energies on specific therapy activities. Another reason for not beginning intensive speech therapy programs in the early weeks is that many of the symptoms observed may be only temporary and the patient will recover spontaneously. As shown by the recovery curves in Figure 8-3, the early post-onset months show the greatest rate of improvement. This is referred to as the period of "spontaneous recovery." Schuell, Jenkins and Jimenez (1964) state that the period of physiological instability is sixty to ninety days post-onset and do not recommend beginning formal therapy activities until this period has passed. Although it is often heard, there is little empirical support for the statement that the earlier speech therapy is begun the better will be the level of recovery.

Phase II

The second phase of recovery takes place from about two to six months post-onset. After the patient has stabilized progress continues but at a less rapid rate than the earlier period of spontaneous recovery. Often the level or rate of recovery is less than had been hoped for by the aphasic and his family and doubt and discouragement take root. It is in this period that a program of speech therapy will be most effective in insuring that the aphasic's

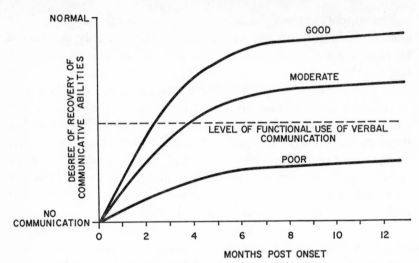

Figure 8-3. Recovery of communicative abilities in aphasia. Recovery curves for good, moderate and poor return of communication are shown. The greatest rate of return takes place in the first phase of recovery (0-3 months) followed by a gradual decrease in rate of improvement in the second phase (3-6 months). The third phase of recovery (post 6 month period) is characterized by a leveling off to an aymptotic curve. The rate of recovery in the first phase can be predictive of the level of functioning at later stages. These curves are based on clinical observation.

"Level of Functional Use of Verbal Communication" refers to the ability to use words to convey meaningful propositions rather than the mere imitative or automatic use of words. At this level communication may still be defective but words are consistently and substantially helpful in exchanging information between speaker and listener.

maximum potential for communication will be achieved. A program of systematic therapy not only provides stimulus for improvement of specific language skills but also provides needed psychological support during a long and difficult period. In discussing his reaction to programmed instruction one recovered aphasic wrote:

> I didn't think it was possible, but step by step, starting with one sound, then a word, then a phrase, and finally the sentence, I did it. It was quite an achievement for me, and it lifted my spirits substantially. With the programmed approach, I could see some progress and felt that I was doing something about my aphasia (Holland, 1968, p. 215).

The "lifting of the spirit" and the "feeling of doing something" about his aphasia is a common response to therapy in general in this phase of recovery and not peculiar to programmed therapy.

It is during the second phase of recovery that indications of long-term prognosis become evident. His pattern of test performances, rate of recovery, response to therapy can indicate the ultimate level of language recovery which can be expected. The family should be involved in therapy activities as much as possible, not only to be shown how to provide additional therapeutic activity and stimulation, but to insure that they are realistically aware of the aphasic's progress and limitations. The family should be gradually prepared for the termination of therapy and planning for the future.

How frequently the aphasic should be seen for therapy depends on many factors. Some types of problems may require daily intensive stimulation if improvement is to be expected (Schuell, Jenkins and Jimenez, 1964) ; other problems may be seen less frequently. A principal determinant of the frequency of therapy is whether there is an interested capable family member who can work with the aphasic under the direction of the clinician. If the clinician can have the family carry out appropriate therapeutic activities, he may need to see the aphasic only as often as necessary to review progress and modify the therapy activities accordingly. The psychological and social needs of the aphasic and his family also influence the frequency of therapy visits.

Phase III

The third phase of recovery generally takes place from the fifth to seventh month post-onset and is marked by a plateauing of progress followed by only small increments of improvement over long periods of time (see Fig. 3) . When the plateauing indicates that the aphasic has reached maximum benefit from therapy activities termination of formal therapy should be made. Some clinicians do not feel that no further benefits can be gained from speech therapy at this point and will continue to provide speech therapy for as long as the aphasic, or his family, is motivated and willing to come.

When termination of speech therapy is indicated it must be done with adequate preparation. Sufficient time through the second phase of recovery should have been alloted to preparation of the family and aphasic for the possibility of eventual termination of therapy without complete recovery. And even though appropriate counselling has taken place through the course of the treatment, it often comes as a shock and disappointment when therapy is actually terminated. It signals the end of hope and forces them to face the unpleasant reality of a difficult future.

> Cold basic facts are indeed difficult for even professional personnel to accept readily. But we are assuredly obligated to be completely honest with the families of our patients even though what we have to tell them may be unpleasant or negative. There are many brain-damaged people who will never be able to show improvement in language despite long and intensive help from the most skilled clinicians. Many of these patients with a poor prognosis never seem to become discouraged. This in itself is often an indication of severe damage to intellectual processes. It may reflect a lack of realistic memory span, or simply the desire to have something other to do than just 'hang around the house' (Buck, 1968, p. 118).

The family may find it difficult to believe that no further improvement can be expected. And even a year or two after onset they will point out small gains which continue to be made as proof of potential for further improvement. The family should be prepared to expect these small gains as part of the natural course of recovery. Natural recovery seems to go on slowly, gradually and almost indefinitely. Even the most severe aphasic can continue to show gains; the gains are usually such things as better automatic speech, increased use of social gesture speech ("hello," "so long"), improved verbal recognition of single words and phrases, copying or writing a few words spontaneously, etc. In other words, the "improvement" is an increased ability in some primitive language skills. However, it is rare that there is a significant improvement in the functional level of communication, that is, in the adequacy to convey propositions or meaning through words.

The family may ask to keep the aphasic in therapy longer, or may seek revaluation and treatment elsewhere. The aphasia clinician should recognize these attempts as probably being therapeutic for the family by reassuring themselves that they are doing everything possible to aid the stricken family member.

It is in the third state of recovery that the vocational or social readjustment demanded by the limitation of communication must be considered. Persons with apparently good recovery of functional language for routine communication may find that attempting to return to positions which require unusual demands on language abilities (e.g. teaching, lawyer, secretary) will be impossible, or will require special adjustment. For example, the trial lawyer may change to specializing in other types of legal work if he has some residual problem in word recall or his rate of general language processing is slower. The patient with no functional language also needs assistance in developing a life style which best suits him as a person. It is possible for him to travel, visit, entertain and enjoy friends even with very limited communication abilities. Schuell, Jenkins and Jimenez (1964, pp. 371-386) and McBride (1969) discuss the needs of the patient with little functional communication.

APPROACHES TO SPEECH THERAPY FOR THE APHASIC

When the aphasic reaches the second phase of recovery and the clinician decides that the patient is ready and can benefit from specific therapeutic activities he must decide on which of a number of possible approaches to take. A variety of publications detailing specific therapy activities are available (Agranowtiz, 1964; Granich, 1947; Longerich and Bordeaux, 1954; Berry and Eisenson, 1956; Schuell, Jenkins, Jimenez, 1964; Wepman, 1951). There are little empirical data derived from controlled studies of the effectiveness of various types of therapy to help the clinician to decide which methods of therapy to use. His choice will ultimately depend on his personal clinical experiences and what he believes to be the nature of aphasia. He must decide whether aphasia is a disturbance of general symbolization, specific language symbolization, impairment of cognitive abilities, or specific agnosic and apractic disorders. His therapy procedures should be logically consistent with his decision about the basic nature of aphasic disorders.

Those who believe that aphasia is a manifestation of some form of cognitive disturbance do not attempt to work directly with speech, reading, writing or verbal comprehension. For example, Bay (1964) who believes that aphasia is an impairment of conceptual actualization and specificity states:

> Therapeutic efforts must aim to occupy and to strengthen his (the aphasic's) conceptual thinking and his concept formation. . . We must employ and exercise his conceptual thinking without the temporal urge of speaking; we must shift our training efforts to nonlinguistic spheres. For this purpose, we can use the performance batteries of intelligence tests (of course, without time limits). Other suitable means are games, either card games or chessboard games (chess or checkers) and, last but not least, drawing or modeling objects from memory (p. 330).

Goldstein believes that some aphasic disturbances are the result of impairment of abstract attitude, an inability to think categorically (conceptually), and therefore an inability to use words as the symbols of these categories. He states that language disturbances which reflect this basic impairment have poor prognosis for improvement with any kind of therapy.

Wepman (1968) states that language recovery is the result of the interaction of three factors: the functional condition of the cortex, the motivation of the aphasic toward recovery and the activities of the clinician (and only the latter two factors are under the control of the clinician). He sees the role of the clinician as primarily one of providing stimulation to use language and to modify it.

> Over the years we have experimented with many different approaches to therapy. We have tried straightforward teaching and have obtained some good results. We have tried rote training for specific function, with less effective results, and also conditioning and more-or-less stimulation of the patient. All these approaches have their place, but we have found the latter method to be the most rewarding . . . We have been more concerned with a good climate for therapy than with the actual techniques or methods to be used . . . There is, to our knowledge, no series of steps that apply to all or even to most patients, no cookbook approaches of merit (p. 23).

Schuell, Jenkins and Jimenez (1964) also believe that stimulation is a desirable approach to therapy. They point out that the aphasic has not "lost" his language abilities but that he is unable to use them as effectively and quickly as previously. Under appropriate conditions language can often be elicited thereby demonstrating that the primary need is to facilitate the recall of language. They stress intensive auditory stimulation as a foundation for improving language functioning in all modalities.

Some therapy approaches stress the need for retraining language skills through the development of the basic elements of language (e.g. phonemes, letters) by drill. Attempts are then made to combine these elements into larger units. For example, individual speech sounds are combined into words which are then combined into phrases and into sentences. This approach to therapy seems to assume that aphasia is the loss of specific motor and sensory abilities and that restoration of these abilities can be obtained by repetitious taxing drills. It is learning to speak all over again; it simulates the language learning of the child. Often associated with this type of therapy is the belief that new areas of the brain or the opposite hemisphere can be retrained to take over the function of the damaged areas.

It appears that in the absence of clear-cut evidence supporting one therapeutic approach over others, the clinician must choose his therapy regime on the basis of his clinical experience and logical inferences about the nature of aphasia.

Group Therapy

Group therapy has been employed with aphasics and their families for all the reasons it is recommended for other problems (Aronson, Shatin and Cook, 1956; Bloom, 1962; Taylor and Meyers, 1952). Group therapy is not used simply to economize on the clinician's time by providing treatment to a number of patients simultaneously. It is generally employed to provide the socialization and identification which can result from the dynamics of group interaction with those who have similar problems. Group therapy sessions with family members have been found to fill a real and great need for sharing, unburdening and drawing strength from others. Participation in group activities following the termination of formal treatment programs is one way to meet the persisting needs of the aphasic and family for socialization, understanding and support.

NOTIONS ABOUT APHASIA

There are several notions about aphasia which are commonly encountered in clinical practice but which have little basis in fact. They often lead to misunderstanding and confusion about a patient's communication problem. One belief is that it is possible for a polylingual person to be aphasic in one language only while his other language (s) remain unimpaired. The other belief is that aphasia will result from damage to the right cerebral hemisphere in left-handed persons.

Aphasia in Polyglot Patients

The belief in aphasic impairments of only one language in polyglot patients appears to be an outgrowth of the early structuralists theories of separate language centers in the brain and is related to the belief that separate language modalities could be independently impaired. As reviewed by Charlton (1964) this theory has three forms:

1. The language learned earliest in life will be the one retained—Ribot, 1906.
2. The language employed in daily life immediately before the onset of aphasia will be retained—Pitres, 1895.
3. The language retained is determined by unconscious emotional factors—Minkowski, 1928.

Most of the literature supporting the separate dysfunction of languages is based on isolated case reports and does not reflect typical clinical findings. Clinical experience indicates that patients generally report equal difficulty across languages.

Misinterpretation often arises in a clinical situation when the examiner is unfamiliar with the second language. If the examination is done by someone familiar with the other language, or when the family is asked to interpret for the patient, the "foreign language" often turns out to be jargon.

Charlton's study is one of the few attempts to systematically evaluate loss of language in polylinguals. He concludes, "It seems clear from this unselective study of bilingual and polyglot patients afflicted with aphasia that it is usual for all languages to be affected to a similar degree."

Aphasia and Handedness

It is commonly believed that one cerebral hemisphere is dominant over the other and is responsible for the coordination of bilateral motor activities, and the dominant hemisphere is opposite to the side of the preferred hand because of the decussation of neural tracts. Therefore, the dominant hemisphere for a right-handed person would be the left, and the dominant hemisphere for the left-handed person is the right. Cerebral language mechanisms reside in only one hemisphere, presumably the dominant one. Therefore, since most people are right-handed it follows that the left hemisphere contains the language mechanisms for most people.

But what about the reported 6 to 10 per cent of the population who are left-handed? Is their language mechanism in the right hemisphere and do they become aphasic if damage is sustained in the right hemisphere? How valid an indication of hemispheric language dominance is handedness? These questions have been discussed since the earliest studies of aphasia and it remains a common clinical belief that the dominant hemisphere for language is opposite the preferred hand. However, in recent years there have been several systematic studies which support the conclusion that the left hemisphere is dominant for language regardless of the handedness of the person.

Schuell, Jenkins and Jimenez (1964) present data on 120 aphasics showing the relationship between handedness and the site of the lesion. Handedness was determined by questioning the patient and his family. The cerebral hemisphere which was damaged was determined from the contralateral signs of neurological involvement particularly of the arm and leg. Bilateral damage was indicated by positive neurological findings on both sides of the body. The data of Table 8-I show that 33 per cent (3 patients) of the left-handed group had indications of right hemisphere damage. Although the percentage may be impressive, the number

TABLE 8-I

DIFFERENCES IN PERCENTAGE OF PATIENTS WITH APHASIA AFTER OPERATION ON THE LEFT AND RIGHT HEMISPHERE (Penfield and Roberts, 1958)

Hand	Total No.	No. With Aphasia	%	Total No.	No. With Aphasia	%	Significance of Difference
R[1]	157	115	73.2	196	1	0.5	<.001
L[2]	18	13	72.2	15	1	6.7	<.001
Total	175	128	73.1	211	2	0.9	<.001

[1]Including predominantly right
[2]Including predominantly left

of left-handed patients is too small to allow for definite conclusions to be drawn. The authors further point out that it is not always possible to rule out bilateral involvement conclusively so that what appeared to be right hemisphere lesions could have had accompanying left hemisphere lesions without positive neurological signs on the right side of the body. It is also to be noted that five right-handed aphasics had right hemisphere damage. It may be concluded from these data that aphasia is more often associated with left hemisphere damage regardless of the handedness of the patient. Aphasia may also be associated with right hemisphere damage and when it is the patient is more likely to be left-handed than right-handed.

Penfield and Roberts (1959) report data on a larger number of patients with more exact determination of hemispheric involvement. They comprehensively review the general problem of handedness and cerebral dominance and report the results of an investigation of the relationship between handedness and aphasia in over five hundred cases. In their study they determined the patient's handedness prior to brain surgery and observed the post-surgical appearance of aphasia in relation to the hemisphere operated on. The results are presented in Table 8-II. The data show no difference in the incidence of aphasia after operation on the left hemisphere between the left- and right-handed. For the left-handed aphasia occurred ten times more often after operation on the left than on the right hemisphere.

Aphasia does occur occasionally from interference from the right hemisphere in both the right- and left-handed. It occurs only

TABLE 8-II

HANDEDNESS AND HEMISPHERE INVOLVEMENT

(Schuell, Jenkins and Jimenez, 1964)

Handedness	Left Hemisphere Lesions		Right Hemisphere Lesions		Bilateral Involvement		Total
	N	Percent	N	Percent	N	Percent	
Right-handed	90	80%	5	4%	18	16%	113
Left-Handed	4	44%	3	33%	2	22%	9
Ambidextrous	1						1

about 1 per cent of the time in the right-handed and less than 10 per cent of the time in the left-handed. Also noted by the authors is that the type of aphasic disturbance which occurs with disease of the right hemisphere is different from that of the left hemisphere. They note that permanent aphasia rarely if ever, occurs with involvement of only the right hemisphere. Dysarthria can, of course, result from damage to either hemisphere and is not to be confused with aphasic language impairments.

Penfield and Roberts conclude their discussion by stating that "there is no significant difference in the frequency of aphasia after operation on the right hemisphere between the right- and left-handed. Dysphasia, is of course, quite rare with involvement of only the right hemisphere. This conclusion is at variance with most of the opinions in the literature. In almost one hundred years, only about 140 cases have been reported with aphasia and involvement of only the right hemisphere. It seems clear that the left hemisphere is usually dominant for speech, regardless of handedness. The reason why the right hemisphere is sometimes dominant for speech remains unclear, but it is not related solely to handedness."

SUMMARY

Aphasia has been of interest to a number of disciplines such as psychology, linguistics and medicine. This chapter has discussed aphasia as a clinical disorder of communication and its management by the speech pathologist. Aphasia is defined as an *impairment in the ability to communicate due to disorders of symbolic language processes.* It is caused by damage to the brain. Apraxia, agnosia, dysarthria and disturbed mental functioning may also be produced by brain damage and result in communication disturbances, however, these disorders are to be differentiated from aphasia.

Although aphasia is usually viewed as a language disturbance, a number of authors have indicated that aphasia may be broadly conceived of as a general difficulty in the use of symbols—nonlanguage as well as language. Others view aphasia as a reflection of a more fundamental disturbance in some aspect of cognitive functioning.

Because aphasia is an impairment of basic language processing all modalities of language usage—speech, verbal comprehension, reading and writing—will show approximately equal degrees of impairment. For the same reason all languages of a polyglot patient will generally be impaired to the same extent.

A number of personality, behavioral and physical disturbances may be produced by brain damage and therefore be associated with aphasia. Aphasia is usually caused by lesions of the left hemisphere (regardless of the handedness of the patient) which produce right hemiplegia and other right-sided neurological symptoms. These associated problems must be carefully taken into consideration by the speech pathologist in the evaluation and treatment planning of the patient.

Several tests of aphasia which provide clinically significant information for treatment and prognosis are available. In the course of his treatment the aphasia clinician must be aware of the changing needs of the patient and his family as he passes through various phases of recovery. Family counselling is an integral part of aphasia therapy. The speech pathologist must choose from a variety of specific therapy approaches which have been proposed for the treatment of aphasia.

REFERENCES

Agranowtiz, A., and McKeown, M.: *Aphasia Handbook for Adults and Children.* Springfield, Thomas, 1964.

Aronson, M.; Shatin, L., and Cook, J.: Socio-psychotherapeutic approach to the treatment of aphasic patients. *J Speech Hearing Dis, 21*:352-364, 1956.

Bay, E.: Present concepts of aphasia. *Geriatrics,* May, 319-331, 1964.

Benton, A., and Joynt, R.: Early description of aphasia. *Brain, 65*:205-222, 1960.

Berry, M., and Eisenson, J.: *Speech Disorders.* New York, Appleton-Century-Crofts, 1956.

Bloom, I.: A rationale for group treatment of aphasic patients. *J Speech Hearing Dis, 27*:11-16, 1962.

Boone, E.: *An Adult Has Aphasia.* Danville, Ill., Interstate, 1965.

Brain, R.: *Speech Disorders: Aphasia, Apraxia and Agnosia.* Washington, Butterfield, 1961.

Buck, McK.: Life with a stroke. *Crippled Child,* 1957.

Buck, McK.: *Dysphasia: Professional Guidance for Family and Patient.* Englewood Cliffs, Prentice-Hall, 1964.

Charlton, M.H.: Aphasia in bilingual and polyglot patients—a neurological and psychological study. *J Speech Hearing Dis, 29:*307-311, 1964.

Darley, F.: *Diagnosis and Appraisal of Communication Disorders.* Englewood Cliffs, Prentice-Hall, 1964.

Eisenhower, D.: *The White House Years: Waging Peace* 1956-1961. Garden City, Doubleday, 1965.

Eisenson, J.: *Examining for Aphasia.* New York, Psychological Corp, 1954.

Geschwind, N.: Non-aphasic disorders of speech. *Int J Neurol, 4:*207-214, 1964.

Goldstein, K.: *Language and Language Disturbances.* New York, Grune and Stratton, 1948.

Goodglass, H., and Kaplan, E.: Disturbance of gesture and pantomime in aphasia. *Brain, 86:*703-720, 1963.

Granich, L.: *Aphasia: A Guide to Retraining.* New York, Grune and Stratton, 1947.

Head, H.: *Aphasia and Kindred Disorders of Speech.* Cambridge, Cambridge Press, 1926, vol. I.

Hirschberg, G.G.; Lewis, L., and Thomas, D.: *Rehabilitation.* Philadelphia, Lippincott, 1964.

Holland, Audrey, and Harris, A.: Aphasia rehabilitation using programmed instruction: An intensive case history. In Sloane, H., and MacAulay, B. (Eds.): *Operant Procedures in Remedial Speech and Language Training.* New York, Houghton Mifflin, 1968.

Horowitz, B.: An open letter to the family of an adult patient with aphasia. *Rehab Lit, 23:*141-144, 1962.

Kann, J.: A translation of Broca's original article on the location of the speech center. *J Speech Hearing Dis, 15:*16-20, 1950.

Longerich, M., and Bordeaux, J.: *Aphasia Therapeutics.* New York, MacMillan, 1954.

McBride, Carman: *Silent Victory.* Chicago, Nelson-Hall, 1969.

Osgood, C., and Miron, M.: *Approaches to the Study of Aphasia.* Urbana, U. of Illinois Press, 1963.

Penfield, W., and Roberts, L.: *Speech and Brain-Mechanisms.* Princeton, Princeton U. Press, 1959.

Porch, B.: *Porch Index of Communicative Ability: Theory and Development.* Palo Alto, Consulting Psychologists, 1967.

Ritchie, D.: *Stroke.* New York, Doubleday, 1961.

Rose, R.: A physician's account of his own aphasia. *J Speech Hearing Dis, 13:*294-305, 1948.

Rusk, H.: *Rehabilitation Medicine.* St. Louis, Mosby, 1964.

Schuell, H.: *Differential Diagnosis of Aphasia with the Minnesota Test.* Minneapolis, U. Minnesota Press, 1965.

Schuell, H.: Aphasia in adults. *Human Communication and Its Disorders—*

An Overview. Bethesda, U. S. Dept of Health, Education and Welfare, 1969.

Schuell, H.; Jenkins, J., and Jimenez, E.: *Aphasia in Adults: Diagnosis, Prognosis, and Treatment.* New York, Harper and Row, 1964(a).

Schuell, H., and Jenkins, J.: Further work on language deficit in aphasia. *Psych Rev, 71*:87-93, 1964b.

Sies, L., and Butler, R.: A personal account of dysphasia. *J Speech Hearing Dis, 28*:261-266, 1963.

Taylor, M., and Meyers, J.: A group discussion program with families of aphasic patients. *J Speech Hearing Dis, 17*:393-396, 1952.

Weisenburg, T., and McBride, K.S.: *Aphasia: A Clinical and Psychological Study.* New York, Hafner, 1964.

Wepman, J.: *Recovery from Aphasia.* New York, Ronald, 1951.

Wepman, J.: *Aphasia and the Family.* New York, American Heart Ass., 1968.

Wepman, J., and Jones, L.: *Studies in Aphasia: An Approach to Testing.* Chicago, Education-Industry Service, 1961.

Wepman, J., Jones, L., Bock, D., and Van Pelt, D.: Studies in aphasia: Backgound and theoretical formulations. *J Speech Hearing Dis, 25*: 323-332, 1960.

CHAPTER NINE

DISORDERS OF HEARING

THOMAS G. GIOLAS

T HE NORMAL development of verbal communication skills depends to a great extent on an intact auditory mechanism. Problems with the normal acquisition of language, speech, educational and vocational skills arise when there is a faulty hearing apparatus. In addition, a hearing impairment can have psychological effects. The severity of these problems depends on what aspect of the auditory pathway is damaged, the amount of auditory deprivation, and when it occurred. Knowledge of the interaction of these three factors is necessary in order to identify and understand the hearing handicapped person. The purpose of this chapter is to provide a general discussion of these factors. Where important, the reader is referred to more extensive discussions of certain issues. It is hoped that the discussions will stir the reader's interest sufficiently for him to pursue many of the areas in depth. The relationship of *speech pathology* and *clinical audiology* is emphasized as both fields play significant roles in the rehabilitation of the hearing handicapped.

Damage to the auditory pathway is the initial factor contributing to hearing impairment. This is commonly referred to as *types* of hearing disorders and these are best divided into five categories. They are *conductive, sensori-neural, mixed, central* and *nonorganic disorders.*

CONDUCTIVE HEARING DISORDER

Chapter Two has dealt with the nature of sound generation and the normal process of sound reception. It was established that the basic function of the middle ear was to transmit sound to the inner ear and by so doing increase the inner ear's *sensitivity.* This results in an increase in the loudness of the auditory signal being presented to the inner ear. Any breakdown with the middle ear's sound conduction process would, therefore, cause a loss of hearing sensitivity commonly referred to as a *Conductive Hearing Disorder.* This section deals with some of the medical problems of the outer and middle ears, which can cause a conductive disorder.

Outer Ear

The contribution to hearing sensitivity of the outer ear, while significant in animals and, perhaps, prehistoric man, is minimal in modern man. However, medical problems of the outer ear are often indicative of deeper structure malformations and, consequently, warrant mention here. Medical problems of the outer ear can be categorized as stemming from congenital malformations, blockage of the *auditory meatus* and *external otitis.*

Congenital malformations of the outer ear usually consist of some degree of deformed *Pinna* or closure *(atresia)* of the auditory meatus. While such deformities are often accompanied by middle ear structure problems, a loss of the pinna and auditory meatus alone produces little or no hearing loss. However, reconstruction of these structures is often done through plastic surgery for cosmetic reasons. In some cases where deeper anatomical structures are involved and a hearing aid has been recommended, it may be necessary for the auditory meatus to be reconstructed so that an ear mold can be properly fitted.

In some cases a minor hearing loss has been detected because of some obstruction in the auditory meatus. This blockage can occur because of excessive wax *(cerumen)* or, in the cases of children, the insertion of a foreign body. With the removal of this blockage by a physician, the hearing usually returns to its natural state. The danger of removing excessive wax, or other blocking substance (s) , from the auditory meatus by yourself is that you run the risk of scratching or scraping the walls of the canal. Such irritations can become infected and produce an inflammation called *external otitis.* External otitis can also occur because of sudden weather changes which allow the growth of bacteria and fungi, as well as pimples and styes usually found at the mouth of the meatus. Treatment for external otitis consists of some form of sulfur and mycin drugs to prevent the infection from spreading.

Otitis Media

Etiology. One of the most common diseases of the middle ear and causes of a conductive hearing disorder is *otitis media*. It usually develops as part of a general upper respiratory congestion (a head cold) and manifests itself in the form of *fluid* in the middle ear. Consequently, otitis media is often referred to as a "cold in the ears." Fluid in the middle ear is formed in one or a combination of two ways. Because of general infection in the nasopharynx region and at the mouth of the *eustachian tube* infection is transferred through the eustachian tube to the middle ear. The mucous membrane lining of the middle ear and adjoining structures *(mastoid air cells)* become infected causing them to drain— as in the early stages of a running nose. Other medical problems which can cause the mucous membrane lining to drain are measles, mumps, virus infections and, to a lesser degree, some forms of allergies. A second common cause of fluid in the middle ear is an improper supply of oxygen to the middle ear. One of the most important functions of the eustachian tube is to maintain the proper oxygen balance in the middle ear. The eustachian tube, which is normally closed, is opened periodically to allow for additional oxygen to enter the middle ear. This function can be impeded through blockage of the eustachian tube passageway by accumulation of infection or a collapsed tube due to sudden atmospheric pressure changes, such as can occur in some airplane flights. The existing oxygen is absorbed by the middle ear blood supply and when no new oxygen is supplied the mucous membrane linings react by emitting a fluid substance.

The fluid found in the middle ear during a bout of otitis media can take one of two forms. It can be a clear nonbacteria substance, which if it remains in the middle ear too long becomes thick and gluey producing a condition referred to as "glue ears." Otitis Media of the clear fluid type is called *nonsuppurative serous* or nonpurulent otitis media. It usually occurs in the early stages of otitis media and is accompanied by a retraction of the tympanic membrane. This retraction is primarily due to the reduced air pressure in the middle ear cavity in comparison to the air pressure in auditory meatus at the tympanic membrane. Otitis media fluid can also be pussy, reddish and, due to direct inflammation of the mucous membrane lining, contain bacteria. When this occurs the tympanic membrane is distended and the condition is referred to as *suppurative* or *purulent otitis media.*

Treatment. In order to minimize the damaging effect of otitis media, the fluid must be removed as soon as possible. Antibiotics such as sulphur or penicillin are quite effective. It also often becomes necessary to surgically puncture the tympanic membrane to allow the fluid to drain out. This procedure is referred to as a *myringotomy* and involves making a neat incision on the tympanic membrane in a strategic spot, allowing for the most efficient draining and healing. In cases where there is repeated reoccurrence of fluid, plastic tubes are placed in the tympanic membrane to allow for continued drainage and proper oxygen equalization in the middle ear cavity. In cases where the fluid has become thick it must be suctioned out. Often the fluid is of sufficient amount and under extreme pressure causing a hole to burst in the tympanic membrane, and the fluid drains naturally. This is not a desirable course but is often not avoidable. In order to prevent this, the drum is often punctured surgically.

In most cases the self-punctured tympanic membrane will self-heal. However, in cases when it doesn't (perhaps because of repeated ruptures) the hole must be closed surgically employing a procedure referred to as a *myringoplasty.* If more damage to the middle ear has occurred it may become necessary to perform a *tympanoplasty* in which some reconstruction of the middle ear structure is performed to allow for a new rerouting of sound. When the disease has become more extensive and has involved the mastoid cells it is often necessary to clear up the disease process with a surgical procedure called a *modified radical mastoidectomy.* This procedure is done without sacrificing the middle ear structures and seldom causes a permanent hearing loss. In other cases a more involved procedure is indicated which involves removal of some middle ear structures and some permanent hearing loss. However, there are those who feel that the disease was so advanced that the observed loss of hearing was present prior to the surgery. In any case, this surgery is performed as a life-saving measure guarding against such complications as a cholesteotome growth, which can attack the brain covering and cause meningitis. In special cases an artificial tympanic membrane prosthetic device is used to restore middle ear function. Other medical procedures involve removal of diseased tissue around the eustachian tube surgically and/or with radiation and inflation of the eustachian tube to replenish the middle ear with oxygen until the normal function of the eustachian tube can be restored.

Otosclerosis

Otosclerosis is a disease which attacks the hard bony shell of the cochlea. The disease takes the form of a new spongy bone growth typically centered around the oval window. The new spongy bone growth hardens and fixes the foot plate of the stapes into the oval window reducing its movement. The reduced movement of the stapes reduces the sound transmission efficiency of the middle ear and a conductive hearing disorder occurs. Sometimes more of the cochlea is involved, especially in the advanced stages of the disease, and a sensory-neural disorder (to be discussed in the next section) is also present.

The specific cause of otosclerosis is unknown. It has been found to be hereditary and is more prevalent in women than in men, and in the Caucasian race than in black people. It is typically noticed between the ages of thirteen and the late twenties. The hearing loss associated with otosclerosis generally appears gradually, seldom reaches more than 60 dB in degree and has been found to be heightened by pregnancy. However, this is not always true and physicians do not routinely advise avoiding pregnancy because of possible otosclerotic hearing loss. Clinical diagnosis of otosclerosis is typically made on the basis of the following observations: (a) a familial history of hearing loss, (b) no history of ear infections and a negative otological examination revealing normal tympanic membranes and (c) a gradual mild-to-moderate loss of hearing of a conductive nature demonstrated audiometrically.

Fortunately, the primary symptom of otosclerosis (diminished hearing) can be treated surgically with often resultant hearing within the normal range. The most current and popular surgical procedure is the *stapedectomy*. This operation is performed through the auditory meatus and under a local anesthesia. Briefly, it involves lifting the ear drum and removing the complete stapes, replacing the stapes with a plastic strut or wire and covering the oval window with a vein graft or fatty body tissue. Near normal sound transmission is restored in most cases. The procedure involves two-to-three days hospitalization and once healing has taken place the postoperative care is minimal. Other surgical procedures for otosclerosis include the *fenestration,* which involves rerouting the sound waves through a new window made in the horizontal canal, and the stapes mobilization, which consists of partially or completely freeing the stapes from the spongy growth fixing it in the oval window. The results from these latter procedures have not been as consistently satisfactory as the results obtained with the stapedectomy procedure.

As mentioned earlier, the hearing loss associated with otosclerosis is primarily conductive in nature. Consequently, the person with this disease can be helped considerably from amplification as is provided by the hearing aid. The amplification provided by the hearing aid overrides any reduced function of the stapes and the fluid of the cochlea is stimulated. In cases where surgery is medically contraindicated, a hearing aid is the best solution for improved hearing.

SENSORI-NEURAL HEARING DISORDER

The basic function of the inner ear is to code the frequency and intensity components of the auditory signal, thereby, contributing not only to the sensitivity of the signal but to its *understandability (intelligibility)* as well. In this section the inner ear refers to the area beyond the middle ear through the cochlea to the brain stem. The problem, therefore, can lie in the cochlea (sense organ) or along the VIIIth (auditory) nerve. Consequently, any abnormality or disease involving these structures can cause a sensori-neural hearing disorder. The etiology of a sensori-neural disorder can be either congenital or acquired.

Congenital Causes

The two common causes of a congenital sensori-neural hearing disorder are hereditary and damage to the embryo. A hearing problem is considered to be congenital if it is present at birth or occurs prior to when the child learned to speak. Little is known about hereditary cause of hearing problems. It has been observed, however, that a hearing impairment of hereditary origin can occur at any time during one's life and it is usually a sensori-neural disorder of any degree of severity. The damage is usually specific to the auditory nerve and other anatomical structures are not involved. Furthermore, statistics have shown that children of deaf parents who have true hereditary deafness are also likely to be born deaf. This is not true of children born of parents with a hearing problem due to nonhereditary causes. This observation is sufficiently stable to warrant appropriate marriage counseling of all deaf persons. Congenital malformations of the external and middle ear may also be hereditary.

Diseases contracted by the expectant mother during the early stages of pregnancy (first three months) while the ear is in its developmental stages can cause severe damage to the embryo and interrupt this developmental process. These diseases include (a) *viruses* such as *mumps* and *influenzas,* (b) *German measles* (rubella) and (c) *Rh blood incompatibility.* Erythroblastosis due to Rh blood incompatibility will be discussed later. In general, however, these diseases produce a toxic effect on the embryo and the damage results in one or a combination of congenital problems. Expectant mothers are encouraged to contact their doctor if they feel they have been exposed to persons who have an active case of any of these diseases.

Acquired Causes

Probably the most common cause of a sensori-neural hearing disorder is advancing age. This hearing problem is referred to as *Presbycusis.* It is caused by the natural atrophy of the organ of corti, which begins between the ages of thirty to forty years. The hair cells near the base of the cochlea begin to degenerate and have even been observed to vanish. The impairment manifests itself initially in the high frequencies and gradually progresses to the lower frequencies. As is true with most sensori-neural hearing disorders, presbycusis produces a permanent hearing problem. It is not medically reversible. This is because when there is actual sensory cell or nerve fiber degeneration or destruction no medical assistance can restore the lost hearing. However, we will discuss later how persons with presbycusis and other sensori-neural hearing disorders can be helped to compensate for their hearing difficulty.

Several diseases and drugs can cause a sensori-neural hearing disorder. The hearing problem occurs in one of three ways: (a) through the absorption of toxins (poisons) produced by a particular disease, (b) a high fever and (c) through the use of certain drugs necessary to combat the disease but detrimental to the sense of hearing. All three of these conditions contribute to the destruction of the auditory nerve. An example of such a disease is *meningitis,* which is an infection of the membrane surrounding the brain (meninges). The spinal fluid becomes infected and eventually the cochlea is attacked causing a hearing deficiency through destruction of auditory sensory structures. Damage to the cochlea can also occur through the high fever associated with meningitis and the drugs often used to combat the disease—streptomycin, kanamycin.

It should be pointed out that knowledge of the effect of these drugs on hearing is well known and they are only used in cases where it becomes necessary to save a life. Other diseases such as measles, scarlet fever, diphtheria, whooping cough, influenza and virus can adversely effect hearing through toxic absorption. Middle ear problems may also be associated with these diseases.

Special mention should be made of the effect of mumps on hearing. In some cases, mumps cause an infection of the brain, unlike meningitis, and attack the tissues of the cochlea. A severe loss of hearing occurs. Fortunately, the hearing deficiency is almost always in one ear and hearing for communication efficiency is not impaired dramatically.

A sensori-neural hearing disorder is also caused by a disease called Menieres. The symptoms of this disease include vertigo (dizziness), tinnitus (ringing in the ears), nausea and a loss of hearing. The symptoms are said to be a result of the endolympha- tic fluid having been placed under pressure due to vascular changes. The vascular changes are considered to be a result of intermittent interruption of blood supply, certain allergies or psychosomatic. If the blood supply to the inner ear becomes ex- tensive (a few hours) a permanent severe loss of hearing can occur referred to as a "sudden deafness."

Medical treatment varies from physician to physician. Further- more, because of the high frequency of psychological correlates governing the symptoms, the response to medical treatment has a wide range of success. Generally, however, a vasodilator drug such as *nicotinic acid* or injections of histimine, with often a *procaine* drug to increase blood flow, is prescribed Some physicians also prescribe a salt-free diet. It is usually felt that the treatment pro- gram should begin quite early after the onset of the symptoms to be effective.

In some cases a Meniere's attack can be completely incapaci- tating while it lasts. The patient experiences severe dizziness and loss of balance, accompanied by acute nausea. During these at- tacks he may not be able to maneuver independently. Further- more, the onset of these attacks is sudden and without warning. When these severe cases do not respond to medication, surgery designed to destroy the labyrinth is considered to eliminate the incapacitating symptoms. Medical treatment for patients acquir- ing a *sudden loss* is quite similar to the treatment for Meniere's, with the addition of an anticoagulant drug in some cases.

Tumors in the region of the VIIIth (auditory) nerve can also cause a sensori-neural hearing disorder due to pressure on the nerve fibers. If the tumor is present for an extensive period of time some nerve fibers can actually be damaged and a permanent hearing impairment occur. Often, however, the hearing returns to normal when the tumor has been removed. A tumor of the auditory nerve is usually nonmalignant. If the tumor is not re- moved there is the danger that the pressure may spread to other vital areas in the brain.

Exposure to sufficiently intense noise can also cause a sensori-

neural hearing disorder. This impairment can be either temporary or permanent, depending on several things including (a)
the intensity of the noise, (b) the amount of exposure time, and
(c) the rest periods during the exposure. The hearing impairment
usually begins in the high frequencies and progresses to the low
frequencies. There is considerable variability concerning the degree to which persons are susceptible to *noise induced hearing
loss.* However, at present there is no reliable measure of one's
susceptibility. Many industries have taken several precautions to
minimize chances for employees incurring a hearing loss due to
noise exposure. These precautions include (a) minimizing overall
environmental noise levels, (b) rotating employees out of noisy
environments on a regular basis and (c) routine hearing tests to
be aware of any changes in an employee's hearing level.

It should be mentioned that it is possible for a person to have
a combination of both a conductive and sensori-neural disorders.
This is referred to as a *mixed hearing disorder.*

CENTRAL AUDITORY DISORDERS

Auditory disorders involving the auditory pathway from the
brain stem on up to and including the cortex are referred to as
central auditory disorders or *central deafness.* This type of hearing impairment is usually caused by damage to the brain through
(a) a brain tumor or abscess, (b) vascular changes or (c) *erythroblastosis* with associated Kanicterus. Erythroblastosis is a result of
blood incompatability between the mother and the infant and results in the destruction of the infant's red blood cells and subsequent deposition of blood pigments in the brain stem. The blood
incompatability occurs when a mother with RH negative blood
type and a father with an RH positive blood type produce a child
with an RH positive blood type. In addition to hearing impairment, other problems such as cerebral palsy and mental retardation can emerge. The damage usually occurs right at birth, but
damage can also occur prenatally. Treatment involves careful pre-
natal care and transfusion of the infant's blood at birth to eliminate or at least minimize, any real blood cell destruction. This
treatment is quite successful.

NONORGANIC HEARING DISORDER

It has been found that on occasion persons will simulate hearing difficulty for emotional reasons. These persons can have normal hearing or actually have an organic hearing disorder which they are exaggerating. The motivation for creating a *nonorganic hearing disorder* may be conscious or unconscious. If the motivation is on an unconscious level, the apparent hearing loss is often referred to as a *psychogenic hearing loss* or *hysterical conversion* and is believed to have a psychological etiology. The simulated hearing problem is viewed as a symptom of a deep-seated emotional problem and treatment requires intensive psychological counseling. Furthermore, because the hearing problem is simulated unconsciously, it is difficult to detect audiologically. On the other hand, hearing losses simulated consciously (outright *malingering*) can be detected much easier. Utilizing several psychoacoustic principles, tests have been developed which can estimate a person's organic level of hearing even though he is attempting to conceal this level. The consciously simulated nonorganic hearing disorder is also considered to have a psychological base, but mostly to a much lesser degree of severity. For example, the child may be having difficulty in school and wish to blame it on something organic like a hearing impairment. Treatment would consist of helping the child understand his motivation and develop more acceptable ways of dealing with his frustrations. Another example is the person who is interested in collecting financial remuneration from an insurance company by pretending that the automobile accident he was in caused some permanent damage to his sense of hearing. The object of the treatment program in this situation is to assess how much, if any, loss of hearing occurred and compensate accordingly. A comprehensive discussion of medical problems of the ear can be found in DeWeese and Saunders (1964).

BEHAVIORAL SYMPTOMS

Conductive and sensori-neural disorders often manifest themselves in observable behavioral symptoms. While many of these symptoms can be associated with a number of clinical problems and cannot be used independently for diagnosis, they can be used as guides for further referral. Furthermore, they offer some insight into the kinds of communication problems experienced by persons with these types of hearing disorders.

It has been observed that a person with a conductive disorder often speaks in a relatively quiet voice. This is true even in noisy situations where persons with normal hearing tend to increase the intensity of their voices to be heard over the environmental noise. It is assumed that because of the loss of sensitivity associated with the conductive disorder, the person with this type of disorder is not aware of the extent to which the environmental noise is interfering with his speech and, consequently, does not raise his voice. Furthermore, as the inner ear is presumably intact and we hear ourselves partially by bone conduction, he hears himself fairly well and has no clue to speak louder. On the other hand, a person with a sensori-neural disorder tends to speak louder than is appropriate for the particular situation. This is thought to occur because his hearing impairment involves the inner ear. Unlike a person with a conductive disorder, he cannot take advantage of hearing through bone conduction and must speak louder in order to hear himself.

A second symptom of conductive disorders is that speech discrimination is quite good as long as it is loud enough to be heard. A typical statement made by persons with a conductive disorder is, *I don't have any trouble understanding people as long as they talk loud enough.* This phenomenon is again hooked to the fact that conductive disorders predominately involve a loss of sensitivity and not the sound analysis process of the cochlea. This also explains why this person also heard better in noisy situations (*paracusis willisiana* or *willisii*). Those talking to him tend to speak louder to override the environmental noises and the increased volume helps the person with a sensitivity loss. As speech discrimination is unimpaired, the message is properly analyzed when it is received. Such is not the case with persons having a sensori-neural hearing disorder. Speech discrimination ability can be impaired. The sound analysis process which takes place in the inner ear is damaged and sound is not transmitted to the brain in its entirety. Aspects of the message have not been coded. The result is an incomplete or unclear message resulting in poor speech discrimination. While it is often enough to just speak louder to the person with a conductive disorder, it is often necessary to slow down, enunciate clearly and repeat statements for the person with a sensori-neural disorder. A typical statement concerning speech discrimination by a person with a sensori-neural disorder is, *I hear people all right, I just can't understand what they're saying.*

With a conductive disorder one can tolerate sounds of much greater intensitives than can persons with normal hearing or a sensori-neural impairment. The loss of sensitivity removes some of the energy of the signal being heard and the signal is not perceived as loud. It, therefore, takes much greater overall levels of intensity for sounds to reach discomfort levels. This is only true at intensity levels below 130 dB. The situation with sensori-neural disorders can be quite different. In many cases, the reverse is true and there is an *abnormal growth to loudness* (commonly referred to as recruitment). This is exhibited by observing that once threshold is reached with persons with a sensori-neural disorder, an increase in intensity of the sound is perceived with considerably greater loudness than the same increase in intensity above threshold for persons with normal hearing. While their thresholds for a given sound differ (0 dB for the person with normal hearing and 60 dB for the person with a sensori-neural disorder), at a certain point the person with a sensori-neural disorder will perceive the sound equally as loud or louder than the person with normal hearing. It is this abnormal growth to loudness that creates the situation in which a person is unable to hear speech at one point and with a slight increase of intensity the speech is perceived as much too loud. Recruitment is thought to be a result of damage in the cochlea, rather than along the VIIIth nerve.

Sudden behavioral changes are often symptoms of a hearing problem. A person may experience a temporary reduction in hearing due to otitis media. He may begin asking to have statements repeated, watching the talker's face more closely and appear to miss a lot of what is being said. His hearing, of course, will improve when the ear infection is no longer present and this change in hearing level is a good sign that the disorder was conductive. This cycle can repeat itself several times if the otitis media is chronic.

Inconsistent responses to auditory stimuli on a long term basis, however, may suggest a mild-to-moderate hearing impairment of a more permanent nature. Persons with a sensori-neural impairment typically hear low frequency sounds better than high frequency sounds. This is true for most sensori-neural impairments regardless of the extent of the loss. Furthermore, in mild cases, it is possible for hearing for the lower frequencies to be within the normal range, with considerable difficulty hearing the higher frequencies. As speech includes sounds with low frequencies (vowels) and high frequencies (consonants), persons with a high frequency hearing impairment do not often hear all parts of the speech message. Their responses to speech may often seem inconsistent because they hear some, but not all of the message.

Special mention should be made about problems encountered with a unilateral hearing impairment. Because persons with hearing in only one ear have functional hearing for the acquisition of speech, language and academic skills, the communication problems they exhibit in many situations have been minimized. The observable problems include (a) localizing from which direction sound is coming, (b) understanding speech when the speaker is located on the side of the poor ear or when there is any extraneous noise, such as an air conditioner, music, other talkers as in a party situation. Interviews with persons with a unilateral hearing impairment revealed that they are extremely aware of their hearing problem and feel they must constantly make special arrangements to insure that they will hear optimally.

MEASUREMENT OF HEARING

Chapter Two contains a discussion concerning how environmental sounds are produced and how the ear normally receives and transmits the acoustic message to the brain. The preceding section of this chapter discussed how the normal sound reception process can be interrupted through disease and/or faulty anatomical structure. The discussion to follow is concerned with how the hearing function is measured, with the purpose of determining the presence or absence of a hearing impairment and what remedial program is indicated.

If a hearing impairment is detected, three basic questions are asked about the nature of the impairment. One question deals with how much energy or intensity is lost from the perceived auditory message. This is referred to as the *extent* of the hearing loss. In this chapter the term *hearing loss* will always refer to a loss of intensity (measured in decibels). The term *hearing impairment* has been used as the more general term referring to a problem of hearing of a nonspecified nature. A second question deals with what *type* of hearing disorder is present, that is, whether it is primarily conductive, sensori-neural, or the result of damage to some other site along the auditory pathway. Finally, investigation is made of the degree to which a person's extent and type of impairment combine with his basic abilities and personality to cause a handicapping effect.

This information is secured through several test procedures. These procedures will be described and their contribution to the total diagnostic picture discussed.

The primary goal of any hearing evaluation procedure is to obtain consistent responses to known auditory messages which were presented to the listener in a standardized manner. This requires trained personnel, employing calibrated equipment used in a relatively noise-free environment.

PURETONE AUDIOMETRY

One of the basic test procedures used to evaluate hearing is the *Puretone Audiometric Test*. Puretone audiometry consists of presenting the listener with a series of calibrated pure tones at different frequencies and intensities. The acoustic components of a pure tone have been discussed in Chapter Two. Simply, it consists of an auditory stimulus with a known frequency, intensity and phase. The tones are produced by an *audiometer* which includes, among other things, a *frequency generator, intensity attenuator* and *tone interrupter switch* for presenting and terminating the pure tones. The intensity of the pure tones can be manipulated through the attenuator, which acts similar to a volume control switch on a radio. The goal is to determine the lowest (softest) intensity needed to obtain a response 50 per cent of the time. Briefly, the procedure consists of presenting the tone at an intensity level sufficiently loud for the listener to hear it. He is asked to respond, typically by raising his hand, each time he hears the tone. The tone is then systematically decreased in intensity until the listener no longer indicates that he hears it. This is referred to as obtaining a listener's *threshold* for pure tones.

There are several procedural considerations to be made when searching for a listener's threshold. These include (a) the length of time the tone is presented to the listener, (b) the length of time between tone presentations, (c) whether the tone progressed from audibility to inaudibility (as described earlier) or in reverse order and (d) the kind of listening instructions given. Each of these factors can alter the threshold obtained. An excellent discussion of these factors, as well as a detailed discussion of a preferred test procedure, can be found in Carhart and Jerger (1959).

The measured threshold is compared to a standard threshold for normal hearing for pure tones (Davis and Kranz, *J Speech Hearing Res,* 1964). The degree to which the listener's hearing varies from the standard for normal hearing is viewed as his *hearing loss* for that frequency. The attenuator is generally calibrated in 5 dB steps, making it possible to state the extent of the hearing loss in decibels. The tones are presented through ear phones so that the hearing in each ear is measured separately.

Thresholds are obtained for several pure tone frequencies. They are 125Hz, 250Hz, 500Hz, 1000Hz, 2000Hz, 6000Hz and 8000Hz. The average of the thresholds for three of these frequencies (500, 1000, 2000 Hz), which have been found to contribute the most to the reception of speech and are known as the *speech frequencies,* is often obtained. This average is then used to express the *extent* of a person's hearing loss.

An *audiogram,* such as the one shown in Figure 9-1, is typically plotted. An audiogram simply consists of a diagram of the listener's threshold of hearing for each frequency tested. Figure 9-1

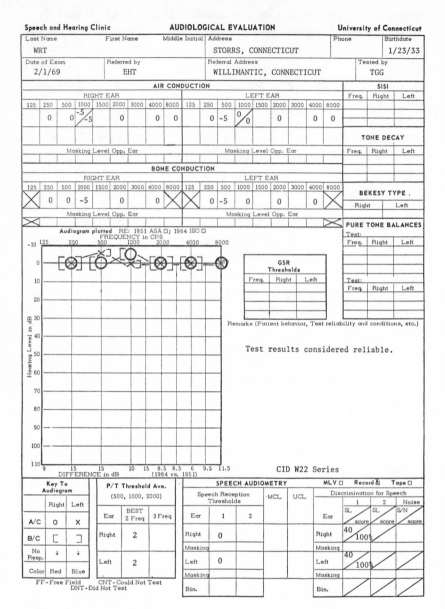

Figure 9-1. Typical audiologic record demonstrating normal hearing.

represents an audiogram of a person with normal hearing or thresholds obtained at Zero dB (0dB) *Hearing Level* (H.L.). 0dB Hearing Level is defined as a point at which most persons with *normal hearing* yield thresholds 50 per cent of the time. 0dB Hearing Level is designated on the audiometer intensity dial and all subsequent intensity markings (5dB, 10dB, 15dB, etc.) are in relation to this reference point. A threshold of 40 dB Hearing Loss for a given person at a given frequency would be interpreted to mean that the person being tested has a threshold which is 40dB poorer than a person with normal hearing.

In addition to measuring the extent of the hearing loss, it is also desirable to obtain some indication of where the locus of the hearing difficulty lies from the standpoint of anatomical structures and physiological processes. This is referred to as determining the type of hearing disorder and is secured by comparing *bone conduction* (b/c) thresholds to the air conduction (a/c) thresholds which are obtained through earphones. Bone conduction thresholds are obtained by presenting the test frequencies through a vibrator which is placed directly on the head. Bone conduction thresholds are obtained by the same test procedure as air conduction thresholds. Audiometers can be equipped to test for either mode of tone presentation. Tones presented by bone conduction are considered to by-pass the outer and middle ears and stimulate the cochlea directly. Therefore, if the bone conduction thresholds reveal more sensitive hearing (by 10dB or more) than the air conduction responses for the same frequencies, the hearing problem is considered to have a conductive component. On the other hand, identical threshold losses for air and bone conduction suggest the problem lies in the inner ear or along the auditory pathway to the brain and the loss is considered to be sensori-neural. Figures 9-2 and 9-3 are examples of pure tone audiometric test results of conductive and sensori-neural losses, respectively.

Sweeptest Audiometry

Pure tone audiometry can be used as a screening test for identifying persons with a hearing loss. For example, the intensity dial on the audiometer can be set at a constant level, which is

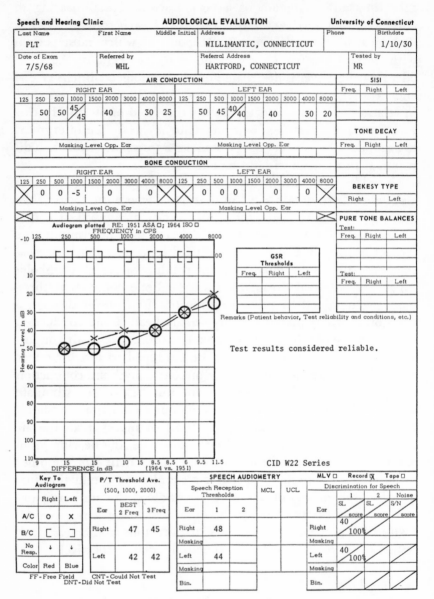

Figure 9-2. Typical audiologic record demonstrating a conductive hearing disorder.

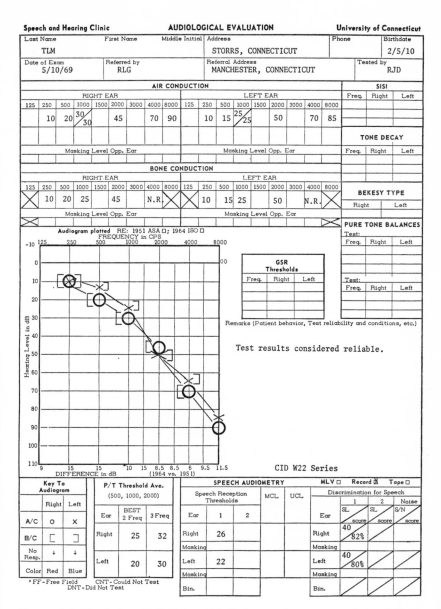

Figure 9-3. Typical audiologic record demonstrating a sensorineural hearing disorder.

considered to be at the lower end of the range of normal hearing. A check is made of the listener's hearing by *sweeping* across the test frequencies at this level. The listener indicates whether he has heard the tone at each frequency by raising his hand. If the listener does not hear a significant number of the test frequencies at this screening level, he is referred for a complete pure tone threshold test. This is the basic procedure used in many public school, community and industrial hearing conservation programs. A complete discussion of hearing screening programs can be found in Darley (1961).

SPEECH AUDIOMETRY

The handicapping effect of a given hearing impairment is viewed as closely related to the ability to *receive* and *understand* speech. A major portion of human communication and interchange of information is conducted verbally. Consequently, the degree to which a hearing impairment has interfered with a person's ability to follow everyday conversational speech can be used as an indication of his hearing handicap. While an average of the pure tone *speech frequency* thresholds offers some insight into speech reception efficiency, it is only a prediction. A more direct measure of this skill uses speech rather than pure tones as the auditory message. *Speech Audiometry* was developed to obtain this measure. The two basic measures obtained in speech audiometry are (a) a speech reception threshold (SRT) and (b) a speech discrimination score (SDS).

Speech Reception Threshold

The SRT represents an estimate of the extent of the hearing loss for speech. The threshold is defined as the point at which a listener can understand 50 per cent of the speech message presented to him. It is assumed that at this point he can just follow the gist of connected speech (Silverman, 1950). The most common clinical test items are standardized lists of disyllabic words (spondees) which can be spoken with equal stress.

Specific lists designed to measure the threshold of speech for children have been developed. They employ items such as the standard spondiac words, simple commands, and monosyllabic words. These procedures consist mostly of presenting picture representations of the test items. These modifications correct for problems encountered with children whose speech and langauge limitations prohibit the use of adult lists and standard "repeat the word" mode of response.

The SRT is usually obtained by presenting a series of words, either monitored live voice or recorded, through an electrical system which controls intensity. The intensity at which the words are presented is progressively reduced until threshold is reached. Tests for the threshold of hearing for speech are regarded as quite reliable and the various formal techniques developed to obtain the SRT are roughly equivalent.

The major contribution of the SRT is two-fold. One, it is a more valid measure of hearing loss for speech in that it uses speech rather than pure tone signals. Secondly, because of its close relationship with pure tone thresholds, the SRT serves as a corroborator of the pure tone audiogram. For example, if the pure tone thresholds for the speech frequencies are relatively similar in extent, the SRT and the average of these frequencies will closely approximate each other.

Speech Detection Threshold

When standard or slightly modified speech reception threshold procedures are not applicable because of extremely poor speech and language skills, it may be necessary to obtain a speech detection threshold. A speech detection threshold does not assume that the child is able to understand the speech presented at threshold or near threshold levels. It simply assumes that he was aware that something was being said. It is, therefore, possible to approximate the SRT from some pure tone thresholds and the speech detection threshold and make inferences about the extent of the hearing loss.

Speech Discrimination Score

Normal conversational speech does not typically occur at threshold levels, but rather it occurs at suprathreshold levels. Further-

more, difficulty with understanding speech at these normal conversational levels will certainly influence general communication
efficiency. The speech discrimination score (SDS), therefore, was
developed to measure the ability to reproduce a speech message
which is presented sufficiently loud to be heard comfortably.

Current clinical procedures which evaluate the ability to
understand speech at suprathreshold levels include the use of
monosyllabic word lists. The word lists are considered to be representative of conversational speech in that they consist of highly
familiar words and contain a phonetic composition similar to that
found in the English language.

The general clinical speech discrimination procedure consists
of presenting the words at a given suprathreshold intensity. The
score is the percentage of words repeated correctly from a prede-
termined sample. In addition to giving some indication of how
well a person understands speech when it is presented to him
under amplification, it often differentiates between types of hearing disorders. A high discrimination score is usually associated
with normal hearing or a predominantly conductive disorder. A
low score is indicative of a sensori-neural or central involvement.

Where formal testing is not possible, it is often valuable to observe the listener's responses to comfortably loud speech as predicted from the speech detection threshold and presented through
a loudspeaker in a sound field. With children who do not respond
verbally in the test setting, speech audiometry provides an opportunity to observe the child in a controlled environment. The
child may be observed while playing in a sound-treated room into
which auditory signals of known intensities are introduced. Such
responses, while certainly not threshold responses, suggest the degree of the loss and help in deciding if speech and language difficulty may be attributed to a hearing problem. A detailed discussion of speech audiometry from the standpoint of necessary
equipment, test administration and interpretation of test results
may be found in Newby (1964).

SPECIAL AUDIOLOGICAL TESTS

Pure tone and speech audiometry will serve as adequate tools
for measuring the auditory process of most persons with a hearing

impairment encountered by speech pathologists in the clinical setting. Given a cooperative listener and responder, these measures can usually establish the extent of the hearing loss, put the site of lesion in a general category of a conductive or sensori-neural hearing disorder and suggest prognostic hunches concerning the kinds of communication problems the listener may encounter. This information, along with a medical opinion concerning the medical reversibility of the impairment, is usually sufficient to determine appropriate referrals or to initiate a treatment program.

The *clinical audiologist*, however, is frequently called upon to participate (usually with otology) in making finer discriminations concerning the site of lesion causing the hearing difficulty. A battery of auditory tests have been developed which pinpoint with varying degrees of accuracy where along the auditory pathway the hearing process has been disrupted. For example, is the damage in the cochlea (Meniere's Disease), along the VIIIth auditory nerve (tumor), or involve brain stem or cerebral lesions? In addition, auditory problems with a nonorganic component are routinely encountered and diagnosed with the aid of special tests designed to obtain the organic level of hearing of listeners who have a tendency to simulate or exaggerate a hearing loss. Newby (1964) also contains a comprehensive discussion of these special audiological tests.

HEARING IMPAIRMENT AND HANDICAP

Previous sections of this chapter have been concerned with the disorders of hearing and the measurement of hearing loss. However, in the final analysis it is the effect that a hearing impairment has on functional behavior that is of major importance. How has the hearing deficiency affected communication behavior? Has the normal process of speech and language acquisition been impeded? Has there been interference with the learning of educational skills? Is the hearing impairment socially and/or vocationally handicapping? The answers to these questions depend upon a number of factors. The purpose of the next two sections is to discuss (a) the handicapping effect of hearing impairment and (b) rehabilitation considerations.

Hearing handicap is defined as . . . *any disadvantage in the activities of everyday living which derives from hearing impairment.* (High *et al.*, 1964) . One of the primary factors contributing to the handicap is the extent of hearing loss. It is fairly obvious that the greater the extent of the hearing loss, less of the auditory signal is received and the greater the handicapping effect. This is so because the normal acquisition of basic communication and academic skills is predominantly learned through the auditory modality. Although the intensity of speech varies from situation to situation, it is generally accepted that conversational speech is heard at approximately 40 dB-50 dB H.L. (62 dB-72 dB SPL). If a person had an audiometrically measured hearing level of 50 dB (International Standard Organization) he would be receiving normal conversational speech quite faintly, missing faint speech altogether and only receiving loud speech at a comfortable loudness level. This level represents listening in a quiet setting; typical environmental noisy settings would create an even more difficult listening task for the hearing impaired person. This listening condition would cause the listener considerable difficulty in many talking, learning and working situations.

Extent of loss is often used as a partial guide to establish some of the educational needs of children with a hearing impairment. While these decisions are never based on extent of loss alone, the following classifications established by Davis and Silverman (1970) are quite descriptive. They are based on hearing levels for speech.

Class 1: Better than 40 dB. These children should be given the benefit of favorable seating in regular classrooms and may be assisted by special instruction in speechreading.

Class 2: 41 to 55 dB. These children should wear hearing aids and be given training in their use. They should be taught speechreading and also be given the benefit of speech correction and conservation of speech. They should also have the advantage of favorable seating in classrooms.

Class 3: 56 to 70 dB. Hearing aids and auditory training, special training in speech, and special language work are all essential. With such assistance and with favorable seating, some children can continue in regular classes. Others may derive more benefit from special classes.

Class 4: 71 to 90 dB. These children should be taught by means of educational procedures for the deaf child which were described in the preceding chapter, with special emphasis on speech, on auditory training, and on language. After a period of such instruction it is possible that these children may enter classes in regular schools.

Class 5: Worse than 91 dB. These are deaf children who require the special educational procedures described in the preceding chapter. Some of these children, however, eventually enter high schools for the hearing.

The types of educational settings designed for hearing handicapped persons will be discussed later.

A second factor influencing the nature of the hearing handicap is when the loss occurred. If the loss occurred prior to the age when speech is usually learned, the eventual speech and language status even with good remedial work will be quite different than if the loss was acquired in later years. It is much easier to maintain existing language and speech and to teach new verbal communication skills when there is a language foundation which was learned through the normal hearing process. Consequently, the later the *onset* of the hearing impairment the less the resulting handicap.

Hearing impairment invariably causes some degree of psychological disruption and adjustment. So much of human interaction and learning depends on good hearing, that the disadvantage at which a hearing handicapped person is placed is bound to affect him adversely. The psychological problems seem to manifest themselves in varying degrees of inadequacy due to (a) missing so much of what is being said, (b) feelings of being talked about, and (c) actually reduced communication skills.

It also seems that persons who have heard prior to acquiring a hearing impairment have more adjustment problems than those whose hearing impairment is congenital. The loss of something once had has greater consequences than not having had it at all.

The intellectual status of the person with the hearing impairment must be included in all considerations concerning the relationship between hearing impairment and handicap. Certainly, the person with good learning potential will be able to supplement and compensate for his hearing impairment much more readily than the person with lesser intellectual ability.

Looking at the total picture, it can be said that a hearing impairment has many far-reaching implications for a person's life style. It seems to be an interaction between intellectual ability, motivation to improve, onset of loss, extent of loss, type of impairment and, of course, the effectiveness of the remedial program available.

AURAL REHABILITATION

The process of helping a person function optimally with a hearing impairment takes several forms and involves a variety of professional persons. Because so many hearing problems are medically reversible, the otologist plays an extremely important role in the treatment program. All persons demonstrating a hearing loss audiometrically or suspected of having a problem because of reported symptoms should be referred for a complete otological examination. The role of audiology in this instance is to (a) serve as an otological referral source based on audiometric findings, and (b) assist in assessing the progress of medical treatment programs through audiometric revaluations. Periodic audiometric checks are vital in that very often a hearing loss is still present, but not noticeable to the listener. However, if such a hearing loss goes untreated, it can increase in severity and possibly cause some permanent damage. The wise otologist combines otologic and audiologic data when assisting the patient's response to a medical treatment program. If the otological examination reveals that the hearing loss cannot be reversed medically, the hearing handicapped person must be helped to function optimally with the hearing he has through a nonmedical audiological rehabilitation program.

Auditory Training

As indicated earlier, very few persons have a total loss of hearing; some residual hearing always exists. Probably the most important aspect of an audiological rehabilitation program is helping the hearing handicapped person make optimal use of his residual hearing. This clinical process is typically referred to as *auditory training.* The specific clinical activities vary depending on several diagnostic factors, but primarily on the amount of residual hearing present, the age of the listener and, perhaps, on the onset of the hearing loss. For example, if the hearing loss is severe (minimal residual hearing), auditory training activities could begin with learning to auditorially discriminate between grossly different acoustic signals such as a horn, drum, bell or speech. On the other hand, a person with a mild loss of recent onset may only require work in refining his ability to discriminate between speech messages of quite similar acoustic patterns, i.e. thin-fin, tin-pin, or sat-fat. The motivating devices used will, of course, depend on the age of the listener. It is obvious, therefore, that the specific goals and activities of an auditory training program depend on a thorough audiological evaluation and often do not completely emerge until after therapy has begun.

Auditory training activities are naturally conducted under ample amplification to provide the listener with the auditory message at a relatively comfortable loudness level. This is usually accomplished through *group auditory training units* which produce fidelity amplification through earphones worn by the listeners. The intensity level for each individual earphone headset can be set separately so that it can be adjusted to each listener's specific amplification needs. The levels are typically set by the listener himself. The listener is usually asked to attend to speech messages on a look-listen basis, but he is also challenged to listen to auditory signals alone.

Hearing Aids

One important aspect of an auditory training program is the use of a *hearing aid.* A hearing aid is actually a small individualized version of a group auditory training unit. The earphones have been replaced by an *ear mold* and *receiver* (one for each ear in a binaural fitting) which fits into the outer ear. Because of the amplifier size reduction and the elimination of earphones, some fidelity and amplification capacity is lost. However, if properly fitted, much can be gained by wearing a hearing aid.

A hearing aid is basically an amplifier and its sole function is to make speech and other desirable auditory signals louder. The degree to which it helps an individual is directly related to the degree to which the hearing problem is one of sensitivity loss. If the hearing problem is due to a conductive middle ear impairment, an appropriately selected hearing aid will be of great benefit. Since the coding properties of the cochlea will be intact and the hearing aid has overridden the volume loss due to middle ear damage, the message is received, coded and sent to the brain. The auditory training program consists primarily of hearing aid selection and orientation. It can be said, therefore, that persons with a conductive hearing disorder can benefit considerably from an appropriate hearing aid. It should be restated, however, that persons with a conductive disorder can usually be helped medically. Since this can only be determined by a medical person, that avenue should be pursued prior to any hearing aid considerations. As a matter of fact, no hearing aid should be fitted regardless of site of lesion until it has been determined that there is no medical reason why a hearing aid could not be worn.

The situation is somewhat different with persons having a sensori-neural impairment. With this type of disorder there may or may not be a significant sensitivity loss for crucial speech reception frequencies, but there usually is a coding problem manifesting itself in poor speech discrimination ability. It should be remembered that a hearing aid only amplifies. Consequently, while speech will be made louder and, thus, easier to detect, it does not necessarily make speech any clearer. The new hearing aid wearer with a sensori-neural hearing impairment discovers this and becomes initially discouraged. It is the role of the auditory training program to prepare the new hearing aid wearer for this initial experience and through systematic listening activities help him make the most use of the amplification provided him by his hearing aid.

It should be emphasized that not all prospective hearing aid wearers experience the same difficulty in adjusting to a new hearing aid. It depends on a host of audiologic findings such as extent of loss, audiometric curve, speech discrimination scores, as well as nonaudiometric factors such as motivation, need and basic adaptability. It is quite wise, therefore, to seek the assistance of an audiologist in considering the purchase of a hearing aid. The audiologist does not sell hearing aids; that is the function of a hearing aid dealer. He does help, however, in making the selection of an appropriate hearing aid for the particular hearing loss demonstrated and conducts proper follow-up hearing aid orientation programs.

Speechreading

A second area of aural rehabilitation deals with helping the hearing handicapped person make better use of visual clues available to him. This process is commonly referred to as *lipreading* or *speechreading*. The term *speechreading* is preferred in this chapter because it suggests the goal (understanding speech) rather than the process (watching lip movements). Furthermore, speechreading is a broader term, which includes lipreading as well as observing all other visual clues used in the verbal communication process. These clues include such things as gestures, facial expressions, situational cues, and knowledge of the talker's speaking habits. The listener is helped to become aware of how he can augment his hearing with these visual clues. Speechreading activities *per se* include a considerable amount of observation of speakers. The speech material used by the clinician is graded with regard to varying degrees of difficulty. Some time is also spent demonstrating sound production, words that look alike on the lips *(homophenes)* and the use of contextual clues.

Speechreading is a learned skill (O'Neil and Oyer, 1966) and performance can be improved with proper training. The nature and amount of speechreading lessons required are quite individualized and depend on many of the same parameters governing the planning of an auditory training program. Furthermore, speechreading and auditory training activities are often combined and self-reinforcing.

Speech and Language

Speech and language problems often accompany hearing impairment. This is certainly true for persons with a severe hearing

No opotunitys to hear speech in order to learn speech [handwritten annotation]

loss of a congenital origin. For them learning language concepts and functional verbal skills requires special help for most of their developmental years. This assistance comes in the form of special speech, language and educational programs designed to take into account the hearing impairment.

Educational Settings

Preschool programs for hearing impaired children are now available in most communities on a local or at least a regional basis. Based on the assumption that early preparatory training is vital to developing effective communication and academic skills, children are enrolled as early as three years of age. The basic goal is to provide the child with substantial and systematic speech and language stimulation, as well as to provide readiness activities for the acquisition of academic skills. The number of children in each class is usually between six and eight and they are divided into work groups according to their speech, language, and social maturational level. Parent education is also a vital and integral part of these programs. The preschool program for hearing impaired children provides the best opportunity to obtain a solid foundation for developing functional communication and academic skills.

For persons with milder hearing losses, speech production problems may consist of a few distortions or omissions of the sibilant sounds. Work with these persons is usually carried out by the speech clinician in either the public school setting or at a speech and hearing center in the community.

In addition to the preschool nursery programs special educational facilities are necessary at the elementary and secondary school levels to help the child with a severe hearing loss to compensate for his hearing impairment. In many public school systems special classes have been established. These classes are actually extensions of the preschool programs described earlier in which academic work is presented with the necessary modifications appropriate for the hearing loss.

Modifications are not only in the teaching methods used, but also in providing some form of classroom amplification system in addition to individual hearing aids. If enough of these classes exist at multieducational levels, the system can actually be said to have a *day school for the deaf*. Day schools are usually located in metropolitan areas and allow the children to live at home. They may or may not be a part of a public school program for normally hearing children. Their counterparts are *residential schools for the deaf* which maintain dormitory systems and are actually more numerous than the nonresidential programs. They often provide for the complete range of preschool, elementary and secondary educational needs of the hearing-impaired child.

For children who develop to the point where they can be partially integrated into the hearing classroom (including children with mild losses), *public school resource classes* have been established. These are designed to provide the special tutoring the child requires. They assist in making a smooth transition from the special classrooms to complete integration into the classrooms for normally hearing children.

Counseling

A complete aural rehabilitation program includes provisions for responding to the psychological correlates of hearing impairment. Counseling is, therefore, an integral part of such programs. An attempt is made to deal with feelings and frustrations usually accompanying hearing loss. The nature of this counseling takes various forms, from being an integral part of the daily communication skills activities to specific activities designed to stimulate discussion of psychological problems, i.e. role playing. In some cases the psychological problems are sufficiently troublesome to warrant referral to a psychological clinic.

Counseling with parents of hearing impaired children is also extremely important. The audiologist is frequently one of the first professional people to see the deaf child and his parents. Most often, the parents have just recently learned that there is no medical means of restoring their child's hearing, but have not fully realized the implications. The audiologist is, therefore, not only in the position of pin-pointing the level and nature of the child's hearing impairment, but he must also help parents get through their early (and sometimes delayed) reactions to the news that their child has a severe hearing loss. He must be prepared to answer the parents' questions concerning why medical treatment is not indicated, what bearing this has on speech and language development (will he ever talk), what are the educational implications of such a hearing impairment, and most importantly, the audiologist is the one who very often guides the parents through their initial feelings of disappointment, self-pity and guilt. Actually, the degree to which he is a skilled and effective counselor will determine the response of the parents to the rehabilitative program being planned. A considerable amount of counseling is done during the initial contact with the parents. Parent groups are also formed to provide parents with long-term support through each new rehabilitative stage, such as selecting a hearing aid, accepting realistic speech, language, academic and vocational goals. The reader is referred to Ross (in press) for a more comprehensive discussion of the aural rehabilitation procedures employed with the hearing handicapped.

THE SPEECH PATHOLOGIST AND THE HEARING HANDICAPPED PERSON

One of the primary functions the speech pathologist serves with the hearing handicapped person is to identify possible hearing difficulty and make the appropriate referral for final confirmation. Because of the close relationship between hearing and the development of speech and language, many persons seeking help for communication problems may also have a hearing deficiency. Conseqeuntly, a thorough speech pathology diagnostic work-up includes some formal evaluation of hearing acuity. This is usually accomplished through the use of pure tone audiometry and requires that the speech pathologist be competent in obtaining accurate air and bone conduction thresholds. It is also necessary for the speech pathologist to have a complete appreciation of when and how to mask the opposite ear to obtain valid thresholds and of what kind of results can be expected if masking is not used. In other words, the speech pathologist must be well versed in the administration of pure tone audiometry and in the interpretation of the test results. When a hearing loss is uncovered an otological and audiological referral should be made for further testing and confirmation of the loss.

In the public schools the speech pathologist is called upon to perform several tasks in connection with the hearing handicapped child. For example, he is often asked to interpret otological and audiological test results and recommendations to the child's teacher and other school personnel. It is usually the speech pathologist's function to help the teacher understand the implications of having a hearing impairment and what kinds of activities the teacher can do in the classroom to help hearing handicapped children. If a resource classroom for the hearing handicapped child is not available, the speech pathologist may be asked to help the child learn to use his hearing aid and troubleshoot when problems arise with the aid. In addition to helping the child with any speech problems he may have, the speech pathologist may also need to provide speechreading and auditory training activities as part of his total speech therapy program. While the schoolwide hearing screening program is typically administered by the school nurse, the speech pathologist's services are often enlisted to assist in testing the children who fail the screening test. Furthermore, the nurse and speech pathologist often work closely together in determining the procedures to be followed with the children who demonstrate a hearing loss audiometrically. In some cases, the speech pathologist may organize the total hearing screening program.

In summary, the speech pathologist plays an important role in the diagnosis and rehabilitation of hearing handicapped persons. This role is primarily one of identification, referral and follow-up activities once the hearing impairment has been confirmed. As a result, the speech pathologist must (a) be acquainted with normal auditory process and what medical problems can cause faulty hearing, (b) be competent in the administration and interpretation of a basic hearing test for identification and referral purposes and (c) have an understanding of the nature of an audiological evaluation and the therapeutic implications of the various test results.

REFERENCES

Carhart, R., and Jerger, J.: Preferred method for clinical determination of pure tone thresholds. *J Speech Hearing Dis, 24*:330-343, 1959.

Darley, F.D. (Ed.) : Identification audiometry. *J Speech Hearing Dis,* Monograph Supplement No. 9, 1961.

Davis, H., and Silverman, S.R.: *Hearing and Deafness.* New York, Holt, Rinehart and Winston, 1970.

DeWeese, D.D., and Saunders, W.H.: *Textbook of Otolaryngology.* St. Louis, Mosby, 1964.

High, W.; Fairbank, G., and Glorig, A.: Scale of self-assessment of hearing handicap. *J Speech Hearing Dis, 29*:215-330, 1964.

Newby, H.: *Audiology,* (2nd ed.) New York, Appleton-Century-Crofts, 1964.

O'Neil, J., and Oyer, H.: *Applied Audiometry.* New York, Dodd, Mead & Company, 1966.

Ross, M.: Aural rehabilitation. In Halpern, H. (Ed.) : *Communication Disorders.* New York, Random House (in press) .

Silverman, S.R.: The use of speech tests for the evaluation of clinical procedures. *Ann Otol, 54*:688-98, 1950.

CHAPTER TEN

AUDITORY PERCEPTUAL DISTURBANCES

DONALD L. RAMPP

AMONG THE DEVELOPMENTS in speech pathology have evolved more sophisticated methods and materials for assessing behaviors exhibited by children. As speech pathologists we have become sophisticated enough to recognize a constellation of behaviors that allows us to classify a child as auditory perceptually disturbed. It is not a particularly new term; it is one of the subclassifications of "minimal brain dysfunction." This term is defined by Clements (1966) and refers to children of near-average, average, or above-average general intelligence with certain learning or behavioral disabilities ranging from mild to severe. These disabilities are associated with deviations of function of the central nervous system. A number of different terms have been used to refer to children with minimal brain dysfunction including language disturbances, brain-injured, learning disabilities, psychoneurological learning disorders, etc. Children exhibiting auditory perceptual disturbances certainly could be classifiable as having minimal brain dysfunction.

Traditionally, and not just historically, auditory perception has been equated and synonomous with auditory discrimination in both speech pathology and audiology. Certainly auditory discrimination is one area of auditory perception, of that there is little doubt, but it encompasses much more than the unitary ability to distinguish similar spoken consonants.

There are no incidence figures available which reflect the extent of the problem nor its ramifications on the child, his parents, his teachers, his superintendent, his community, or his congressman. We do know it costs, just in economic terms, $696 per school year for each child to be educated in the United States. If 5 per cent of children fail a grade, then the cost approximates $1.7 billion per year (HEW Reading Report, 1969). These children may be of any age level, race, or socioeconomic class. It is not a new disorder; it has been in existence since the beginning of time. The disturbance manifests itself at an early age and is often noticed by observant parents, however, little is usually done until the child begins to have difficulty in reading in the first grade.

The age range seen most frequently in speech and hearing centers and in public school therapy is six to twelve years. Reasons for these ages being predominant are that these are the ages when most rehabilitative efforts are instituted (and often abandoned) and when parents are most concerned about the problem. After the sixth grade, most parents have tossed in the towel and have "adjusted" to the fact that their child is not going to be academically oriented. Clinically, more boys than girls exhibit auditory perceptual disturbances. At Memphis State University's Speech and Hearing Center, this ratio varies from five- to six-to-one, males to females.

AUDITORY PERCEPTION

An Operational Definition

Nissen (1951) pointed out that low organisms begin life as more or less finished products, then or soon thereafter possessing all the behavioral tools that they will ever have. By contrast, however, higher animals and especially humans go through a long period of change. Bones grow, muscles get stronger, bodily proportions change, and motor skills develop. This freedom from physical inferiority has tended to obscure the more important cumulative development of primitive acquisitions that serve as instruments of behavioral adjustments in all later life. One of the most striking examples of this is a child's development of perception.

Somewhere between sensation and conceptualization lies the process of perception. It involves the selection of sensory experiences, that is, the establishment of a relationship or meaning to them. This relationship is an element of identification. Perception is knowing what the sound is and having the ability to relate it to past experiences. Funk and Wagnell's Dictionary (1963) defines perception as *the faculty, process, or product of cognition. In gen-*

eral, furthering the more immediate and seemingly intuitive ways of the senses . . . knowledge, prehension. Myklebust (1954) defines auditory perception as the ability to ". . .structure the auditory world and select those sounds which are immediately pertinent to adjustment (page 158)." Operationally, a more practical definition would be—a capacity for comprehension. This definition implies the ability to receive information, to categorize it, to conceptualize it, and to synthesize it.

Perception is the association of meaning with sensation. The auditory perceptually disturbed child may have trouble selecting one object out of a group, but may be able to select the object individually. Perception is a matter of ordering or orienting rather than knowing, a mental process which gives meaning to stimuli. Little is known regarding auditory perception. Volumes of research are available in the area of visual perception for a variety of reasons that need not be elucidated here. One finds, however, no texts devoted to auditory perception, and the research that has been reported is usually in the area of audiology, again equating auditory perception with the per cent correct of monosyllabic, phonetically-balanced words heard at a specific level above a speech reception threshold. Verbal communication occurs in an on-going continuous sequence of consonants and vowels approaching more of an oral paragraph rather than single words. There is a considerable difference in perceiving one word than perceiving a spoken sentence or sentences.

Methods of perception are inherent and some information is available regarding its characteristics. A perception constitutes a whole; it is intrinsically bound up in memory of past experiences to constitute a whole. This is the basis of Gestalt psychology. One can hear only a portion of a song, and one is able to project and remember all of the song. Second, perception is always a figure against a background; attention and memory are also involved. One receives stimuli as an entity of a background of stimuli. When one receives a stimulus, one associates memory of past experiences to the exclusion of other experiences. Third, perception is developmental, that is, young children initially have poor auditory and visual perception. Perceptual development proceeds in an orderly fashion from simple or primitive to complex. Finally, individual differences exist in perceptual functioning. We all hear the same sound, but our perception of that sound is different. There are auditory, visual, tactile, taste and olfactory differences in perception.

Auditory perception is fundamental and basic in human behavior and language development. Perceptual processes entail on-going sensations, so that when one remembers sensation one is no longer functioning in perception but at a level of imagery (Myklebust, 1954). One functions in perception while and when sensation is present. When a person is perceiving, he must be attending to that sound. Although we are not aware of attending during sleep, it is possible for perception to begin while asleep in regard to warning signals that are usually auditory or tactile in nature. It is always in terms of a given kind of input of one or more than one modality. One must be attending because attention selects. Perhaps there is no perception without selection. Selection can be multisensory.

Attention

Attention is a central concept in perception, and it is also a key factor in communication. No matter how significant the speaker's message, and no matter how strongly he feels about it, it will be lost unless his listeners attend to it. The psychology of listening is predicated on the concepts of attention and perception. When we listen, we attend; we organize a maximum concentration of our sensory receptors upon the spoken words. Only after we attend can we perceive; we are aware of the stimulus symbols and of the objects, conditions, or relationship that they represent. When we both attend and perceive, we respond.

Attention is a preparatory process, leading into perception, and culminating with response, sequentially but almost simultaneously (Attention → Perception → Response). A child cannot give continuous attention; even when he tries very hard to attend, he does not hear everything. Attention comes in spurts. Teachers and parents should appreciate the influence of a child's selectivity upon what he will attend to, the utility of categorization and of suggestion in stimulating both learning and remembering, and specific techniques of impressiveness in assuring retention. It is apparent that not all persons attend and perceive in the same way, to the same degree, or for the same reasons. In addition to such variations, partially explainable by differences in personality, it should be recognized that children may be deliberately selective in exposing themselves to learning opportunities.

Selection

Selection is probably directly related to figure-ground, and is probably not possible without figure-ground. This essentially means the psychological circumstance is structured so that one has the priority of attention-selection-structure. Attention is necessary for selection; selection is a prerequisite for structure. This means that the person has established the operational psychological factors to determine which is figure and which is ground in a given situation. Much of this is innate but obviously some is learned. Stimulation is probably organized in terms of past experience. For example, the differences in perception of the same picture by an African as opposed to an American is based on social perception and experience. Perception accompanies all sensory modalities. It is possible that most perception is synesthesia. Synesthesia may be defined as the ability to draw and integrate from other sensations.

As speech pathologists we must recognize that the stimulus must not only be strong enough to energize sense organs but compelling enough to compete successfully with the other stimuli in the environment. Perceptual learning results from our discriminative understanding of concepts. Concepts are generalizations that remain constant as guides to the meanings of objects, persons, qualities, or relationships. Working from the base of acquired concepts, we perceive a wide range of stimuli. Perception becomes discriminative learning because of differential reinforcement. The reinforcement consists of an incentive for responding in a particular way to a specific stimulus. To be effective the incentive must be related to the satisfaction of need or drive, and differential because it rewards the response to one stimulus, but not another. Thus, perceptual learning involves perception of new concepts, or modification of old ones, about objects, persons, qualities, or relationships resulting from the presentation of reinforced stimuli.

AUDITORY PERCEPTION OF SPEECH

Auditory perception of speech is primarily concerned with how the temporal sequences of the auditory stimulus are processed in the central nervous system. Since speech occurs in on-going acoustic wave patterns, effective perception is dependent upon a normal-functioning auditory processing apparatus. There is a paucity of research information available on the central processing of auditory stimuli.

Although hearing acuity losses may interfere with perceptual processes (Myklebust, 1957), auditory perception presupposes normal auditory acuity. Occasionally threshold variances, produced by internal or external stimuli, may alter perception, but the primary concern is not with hearing acuity as it is traditionally assessed by pure tone and speech reception audiometry, but with hearing for speech.

From the first synapse in the ventral and dorsal nuclei at the level of the medulla to the last synapse in the anterior transverse temporal gyrus, the auditory pathways are complex and certainly not within the scope of this chapter. The reader may find many texts that cover the subject thoroughly in a scholarly fashion (Newby, 1964; Zemlin, 1968). However, certain aspects of the central processing system are of importance in the consideration of auditory perception. The research of Penfield and Rasmussen (1950) indicates that the primary receiving strip for auditory stimuli is located in the Sylvian margin of the temporal lobe, and Luria (1966) reports that the secondary division of the first temporal convolution is responsible for the analysis and integration of sound signals. These authors suggest that the secondary regions may be largely responsible for the systematic deciphering of sound signals necessary for the perception of speech. Luria states:

> . . . the disturbance of discriminative hearing, which can now be interpreted as a disturbance in the analytic-synthetic activity of the auditory cortex . . . may be regarded as the fundamental sypmtom of a lesion of the superior temporal region of the left hemisphere,

and the resulting acoustic agnosia may be regarded as the fundamental source of speech disturbance (pp. 106-107).

The reticular formation and activating system may hold the key to many of the characteristics seen in children with auditory perceptual disturbances. The reticular formation is by definition a net-like series of short interwoven fibers and nerve cells. It extends from just above the decussation of the pyramids in the medulla rostralward through the center of the pons and midbrain, and up into the thalamus to form the reticular nuclei of the thalamus (Woodburne, 1967). It includes a highly complicated network of neurons which may be divided functionally into ascending and descending parts.

Attention was directed toward the reticular formation as a result of experiments showing that transection of the brain stem above the level of the colliculi resulted in a condition resembling sleep or coma. Further studies indicated that the influx of impulses centrally through the stem reticular formation was strongly implicated in the arousal mechanism. As a result of this series of studies, the entire mechanism was referred to as the reticular activating system (Magoun and Moruzzi, 1949). Recorded evoked potentials come from practically all the major sensory pathways to the reticular formation.

The descending influence of the reticular formation is that of facilitating or inhibiting motor activity, chiefly at the level of spinal motor neurons. The facilitary action, and inhibitory as well, are carried out through internuncial neurons. The inhibitory action of the reticular formations arises from stimulation of lower, more caudal, reticular segments, largely in the medulla (Woodburne, 1967). Adler (1964), in discussing the reticular formation, notes:

This system, sometimes called a central transactional core, is neither sensory nor motor, but it affects the activity of most of the other parts of the brain. . . . As spokes radiate from a wheel, so does the varied influence of the reticular core radiate to different parts of the brain. Some of its more important functions are as follows:

(1) It facilitates and inhibits nerve impulses.
(2) It influences incoming messages.

(3) It helps regulate glandular output through its control over the hypothalamus.
(4) It is intimately involved in perception.
(5) It affects motion.
(6) It influences wakefulness and consciousness.
(7) It allows for integration of data (pp. 18-19).

If the inhibitory mechanism of the reticular formation is impaired for some reason, this may account for the distractibility, disinhibition, and hyperactivity in children with auditory perceptual disturbances. If sensory impulses are flooding the cortex, difficulty in selection and attention could be manifest. Because of its unique function and with more and more research establishing a connection with the reticular activating system and inter-and intra-sensory brain function, the role of this system could be directly related to the etiology of auditory perceptual disturbances. Berry (1969) reports:

> . . . the reticular system may be even more important in organizing and focusing the perceptive field of audition since interconnections rich in multisensory convergences are found in this system. Many circuits embracing nuclear masses in the brainstem and cortex send information to the reticular system. . . The reticular system is important; and cogent to our concern in language learning are its activities associated with arousal in drive-setting mechanisms, facilitation, and inhibition, differentiated phasic movements, voluntary motor activity, and perception (pp. 66-74).

A neurological correlate of attention is the alerting mechanism of the reticular activating system. According to Hebb (1949), this mechanism provides the immediate facilitation from one phase sequence to ensuing ones and this is the way the system "bids the individual 'to attend.' " Berry (1969) posits that reticular facilitation and inhibition can be described by observing their breakdown in children with nervous system involvement. The major sensory pathways are inundated with disorganized impulses and excitability cycles which bear no spatial or temporal relation to each other. She continues to report that disintegrating emotional states also pervade the CNS with inhibition. Further, in many children the alerting mechanism operates too well, but the reticular system is not selective; it cannot inhibit sensory-motor patterns which are not appropriate, resulting in overreaction by the child.

CHARACTERISTICS OF AUDITORY PERCEPTUAL DISTURBANCES

At the outset, it should be made clear that the characteristics to follow do not always occur in all children with auditory perceptual disturbances. The point previously made should again be reiterated, that is, a constellation of characteristics is the important factor. Many so-called "normal" children may exhibit several symptoms of auditory perceptual disturbance. It should also be apparent that several of the characteristics are the same or similar to children exhibiting other forms of *minimal brain dysfunction.*

Since the environment is composed of constant and multiple auditory stimuli, it is a primary function of auditory perception to hold a conglomeration of auditory stimuli in the background of attention while selecting other specific stimuli for purposes of immediate attention and behavior. Many sounds are present, but only a few are pertinent. All sounds have equal importance to the auditory perceptually disturbed child. The child, while attempting to attend to all sounds, is incapable of listening to a given sound. He cannot direct his attention selectively to an expected sound. All sounds to the auditory perceptually disturbed child are foreground sounds simultaneously.

The auditory perceptually disturbed child can comprehend the meanings of words when his total auditory world has been appropriately simplified and structured. His thresholds of responsiveness vary greatly, not primarily because of shifts in acuity, but because of his inability to relate and integrate experientially. Therefore, he is highly variable to all auditory stimuli, his responsiveness is reflective of his inability to integrate. He does not relate his hearing meaningfully to the environment, for example, he might not respond to being called, or to other common sounds, although no hearing loss exists. He does not use his hearing to systematically scan and to keep in touch with the environment; such hearing is dependent upon integration, normal perception, and listening. An auditory perceptual disturbance precludes normal listening ability.

Disturbances in auditory perception, in a majority of children, create difficulty in auditory discrimination, not only in consonant discrimination but also in discrimination of environmental sounds. In addition to auditory discrimination difficulty sound blending abilities are frequently deficient. Characteristically, these children exhibit difficulty going from parts-to-wholes, that is, auditory synthesis. When presented a one-syllable word these children cannot synthesize phonemes into a meaningful unit. It may be hypothesized that if a child cannot synthesize a consonant-vowel-consonant combination, synthesizing a complete sentence or sentences is out of the question.

Related to auditory synthesis, because of the temporal aspects of speech, is the characteristic performance of these children in auditory memory. Regardless of the types of tests given, whether digit, sentence, or nonsense syllable, these children manifest deficiencies. These deficiencies may be observable as young as four years. They seem to be able to perform better with sentences than noncontextual information. It is not unusual to find these children functioning two or three years below chronological age level on tests of auditory memory.

Not surprisingly, these children exhibit difficulty learning everyday concepts that many of us take for granted. The ability to name the days of the week in serial order is a task that most five-year-olds with nursery or kindergarten experience can do with ease. Children with auditory perceptual disturbances at seven and eight years almost routinely exhibit deficiencies in serial memory, for example, the months of the year, the alphabet, and even difficulty with their home address, their telephone number, and their birthdate.

Behaviorally, these children manifest a variety of seemingly unrelated symptoms. Usually they are easily *distractible* and are *disinhibited*. Distractibility is the forced responsiveness to external stimuli, particularly visual and auditory stimuli. Because of the inability to select out of the auditory world the important stimulus, these children may respond to a jet passing overhead instead of listening to the teachers giving instructions. This distractibility is probably related to the deficiencies with background-foreground concepts previously mentioned; that is, all sounds being foreground sounds simultaneously to the auditory perceptually disturbed child.

If disinhibition is defined as the forced responsiveness to internal (mental) stimuli, certain symptoms manifested by these children become apparent. They frequently verbalize whatever comes to mind without appropriateness and whenever they think of it; for example, they are inclined to anticipate situations. If told by his mother on Wednesday that the family is going to the zoo on Saturday, sporadically throughout the rest of the week he will ask if today is the day to go to the zoo. This failure to inhibit internal thoughts is extremely common among the auditory perceptually disturbed.

Perhaps distractibility and disinhibition are what make these children more *hyperactive* or *hyperkinetic* than other children. Whatever the etiology, these children are described by their parents as being overly active. Parents report their child is fidgity and constantly on the move; even when watching television, a foot is kicking or a hand is moving. They appear as many "brain-damaged" children appear, that is, motor driven. One difference, however, perhaps as a compensatory mechanism, these children frequently seem preoccupied and it is hard to get their attention. Probably because of their distractibility and disinhibition, when they can structure their activities or interest, they become totally immersed "in their own little worlds." Parents observe that occasionally they have to call them several times, and in some instances have to walk over and touch them before they will respond.

Related to distractibility, disinhibition, and hyperactivity is the fact that these children appear easily *bored*. They rarely will persevere at one task for any sustained period unless it is of their choosing. This symptom may be associated with attentional factors previously mentioned.

Difficulty with impulse control is another characteristic. They seem to be more emotionally labile and have low frustration tolerances. Not unlike the aphasic child, they frequently respond catastrophically to seemingly minor upsets. This psychological disintegration usually is in response to a lack of environmental structure or an environmental inconsistency. These children tend to require more reassurance than other children. They have poor self-concepts and are extremely anxious to please, and if verbal perseveration is present as a symptom, this is when it usually occurs. Speech pathologists trained in aphasia therapy have been taught that verbal perseveration is a precursor to a catastrophic response, and the proof of the theory is frequently apparent with these children in stress situations when fearful of making mistakes.

The limitation or modification of the child's abstract abilities, or *concretism,* will result in him being more ego-oriented and tied more closely to himself. He will have difficulty in abstracting, projecting, classifying, and getting outside of himself. One example of this concretism may be seen in play situations; these children are frequently unable to "pretend." The play of auditory perceptually disturbed children is very limited, because of an inability to project their personalities into unrealistic situations.

There are a variety of symptoms exhibited by these children realted to motor coordination and dominance. Erratic body control and unequal development seem frequent in these children. There may be a lack of large and/or small muscle control such as that required for cutting or coloring. They often manifest *soft neurologic signs,* such as minor motor incoordination; difficulty with right-left discrimination; mixed dominance, such as right-footed, left-handedness, and right-eyedness; difficulty hopping on one foot or skipping; and, occasionally mirror movements of the opposite hand are apparent when the dominant hand is participating in an activity. These behaviors are observable on the playground or in the backyard by observant teachers and parents.

When parents of auditory perceptually disturbed children are asked what one word most exemplifies their child, that word is usually *inconsistency.* It is not inconceivable when even a few of the aforementioned characteristics are present in any one child. The world of the auditory perceptually disturbed is at best chaotic and confusing. It is difficult for them to see how things relate to each other, to compete in group situations, to understand exceptions to rules, and even more difficult, to understand why they cannot do what their peers do with ease. As this child gets older the problems become magnified and psychological ramifications come to bear. The constant frustration of failure can lead to a variety of emotional symptoms including destructiveness, withdrawal, aggressiveness, poor self-concept, etc.

READING

The most crippling effect of an auditory perceptual disturbance occurs when the child reaches the first grade. Reading is, of course, the most basic requirement of the language arts in elementary education. Everything a child does educationally is directly related to his ability to read; a possible exception to this might be arithmetic which will be dealt with later. Reading English is no simple task; ask any foreign student trying to learn English. Traditional orthography is rampant with exceptions to the rules. For example, in our conventional English alphabet there are more than two thousand variants in the way the twenty-six symbols are used to make the forty-odd sounds of English speech. There are twenty-two separate ways of writing the sound of /i/ in traditional English orthography including: *I, eye, height, pie,* and so on with the exceptions to the rules.

Reading authorities concur that the essential skill in reading consists of extracting the meaning from a printed or written word. According to an HEW Reading Report (1969), the attainment of this skill is directly related to the mastering of many component skills including:

1. The child must know the language he expects to read . . .
2. He must dissect spoken words into component sounds in their temporal order . . .
3. He must recognize and discriminate the letters of the alphabet in their various forms . . .
4. He must respond to the direction in which words are spelled and in order in continuous text . . .
5. He must respond to the patterns of highly probable correspondence between letters and sounds . . .
6. He must recognize printed words from whatever cues he can use—their total configuration, the letters composing them, the sound represented by those letters, and/or the means suggested by the context.
7. The child must learn the printed word signals spoken words and that they have meaning analogous to those of the spoken word . . .

8. The child must learn to reason and to think about what he reads, within the limits of his talent and experience (pp. 25-26).

The report further indicates: "The complexity of the reading process dictates that children who have difficulty learning to read will exhibit a great diversity of symptoms (p. 26)."

One can readily see how a child with an auditory perceptual disturbance would experience difficulty in reading, particularly if taught a phonic approach. To sound out a word from our inconsistent English alphabet is a dream devoutly to be wished for by these children. Reading is primarily a visual symbol system requiring many auditory integrities including the ability to discriminate differences and similarities in sounds, to perceive a sound within a word, to synthesize sounds into words, and to separate them into syllables. It can readily be seen that a child with an auditory perceptual disturbance will not profit from a phonic approach to teaching reading. Myklebust (1957) enumerates some characteristic problems, including the following: (a) numerous auditory discrimination and perceptual disorders which impede use of phonetic analysis; (b) difficulty with auditory analysis and synthesis; (c) an inability to reauditorize sounds or words; (d) disturbance in auditory sequentialization; and (e) behaviorally, these children tend to prefer visual activities.

The reading process is at best abstract, and children with auditory perceptual disturbances have considerable (and probably justifiable) distaste for it. Daily they sit in the reading circle (usually the low group) listening to their friends read orally with effortless ease until it becomes their turn. At this time, while looking at the same words and sentences, no sense can be made of the series of consonants and vowels. He is embarrassed; he does not look up for help from the teacher; his friends giggle quietly; some try to help him; and, to everyone's gratitude, he gives up and says he cannot do it. If reading is hard, spelling is atrocious. How can one spell a word when the consonants and vowels are written differently than they sound? Arithmetic in the early elementary grades is at least more concrete than reading. Children with auditory perceptual disturbances have much less difficulty with the handling of numeric configurations. Why? Because they do not change, they are consistent; a two is always a two, etc. As the child with an auditory perceptual disturbance progresses through the curricula sequences in elementary school, arithmetic changes. Thought problems are introduced along with abstract formulas for multiplication and division. Then, what was formerly enjoyable is pleasant no longer—reading and abstraction is required; grades begin to fall in new areas.

Because these children cannot compete in the classroom, they tend to migrate to areas where they can compete. Rest assured it will not be related to any overt academic activity. It usually is in a performance area requiring the use of the hands. If the motor incoordination problems are not too manifest, these children prefer sporting contests, puzzles, working with wood and tools, etc.

The acquisition of laterality or handedness is usually late in developing in these children. Whereas, in normal children, a preferred hand is evident by eighteen months and firmly established by three years, these children with auditory perceptual disturbances violate the developmental milestones of handedness. Many of them are left-handed, which makes one harken back to the days of Orton (1937) and Travis (1931) and their laterality concepts related to language function.

Children with auditory perceptual disturbances frequently exhibit an inability to comprehend spatial relationships. They do not understand how things go together or how they are related. Teachers frequently report that these children have trouble "finding things." Often they do not understand such concepts as: *inside-outside, top-bottom, yesterday-tomorrow, above-below*, etc. In addition they have a tendency to exhibit *concretism*, that is, difficulty with abstractions. The concept of learning to tell time is usually beyond them until well after their peers have learned.

Not infrequently, auditory perceptually disturbed children will exhibit mild articulatory deviations. Although no characteristic pattern of articulations errors is present, clinical experience suggests an omission pattern of final consonants. Speculating on the etiology of the articulation disorder, one could see the relationship of the auditory difficulties being associated with articulation inaccuracy or perhaps to minor motor incoordinations that are sometimes present as a symptom. These children with auditory perceptual disturbances are occasionally described as having maturational delay which may include an omission pattern of articulation errors.

SUMMARY OF SYMPTOMS

From the rather lengthy characteristics elaborated above, it is not surprising that although a child may have average intelligence with no other gross deviations, a child with an auditory perceptual disturbance is truly educationally handicapped. Teachers often do not understand these children, the apparent intellect, the inconsistency in response, the difficulty with reading, the occasional displays of emotionality all converge, and the teacher tends to view this child as a "spoiled," "stubborn" child. The parents are blamed. Conversely, the parents often indict the teacher for the difficulties in learning that occur. Through it all, the child with the auditory perceptual disturbance is caught in the middle with no place to go and no one to understand him. Is it any wonder when we summarize the variety of symptoms he may manifest?

1. Difficulty with auditory foreground-background stimuli; attention and selection
2. Thresolds of responsiveness vary; disturbances of attention, selection and memory
3. Difficulty with listening; cannot use his hearing in a meaningful fashion
4. Difficulty with auditory discrimination
5. Difficulty in auditory synthesis; sound blending and word attack skills
6. Difficulty in serial memory
7. Distractible, disinhibition, and hyperactivity
8. Difficulty with impulse control; emotionally labile, low frustration tolerance
9. Limitation of abstraction; concretism
10. Soft neurologic signs; minor motor incoordination, handedness confusion
11. Inconsistency

12. Difficulty in reading and all its ramifications
13. Difficulty with spatial and temporal relationships
14. Mild articulatory deviations.

EVALUATIVE PROCEDURES

It would be ideal if children came for behavioral assessment with an isolated or a *pure* type of disturbance. This is very rarely the case. Children come to a speech and hearing center with a variety of reasons for dysfunction, in addition to a variety of symptomatologies. Auditory perceptually disturbed children are frequently classic examples of multiple problems. Many times the behavioral disturbances caused by the constant frustration of failure are of more concern to the parent than the auditory perceptual disturbance. In addition, these children usually have a visual perceptual component that may create an additional interference with learning. Conversely, the same is true with children who have primarily a visual perceptual disturbance, that is, there is usually present some degree of auditory perceptual disturbance. Fortunately, the two primary sensory avenues are rarely equally involved and treatment procedures can take advantage of the less-involved modality.

Language disorders, although not directly related to perceptual functioning, can also occur in conjunction with auditory perceptual disturbances. A child with an auditory perceptual disturbance need not necessarily have a language disorder. However, a child with a language disorder has a high probability of having disturbances of auditory perceptual processes.

The necessity of evaluating all language modalities with informal or standardized tests is important in any behavioral assessment of speech and language. All the clinical and observational tools available to delineate specifics regarding any disorder should be utilized regardless of the type of disorder or of the parents' chief complaint. Only specific items related to the assessment of auditory perceptual disturbances will be presented. This does not suggest that these are the only areas or tests available to be used, nor is it meant to imply that other testing procedures should be disregarded.

Obviously, the behavioral assessment of a child suspected of having an auditory perceptual disturbance requires a thorough evaluation of his auditory abilities. Routine tests of auditory acuity, including traditional pure tone and speech reception audiometry, should be administered with the knowledge that these children frequently have variations in thresholds because of internal and external stimuli. Repeated audiograms are sometimes necessary to establish true acuity for pure tones and speech.

Auditory localization in both silent and noisy surroundings should also be evaluated. Children with auditory perceptual disturbances may be able to localize in a quiet environment but may not be able to identify the direction of speech in a noisy environment. Signal-to-noise ratios, if attainable, are important facets of the evaluation procedure. Frequently a greater stimulus intensity is required before they will respond, therefore, signal-to-noise ratios may give valuable diagnostic evidence of a perceptual disturbance.

Evaluating auditory attention is a complex task compounded by a variety of variables often too numerous to control in most clinical situations. These children exhibit short auditory memory spans. Normative data is available for auditory memory tasks and should be utilized. The use of digits, sentences, or nonsense syllables, etc. will yield information as to whether the child is functioning at age level. The digit subtests from the Illinois Test of Psycholinguistic Abilities (Kirk, McCarthy, and Kirk, 1968), or the Stanford-Binet (Terman and Merrill, 1960) may be employed. Parental and teacher information is important in the child's auditory attention. Questions such as, "Will he follow two- and three-part commands?" may result in clues as to attentional disorders. Children with auditory perceptual disturbances will frequently complete only the first or last request because they are unable to attend to long verbal sequences.

The ability to manage rapidly and slowly presented speech information should be subjectively evaluated since no tests of auditory rate exist that utilize speech sequences. Children with auditory perceptual disturbances have less difficulty with rapidly spoken verbal sequences than those same sequences spoken more slowly. Essentially the same is true for digits; that is, digit memory is better if two digits per second are presented instead of one per second.

Auditory discrimination testing is also appropriate. This area, too, is subject to many variables, but The Wepman Test of Auditory Discrimination (1958), or Goldman, Fristoe, and Woodcock (1970), or the PERC (Drake, 1965), may be used to obtain an estimate of the child's discriminatory abilities. Perhaps one advantage of the second test is that discrimination is tested in both quiet and noisy situations. Auditory perceptually disturbed children are more likely to do poorly in the noise portion because of figure-ground deficiencies often present.

Some estimate should be made of the child's ability to discriminate pitch and rhythm. Many children cannot differentiate pitch differences or changes whether the stimulus is puretones or sustained phonation. Also, many of these children cannot imitate phonated rhythm sequences presented by the examiner or parent. Pitch and rhythm differences are, at best, subjective, but some attention should be directed toward these areas during evaluative procedures.

Synthesis difficulties are to be anticipated in children with auditory perceptual disturbances. The ability of the child to synthesize from parts to wholes may be evaluated through tests of auditory blending. Various subtests from commercially available diagnostic tools can be found, for example, the Illinois Test of Psycholinguistic Abilities (ITPA).

Auditory blending abilities in children with auditory perceptual disturbances are usually poor. These children manifest an inability to perceive sounds within words; they may be able to identify two words that are the same, but may not be able to tell whether sounds within the word are the same. Difficulty in auditory synthesis can be identified through the utilization of tests of auditory blending, such as the subtest from the ITPA. Auditory blending and integration are related because these children are unable to construct words from their sound components, even though they may know all of sounds, they cannot combine them into words. Gates (1936) reported that young children hear words as complete sound units and are not aware that those same sounds occur in different words. Deficiencies in auditory analysis and synthesis are frequently found in these children.

Of course, articulation should be evaluated as it normally would in any speech and language evaluation while assessing auditory abilities of the child. The McDonald Deep Test of Articulation (1964), The Goldman-Fristoe (1969), or other tests of articulation accuracy may be employed, depending, to a large extent, on examiner preference. Again, the pattern of articulation errors may have diagnostic implications; omission of final consonants or final syllables being an added suspicion if other characteristics are present. Cognate confusion is occasionally clinically evident, for example, t/d, f/v, or s/z substitutions.

There are many standardized reading tests that can be used to assess the acquisition of meaning from the printed word. Chall (1967) referred to standardized reading tests currently being utilized.

> I found, however, that most teachers and principals have little faith in the standardized tests now given periodically in every school. The results of these tests are not used, as they might be, as a basis for instruction and for decisions on methods and materials. Further, the standardized reading tests often mask some of the important outcomes of reading instruction because they measure a conglomerate of skills and abilities at the same time (p. 312).

A review of research in central processing dysfunctions in children published by the U. S. Department of Health, Education, and Welfare (1969) indicated that standardized reading tests present various units of visual stimuli. These may be letters, words, phrases, sentences, or paragraphs. Only meager analysis of errors can be completed because of such a limitation of responses and observations. Chall (1967) suggests that the teacher needs simple diagnostic tests and those interested in research need more complex ones. The HEW report described a widely-used five-step procedure for diagnosing children with reading problems: (a) estimating reading potential or capacity, (b) determining reading level, (c) determining behavioral symptoms of faulty reading, (d) analysis of correlated factors, and (e) recommending remedial procedures.

Intelligence testing is usually done to achieve the first step, but since auditory-vocal language is a corollary to reading, language measures should also be included in the testing of reading. Standardized reading tests, such as those of Gray (1963), Durrell (1955), Gates-McKillop (1962), or Gates-MacGinitie (1965) can be utilized to identify the child who is failing in reading. Observation of the child while reading will aid in the determination of behavioral symptoms of faulty reading: how he attacks unfamiliar words; how he blends sounds; how he uses contextual clues; reading rate; comprehension; reversal of letters; omission or addition of sounds; and how he reads silently.

The fourth step is the determination of why the child has failed to learn to read. Medical and intellectual factors should be eliminated first; significant emotional disturbance should also be eliminated. Disturbance in the analysis and synthesis of auditory, visual and haptic information can affect reading acquisition. There is certainly a need for more specific tests measuring perceptual disturbances as they specifically relate to reading disorders, especially when one considers that 15 per cent of children in school today have reading disorders (HEW, 1969, that is, approximately eight million children are doing poorly in school because of reading disorders.

The final step in the behavioral assessment of an auditory perceptual disturbed child with a reading disorder is to prescribe specific treatment procedures. These should be based on the findings obtained on the four steps previously discussed. Recommendations should include a task analysis proposal for remediating the problem, that is, specific methods, materials, and sequence of presentation to remediate the reading disorder.

TREATMENT PROCEDURES

Preliminary to any discussion of a treatment program for children exhibiting auditory perceptual disturbances, perhaps a few words are appropriate regarding the relationship of speech pathology to auditory perceptual disturbances and the reading process. Central processing functions underlie both reading and language. Reading is parasitic to language; this is within the realm of the speech pathologist. If a reading disorder is present as a symptom of an auditory perceptual disturbance, and if time, training, and responsibility permit, treatment procedures can and should be initiated by the speech pathologist. Two of many problems that exist within this conceptual framework are the following: (a) the lack of training in auditory perception that the majority of speech pathologists receive during their clinical and academic programs, and (b), the lack of systematic scientific research to develop specific tests and/or treatment procedures for measuring perceptual disturbances as they specifically relate to reading tasks.

Probably one of the most valuable tools in the evaluation of a child with an auditory perceptual disturbance is the parental interview. Many diagnosticians often forget, or fail to consider, that mothers know more about their children than anyone else, yet this information is often the least considered in the evaluation process. Careful and systematic questioning of the parents can yield crucial descriptions of a child's auditory abilities and his reaction to his environment. This point cannot be stressed too heavily. Most case history forms being used today by speech pathologists do not cover the important points adequately, nor should they necessarily. The kind and quality of questions necessary do not lend themselves to fill-in-the-blank responses. A personal, sometimes lengthy, parental interview is appropriate.

Environmental Manipulation

Parents of auditory perceptually disturbed children can do much to influence the environmental effects on their child. The following suggestions are presented with the knowledge that an *ideal* situation does not exist, and each suggestion must be taken with a large portion of common sense. For example, if their child shares a room with a sibling, this will affect the quality and quantity of the structuring that can be done.

Consistency is the key concept in the treatment approach with children exhibiting auditory perceptual disturbances. Their auditory world has been chaotic and confusing; they have long since learned that what they hear is not to be trusted. They require routine and structure at home and at school. Parents report that during the school week their child is less inclined to emotional outbursts and is less of a behavior problem than on the weekend. One reason is that the school week is routine and structured; they know what is going to happen and when. This is usually not the case on the weekend. The same is true for the academic school year as opposed to the summer months. During June, July, and August, there is little routine except for, perhaps, summer camp or a day program of short duration.

Parents must routinize the daily schedules of these children, including the weekends and summers. They must be as consistent as is practically feasible with the knowledge that parents often have bad days just as their children have. Mealtime should occur about the same time every day. During the meal outside distractions, such as radio and television, should be eliminated. The auditory perceptually disturbed child should not be seated facing a window where outside visual stimuli would distract him from the conversation occurring at the table.

His room probably should be free of bright color contrasts in curtains or drapes and wall color. It would be to his advantage if they were solid colors as opposed to prints, etc. Conglomerations of pictures, posters, pennants, etc. should be kept to a minimum and located in only one area of the room. If he has a study desk, it should be facing a wall or some other placid background so as not to distract him while doing homework assignments.

Study or homework should be done, if possible, at the same time every day—whatever best fits into the family and house routine. It may be after dinner or after school, but it should occur at the same time so he will become accustomed to the routine.

Many times it is necessary for the parents to get down on the floor with these children and "teach" them how to play. Because of the limitation or modification of abstraction often seen in these children, they have difficulty projecting themselves into pretend or play situations. The parents can show these children that cars make "car noises," and that when two cars run together there is a crash or "bang," etc.

Because these children have difficulty with concepts of future, judgment must be exercised in how much advance notice they are given prior to being told when a particular event is going to occur. This is not to imply that they do not require advance warning of a change in their routine; they must be told, but close to the time when the interruption will occur. Because of the difficulty these children exhibit with abstractions, their environments, at least initially, must be concretized and consistent. Disciplinary measures should be as consistent as possible. Parents must learn to be firm, without punishing, and to use patient firmness.

Because these children are not able to associate and make relationships as do other children, they do not profit from the same environment as their siblings or other children do. They are not able to have the same experiences and frequently seem to have a lot of unrelated information about a concept which they are unable to synthesize and integrate meaningfully. Relationships must often be explained and paraphrased again and again before the child will understand. There is much starting and stopping with this type of child, and parents must frequently modify their goals for him in the environmental situation.

The importance of providing successful experiences to the child cannot be overemphasized to parents. The parents must find and provide these experiences, and they must be appropriate and meaningful to the child. The experience probably should be something the child's sibling cannot or does not have; it may be piano lessons, a pet, a household responsibility, etc. In order for it to have meaning, the child must want to do it, enjoy doing it, and succeed at it.

Treatment Suggestions

Many of the concepts discussed under environmental manipulation apply to aiding the auditory perceptually disturbed in the school or clinic situation. Consistent structure and routine are necessary requisites to the treatment process. A sizable number of these children cannot be helped in the regular classroom. A resource room where these children can receive special help for the auditory perceptual disturbance and participate in the regular classroom regime in those areas where they can profit is a preferable alternative (Sabatino, 1971).

Small groups and specially trained tutors are another alternative which may be beneficial to auditory perceptually disturbed children. Behaviorally and academically, these children require greater latitude but with the same responsibility as other children. They must be able to keep up with the teacher's instructions and understand what is expected of them. Individual and group work will both probably be indicated. Again, the importance of success should be emphasized in working with children with auditory perceptual disturbances.

There is little research regarding the most efficient ways to teach children auditory processing tasks. In a publication of the Depatment of Health, Education, and Welfare (HEW, 1969), a table was presented listing seven different auditory tasks that have been identified according to the stimuli presented, the response required, and terms common in the task or failure of the task. This table is, with modification, presented in Table 10-I. The information contained in the table may provide a foundation for the treatment process for children with auditory perceptual disturbances.

Many clinical approaches are described in the literature for teaching a child to attend to auditory stimuli. Intensifying the stimulus with amplification may enhance awareness and attention. Noisemakers, bells, rattles, and other toys, as well as musical instruments can be utilized for training purposes. Sloane and Mac-Aulay (1968) have presented principles of behavior modification to increase a child's attentiveness to auditory stimuli.

The ability to determine whether or not a sound is present is the first step in training in auditory discrimination. The use of pure tones or warbled tones can be used to teach detection and awareness of when sound is present. As previously indicated some of these children have difficulty with sound localization. The ear closest to the sound source should hear the auditory stimulus first, and the time difference between the detection of the stimulus can be used as a clue to detect the source of the signal. Children who have difficulty in sound localization may not learn that different people have different voices or that the voice of one person is specific to that person to the exclusion of others. The therapist will have to invent therapeutic methods and materials for the training of sound localization.

TABLE 10-I—AUDITORY PROCESSING TASKS*

	Stimulus Area	Response of Child	Area of Treatment
1:	Auditory stimulus	Indicate awareness through verval or motor response:	Attentional problem; distractible, disinhibition, hyperactive:
2:	Sound versus no sound	Yes/no	Acuity, detection, awareness:
3:	Sound from several different origins	Indicate direction from which originated	Sound localization:
4:	Sounds varying on one acoustic dimension:	Same/different	Discrimination of pitch, loudness, speech sounds, noises:
5:	Sequences and patterns of speech or nonspeech sounds varying on more than one acoustic dimension:	Reproduce sequence: (a) Imitation, e.g, tapping; (b) speaking; (c) singing:	Pitch, rhythm, melody disturbances, "arhythmical, poor auditory memory."
6:	Sound preselected as "figure" versus sound preselected as "ground."	Select "figure" sound	Differentiation, discrimination:
7:	Sounds from one or more sources	Identify by: (a) Pointing to a visual representation of the sound source; or (b) naming the sound source:	Sound Association.

*Table adapted from NINDS Monograph Number Nine (1969).

Analysis and synthesis of speech sounds are a prerequisite to learning the phonemic structure of language. Thus, discrimination of sound varying on one acoustic dimension is of vital importance for development of auditory memory, articulation, and reading. Sequential training activities are necessary for the auditory perceptually disturbed child. Initially, the maximum contrast between the pairs of sounds to be discriminated should be employed. The gross discrimination of common environmental sounds such as those described by Utley (1950) and Carhart (1961) followed by discrimination of finer sound differences suggested by Mecham (1966) may be employed. Using the rationale of dividing learning behavior into three modes: (a) conditioning discriminative stimuli; (b) differential reinforcement of successive approximations of the desired behavior; and (c) chaining or sequencing behavioral patterns suggested by Mecham *et al.* (1966) may give the clinician ideas for therapy. The review of literature by Reichstein and Rosenstein (1964) also provides information for auditory discrimination in relation to the selection of stimuli and mode of response.

An auditory perceptually disturbed child may have the ability to discriminate one sound from another, but may have severe deficiencies in discriminating rhythmic patterns of acoustic stimuli; the difficulty may be directly related to the temporal aspects of the stimulus. Again, little research is available on the relation of perception of rhythm and rhythmic disturbances. The child with an auditory perceptual disturbance does not seem to acquire an automatic presentation of a rhythmic pattern; this appears true whether the stimulus is reproduction of pitch, acoustic structure, melody patterns, or bodily movements. The difficulty manifested by these children occasionally takes the form of perseveration of a pattern or an apparent lack of inhibition; regardless of the form taken, the result is a lack of integration and analysis. The imaginative clinician may develop a variety of techniques to improve perception of rhythm. The use of counting in rhythm might be one way and, in this matter, the counting response can be controlled by the clinician. Counting and tapping in unison may also be of therapeutic value.

Selecting the appropriate "figure" from the conglomerate of auditory background is another therapeutic avenue that must be traversed. The distractible, disinhibited, hyperactive auditory perceptually disturbed child is a good example of children who attend to irrelevant auditory stimuli. The sequencing and timing of the auditory signal may be an important variable when interference with "figure-ground" occurs. There is a variety of therapeutic techniques that can be devised by the clinician to aid the child in the selection of the significant from the insignificant auditory stimuli.

Sound association, that is, the associating of sounds with their actual sources, is not an uncommon problem for children with auditory perceptual disturbances. The child who cannot select speech sounds from the other auditory stimuli in his environment will undoubtedly have difficulty in auditory perception; he has difficulty relating speech sounds to other auditory experiences, which is similar to, but less severe than, an auditory agnosic. Once again the clinician must exercise imagination and ingenuity to select appropriate methods and materials for sound association, since research is lacking.

The lack of reliable and valid research in the areas described above certainly constitutes a definite handicap for organizing and conducting an efficient therapeutic program for children with auditory perceptual disturbances. The clinician is referred to Berry (1969), Myklebust and Johnson (1967), Davis and Silverman (1961), and other texts and articles to select appropriate therapeutic methods and materials. Selective application of particular techniques to auditory perceptually disturbed children must be kept uppermost in the planning, organization, and execution by the clinician. The purpose of auditory training is to aid the child to make active use of his auditory processing system. This concept has been implemented in therapy with the hard-of-hearing, but not with children exhibiting auditory perceptual disturbances.

Whether the disability is classified as auditory dyslexia (Myklebust, 1967), congenital word-blindness (Hinshelwood, 1895), or analphabetia partialis (Engler, 1917), the reading disorder that accompanies auditory perceptual disturbances is the most devastating and handicapping to the child. There are in existence a multitude of methods to teach reading to children, including the sight, phonic, phonovisual, and multisensory approaches. It should be obvious that the phonic approach is not appropriate, although speech pathologists have been systematically taught to bombard the deficit area in articulatory therapy instead of taking advantage of the child's preferred intact sensory avenues. Thus, the method selected for these children should be visual or a combined visual-auditory approach. The inconsistency of English and traditional orthography creates havoc in the child with an auditory perceptual disturbance.

An approach to teaching reading to children with auditory perceptual disturbances employed at Memphis State University's Speech and Hearing Center has met with a great deal of success. This approach is called the Initial Teaching Alphabet (i/t/a) (Downing, 1962). This approach to the teaching of reading began in the United States approximately eight years ago, in Great Britain approximately twelve years ago, and over a hundred years ago in tradition and philosophy. i/t/a is a tool for the initial teaching of reading, and not a full-blown spelling reform or a language of its own. It is based on a carefully designed, imperfect, phonemic alphabet. The imperfections are carefully built in to facilitate an early transition from i/t/a to traditional orthography (TO). The i/t/a has forty-four symbols, each representing one, and only one, sound (or phoneme) in the English language. Twenty-four of the symbols are traditional, fourteen are augmentations which closely resemble two familiar letters joined together, and six are special symbols. Having learned these symbols and the sound which each represents, a child can read any word written in i/t/a and write any word he can pronounce. It makes each child independent and free of limitation. In the conventional alphabet there are more than two thousand variants in the way the twenty-six symbols are used to make the forty-odd sounds of English speech. These two thousand visual patterns are reduced to fewer than ninety patterns with i/t/a.

The fact that i/t/a is being utilized in many public school

systems as the method to teach reading is testimony to the fact that its usefulness is becoming increasingly popular. Ten per cent of the school systems in the United States now have i/t/a classrooms, including Illinois, Pennsylvania, and California; in New York State, one of every five children learns to read utilizing the i/t/a method.

By contrast with the frustrations of TO in which the child must incessantly disregard analogy and reject the results of observation, the success-motivated "learning by discovery" in applying the rational i/t/a code tends to influence the child's whole attitude toward schooling. Specifically, the application of a visual sound symbol system which bears a one-to-one relationship with the phonemic elements of speech has great potential for children with auditory perceptual disturbances. The i/t/a alphabet's consistency enables continual reinforcement of improving perception, discrimination, association, and directionality; it also stimulates the coordination of learning through the visual, auditory, and kinesthetic areas and at the same time assists the learner in developing improved motivation and an independent attack on language.

Because of its design and consistency, the i/t/a has particular application for children with auditory perceptual disturbances. A pilot project was completed at Memphis State University involving twenty-four children. The children, twenty-two boys and two girls, between the ages of five and twelve years, were diagnosed as having auditory perceptual disturbances, and each had a majority of the constellation of characteristics previously discussed. Utilizing the i/t/a approach to reading, these children were seen twice weekly for one and one-half hours in small groups of between two and five children each. The suggested method for the i/t/a program was modified slightly to specifically meet the needs of these children. For example, writing in i/t/a was not taught nor was it encouraged in the group sessions.

Results of the reading program were most encouraging. Of the twenty-four who began the program, twenty-one completed the i/t/a, including transition to TO, and were reading two grade levels higher than when initially seen for evaluation. Although reading at least one grade level above their original test scores, two were placed in classrooms for the perceptually handicapped because of associated visual perceptual disturbances, and one was removed from the program when the family moved from the Memphis area. All of the improvements noted were completed in less than one year with sessions meeting only three hours per week.

The primary reason i/t/a worked with these children is the consistency of the program. The i/t/a symbols are constant and never change. Once the vowels and consonants have been learned, the child can read. This gives early success to a child who has constantly failed in his previous reading attempts. The i/t/a method has programmed readers with student and teacher workbooks, also, there are commercially available supplementary readers for use in the classroom or at home. Another advantage to i/t/a is that the child begins to feel that he can compete, he can succeed, and he can read. One need only to speak with one of the parents of a child in i/t/a to understand the impact on the whole family of this reading program. One mother stated, "For the first time in Bobby's life, he picked up a book to read for pleasure." While there surely are other reading approaches that can be adapted to these children with auditory perceptual disturbances, none have been found particularly effective, and many have not even been attempted.

The ability of handicapped children to compensate for their deficiencies frequently amazes even the most experienced clinician. Children with auditory perceptual disturbances are sometimes quite proficient at compensating for their disability. Most children with auditory processing deficiencies will become visually-oriented with regard to learning or ordering their environments. A good example of this is seen in normally-intelligent deaf children; they are visually alert and are constantly scanning their visual environment. Children with auditory perceptual disturbances learn that they cannot depend on their auditory modality, and, as a result, tend to compensate with their visual abilities. Compensatory mechanisms are usually evident in these children by the age of seven years and should be observable to the clinician.

In conclusion, the point should again be made that the important aspects in the diagnosis of auditory perceptual disturbances is the constellation of characteristics that the child presents. It is obvious that much more research into the etiology, diagnosis, and treatment of these children is needed. This chapter has primarily been an effort to bring out of a conglomerate "background" of isolated and sometimes confusing information, a "foreground" regarding the characteristics of children with auditory perceptual disturbances.

REFERENCES

Adler, S.: *The Non-Verbal Child.* Springfield, Thomas, 1964.

Berry, M.F.: *Language Disorders of Children: The Bases and Diagnoses.* New York, Appleton-Century-Crofts, 1969.

Carhart, R.: Auditory Training. In Davis, H., and Silverman, S. (Eds.): *Hearing and Deafness.* New York, Holt, Rinehart and Winston, 1961.

Chalfant, J.C., and Scheffelin, M.A.: *Central Processing Dysfunctions in Children: A Review of Research.* NINDS Monograph Number Nine, Washington, D.C. U. S. Department of Health, Education, and Welfare, 1969.

Chall, J.: *Learning to Read: The Great Debate.* New York, McGraw-Hill, 1967.

Clements, S.D.: *Minimal Brain Dysfunction in Children.* Public Health Service Publication No. 11415, Washington, D. C., U. S. Department of Health, Education, and Welfare, 1966.

Davis, H., and Silverman, S. (Eds.): *Hearing and Deafness.* New York, Holt, Rinehart and Winston, 1961.

Downing, J.A.: The i.t.a. (Initial Teaching Alphabet) reading experiment. *Reading Teacher, 18:*105-109, 1962.

Drake, C.: *P.E.R.C. Auditory Discrimination Test.* Sherborn, Mass., Perc. Ed. and Research Center, 1965.

Durrell, D.D.: *Durrell Analysis of Reading Difficulty.* New York, Harcourt, Brace, and World, 1955.

Engler, B.: Uber Analphabetia Partialis: (kongenitale Wortblindheit), *Monat Psych Neur, 42:*119-132, 1917.

Funk, I.K.: *Funk and Wagnall's New Standard Dictionary of the English Language.* New York, Funk and Wagnalls, 1963.

Gates, A.I.: Failure in reading and social maladjustment. *NEA Journal, 25:*205-206, 1936.

Gates, A.I., and MacGinitie, W.H.: *Reading Tests.* New York, Columbia Teachers College Press, 1965.

Gates, A.L., and McKillop, A.S.: *Reading Diagnostic Tests.* New York, Columbia Teachers College Press, 1962.

Goldman, R., and Fristoe, M.: *Test of Articulation*. Circle Pines, Minn., American Guidance Service, 1969.

Goldman, R.; Fristoe, M., and Woodcock, R.: *Test of Auditory Discrimination*. Circle Pines, Minn., American Guidance Service, 1970.

Gray, W.S.: *Gray Oral Reading Tests*. Manual of Directions. New York, Bobbs-Merrill, 1963.

Hebb, D.O.: *The Organization of Behavior: A Neurophysiological Theory*. New York, Wiley, 1949.

HEW National Advisory Committee on Dyslexia and Related Reading Disorders: *Reading Disorders in the United States*. Chicago, Developmental Learning Materials, 1969.

Hinshelwood, J.: Word-blindness and visual memory. *Lancet, 2:*1564-1570, 1895.

Kirk, S.; McCarthy, J., and Kirk, W.: *Illinois Test of Psycholinguistic Abilities*. Urbana, Ill., U of Illinois Press, 1968.

Luria, A.R.: *Higher Cortical Functions in Man*. New York, Basic Books, 1966.

Magoun, H.W., and Moruzzi, G.: Brain stem reticular formation and activation of the EEG. *Electroenceph Clin Neurophysiol, 1:*455-473, 1949.

McDonald, E.T.: *A Deep Test of Articulation*. Pittsburgh, Stanwix House, 1964.

Mecham, M.J.: Shaping adequate speech, hearing and language behavior. In Mecham, M. J.; Berko, M. J., and Palmer, M. F. (Eds.): *Communication Training in Childhood Brain Damage*. Springfield, Thomas, 1966, 115-143.

Mecham, M.J.; Berko, M.J.; Berko, F.B., and Palmer, M.F. (Eds.): *Communication Training in Childhood Brain Damage*. Springfield, Thomas, 1966.

Myklebust, H.R.: Aphasia in Children. In Travis, L. (Ed.): *Handbook of Speech Pathology*. New York, Appleton-Century-Crofts, 1957.

Myklebust, H.: *Auditory Disorders in Children*. New York, Grune and Stratton, 1954.

Myklebust, H.R., and Johnson, D.J.: *Learning Disabilities*. New York, Grune and Stratton, 1967.

Newby, H.A.: *Audiology: Principles and Practices*. New York, Appleton-Century-Crofts, 1964.

Nissen, H.S.: Phylogenetic Comparison. *Handbook of Experimental Psychology*. New York, Stevens, Wiley, 1951.

Orton, S.: *Reading, Writing, and Speech Problems in Children*. New York, Norton, 1937.

Penfield, W., and Rasmussen, T.: *The Central Cortex of Man*. New York, Macmillan, 1950.

Reichstein, J., and Rosentein, J.: Differential Diagnosis in Auditory Defects; A Review of Literature. *Except Child, 31 (2):*73-82, 1964.

Sabatino, D.: An evaluation of resource rooms for children with learning disabilities. *J Learn Dis, 4*:84-93, 1971.

Sloane, H.N., and MacAulay, B.D.: Teaching and the environmental control of verbal behavior. In Sloane, H., and MacAulay, B. (Eds.) : *Operant Procedures in Remedial Speech and Language Training.* Boston, Houghton Mifflin, 1968.

Terman, L.M., and Merrill, M.A.: *Stanford-Binet Intelligence Scale.* Boston, Houghton Mifflin, 1960.

Travis, L.E.: *Speech Pathology.* New York, Appleton, 1931.

Utley, J.: *What's Its Name: A Guide to Speech and Hearing Development.* Urbana, Ill., U. of Illinois Press, 1950.

Wepman, J.M.: *Auditory Discrimination Test.* Chicago, Language Research Associates, 1958.

Woodburne, L.S.: *The Neural Basis of Behavior.* Columbus, Merrill, 1967.

Zemlin, W.R.: *Speech and Hearing Science: Anatomy and Physiology.* Englewood Cliffs, N.J., Prentice-Hall, 1968.

CHAPTER ELEVEN

ISSUES IN DIAGNOSIS OF COMMUNICATION DISORDERS

CLYDE L. ROUSEY

DIAGNOSIS usually implies both a predicted outcome of a given physical or psychological state and a commitment to a theoretical position. Of necessity, diagnosis in this fashion also dictates the form of treatment for a problem. Accordingly, the giving of a diagnosis is not something to be done lightly nor casually and to the informed observer it is a clear indication of the quality of the professional care which has been given.

Numerous treatises have been written about diagnosis. In the past the whole issue of diagnosis has reflected predominantly the so-called medical model inasmuch as this has been the discipline which has most been concerned with treatment. The state of knowledge of the various medical specialties was often reflected by the quality of the diagnosis which was made. For example, the capacity for successful treatment of mental illness was poor at the turn of the century when nearly every mental patient was given the same diagnosis (Menninger *et al.*, 1963). The field of speech pathology is now somewhat similarly affected. That is, we still tend to think diagnostically of speech problems as bits of objectionable behavior which have for the most part been mislearned according to one set or another of learning theories. Put another way, just as all mental illness used to be called a dementia praecox many of our colleagues now categorize most speech problems as articulation or voice problems. Such diagnostic labels conceptually imprison us in our diagnosis, treatment and research. Hence, we cannot think of speech behavior as symptomatic of any underlying psychic phenomena which is symptomatic of unconscious conflicts but rather must think that the speech of a person reflects the rational tenets of learning theories and neurophysiology.

Consequently, it is not surprising that many view diagnosis as nonfunctional and time-consuming since essentially the treatment will be the same irrespective of the diagnosis. Perhaps the current propensity in some circles for making an evaluation rather than a diagnosis is one manifestation of this problem. Certainly, the theoretical stance of the Skinnerians in clinical work is representative of the trend away from diagnosis.

Perhaps of even greater significance is that this scotoma not only affects our diagnosis and treatment of clients but is passed on to our graduate students who enter into graduate programs unaware of a given institution's theoretical biases and how these biases will affect their training. Indeed, the very essence of how most graduate students are picked clearly reflects the disinterest in theoretical diagnosis and emphasis on surface phenomena by the field of speech pathology. That is, potential students are given tests emphasizing their capacities for reasoning and operating with abstract entities, while little attention is given to obtaining any diagnostic impression of their emotional health and well-being and its influence on the potential client with whom they will come in contact. It should be noted there is no reason for this scotoma to be an issue if one sees the changing of speech behavior as something which obeys the laws of learning rather than expresses the irrational feelings with which mankind contends.

We have never struggled as a field about whether the problems with which we routinely deal really are manifestations of educational problems, medical problems, emotional problems, some combination of these, or some other entity. Rather, if by happenstance we have been professionally sired in Europe, speech problems are often thought of as otolaryngological problems or if by happenstance we have been sired in America speech problems are thought of as diction or educational problems or in current parlance as expressions of learning disabilities.

Accordingly, treatment has expressed these parochial views. Put even more broadly, there is no general theory of speech and/or speech disorders which is generally accepted or readily understood by many professional personnel on which we can base any consistent diagnostic process. Rather, we call ourselves eclectic and borrow from numerous related fields in order to attempt to meet and solve the clinical problems which confront us. An eclectic position is never a strong diagnostic or theoretical position. It is only a piecemeal attempt at explaining diversity. A single theory is far more effective in providing a unified diagnosis. With such a position, diagnosis can become ". . . not a search for a proper name . . . or an affliction but rather . . . understanding just how the patient is ill and how ill the patient is, how he became ill and how his illness serves him" (Menninger *et al.*, 1963).

Systems which talk about contingencies (McReynolds, 1970), reinforcement (Weston and Irwin, 1971) or stimulus method (Milisen, 1954; Van Riper, 1963) basically reject the notion and necessity for diagnosis as we have chosen to define it. For this writer, baldly put, a deviation in speech behavior in the absence of obvious neurological and physical difficulties is a reflection of an individual's psychological state, both healthy and unhealthy. Thus, the consideration of the individual's "normal" speech patterns becomes as important as consideration of his deviant speech patterns. Thus, both pathological and normal speech behavior can serve as the basis for understanding ". . . how the patient is ill and how ill the patient is, how he became ill and how his illness serves him" (Menninger *et al.,* 1963).

To illustrate the consequences for diagnosis and treatment of such a position, I propose to present and discuss in detail the diagnostic understanding based on variations in speech and hearing of five clients (four of whom were referred for psychiatric complaints).* The interested reader can consult the numerous expositions which explicate this position (Rousey and Moriarty, 1965; Filippi and Rousey, 1968; LaFon and Rousey, 1969; Filippi and Rousey, 1970; P. Kernberg and Rousey, 1969; Mehrhof and Rousey, 1970; Norris, 1969; Rousey, 1969; Rousey, 1970). In

---

*The reader should not be mislead into thinking these are clients who are markedly different from what is seen in the usual speech clinic. The only uniqueness is that they were with one exception referred initially for psychiatric complaints and all five were examined in a total way by a speech pathologist and audiologist, a neurologist, a psychiatric social worker, a child psychologist, and a child psychiatrist (The Menninger Clinic, Children's Division, 1969). Of further significance is the number of adults included. Rarely are communication handicaps considered in adults unless some blatant degree of organicity is present, e.g., a CVA or laryngectomy.

brief, the sounds of speech (vowels and consonants) are conceived of as primarily expressions of an individual's emotional relationships with fathering and mothering figures throughout his formative years and include such developmental issues as nurturance, developing of object relations, toilet training, and resolution of oedipal struggles. The manner in which the individual discharges his aggressive and libidinal drives is further inferred from the sounds of speech. The presence of a speech deviation* thus clearly signifies unusual conflict.

EXAMPLE NO. 1

The patient is a forty-five-year-old professor of history, who comes with the complaint that for the past two years he has suffered from a complex of something that included nightmares, fugue-like states, and "psychotic episodes." During this period, he also felt as if he were increasingly depressed and feared that some attempt would be made on his life either by himself or others. The patient is the second of six children. He was the oldest son and lived in poverty during his childhood because of alcoholism on the part of his father. The mother is described as being cruel. There is reason to question whether or not the patient exaggerates some of his descriptions of his parents' pathology. His sister died in a state mental hospital after suffering a lifelong mental illness. The neurological examination suggests "bi-temporal spike and wave dysrhythmia, predominantly in the left temporal area." It was also felt that there might be some mild to moderate frontal lobe atrophy suggestive of alcoholism and some degree of cerebral arteriosclerosis.

During his psychological testing, the patient was described as being polite to the point of being ingratiating. The patient saw himself during projective tests as an unappreciated genus. He experienced the world as requiring "cunning manipulation and careful suspicion in order to survive." He seemed bound into the use of "paranoid-like and phobic-like projections." He also described being frequently depressed over the injustices of his life and a lack of nurturance. He sees himself as a special Don Juan who at least in fantasy has numerous affairs. Psychological tests revealed few suggestions of central nervous system dysfunction, although the possibility of some epileptic-type organic impairment could not be dismissed. His I.Q. is 136 on the verbal scale and 123 on the Performance scale of the Wechsler-Bellevue Test. The patient is considered as being a paranoid personality with a depressive syndrome of recurrent nature.

*This should be clearly understood as omitting all language problems whether they be organically or culturally based.

The examination of the patient's articulatory patterns disclosed no errors. The singing pitch range to his voice was constricted, being only eight notes in spread. There was also a tongue thrust present in his swallowing pattern. He has a mild to moderate bilateral sensorineural loss beginning at 4000 Hz. However, his speech reception thresholds are essentially within normal limits. His speech discrimination ability was normal on the W-22 recorded lists but showed a borderline degree of dysfunction in terms of the Rush-Hughes difference scores for the left ear. During the test of intracranial sound localization, the patient perceived a simultaneously and binaurally presented pure tone as emanating from one ear, both ears, or from one foot over his head.

When one thinks of the speech and hearing examination in the diagnostic sense described in the aforementioned publications by Rousey *et al.*, one can make the following inferences about this patient. The constricted pitch range which the patient manifests is viewed as a constriction in affect and inferentially an indicator of depression. This finding is abundantly confirmed by the psychiatric examination. Clinically, a depression of such an extent as is inferred on the basis of this test material would be suggestive of some disturbance in thought processes. The possibility of a thought disturbance is similarly reflected by the patient's deviant perceptions during the test of intracranial sound localization. If one views the tongue thrust as reflecting inappropriate competitiveness and striving, this patient's capacity for impulse control and expression of anger would likely be seriously impaired. This inference again is confirmed by the clinical data obtained during the psychiatric test and psychological evaluation. Finally, of interest to this patient's diagnosis is the disturbance in cortical functioning which would be hypothesized on the basis of the borderline difference score obtained for the left ear. The EEG findings in this case are corroborative of a possible epileptic disturbance.

In retrospect then, as one looks over this patient's speech examination, one becomes acutely aware of the diagnostic implications which are present in the usual speech and hearing examination. Conventional psychological testing and psychiatric interviews strongly support the dynamic interpretation which has been given to the findings of the speech and hearing examination. It is obvious that such a patient would be unlikely to be referred to the average speech clinic since his main presenting symptoms were psychiatric rather than speech. It is possible that because of his hearing loss he might have been referred for an audiological study, which, if it had concentrated solely on his pure tone responses and his speech discrimination ability for material as found on the W-22 recorded word lists and had failed to understand the dynamic meanings which were reflected in his speech, would have surely missed understanding the psychological life of the patient. With the increasing emphasis on routine testing of hearing by subprofessionals or indeed even by professional personnel who have little or no theoretical understanding of complex psychological conditions, one might easily have missed referring this person on for additional psychiatric help.

EXAMPLE NO. 2

The patient is a ten-year-old girl who comes with the complaint of having in the past been described as being developmentally slow with problems of motor coordination, being emotionally disturbed and functioning at a borderline intellectual level. She throws temper tantrums and still soils herself and is in a special education class in school. The child is described as being extremely demanding of her parents. Feelings that this child was unusual date from the beginning of the pregnancy. Developmentally she is described as not sitting by herself until one year and not walking completely alone until twenty-four months of age. Her gait is described as being very unsteady. She has had surgery on her eyes for a plugged tear duct. In her early childhood, she is described as being undemanding and extremely easy to care for. Professional people who saw the child thought that she was retarded. Accordingly, she was placed in a preschool nursery for the retarded when she was 4½ years of age. Shortly after this, she was entered into special classrooms for brain damaged and emotionally disturbed. Even at her present age, toilet training has not been successfully completed for both bowel and bladder control. The current neurological examination revealed a mild degree of microphthalmia. There was mild awkwardness of skilled and rapid movements of the hands, fingers and legs, and her handwriting was deemed to be awkward although legible. The neurologist felt the child sustained profuse congenital encephalopathy. The electroencephalogram completed on this child was mildly abnormal with consistent evidence of a negative and slow wave discharge disturbance in the right hemisphere.

The results of the psychological testing revealed the patient to be hypersensitive to any criticism and to be fighting against a sense of depression. Her mood shifts were sudden and unexpected. At times she indicated that she would have to kill herself if any expression of hostility was allowed to surface. She has a great deal of difficulty in separating reality from fantasy. In a similar manner, her self-concept is distorted, being fragmented as well as disjointed in terms of her actual height and weight. Her intellectual capacities showed a good many inconsistencies with her Verbal Intelligence Quotient being in the dull normal range and her Performance Intelligence Quotient being in the defective range on the Wechsler Intelligence Scale for Children. Her looseness in thinking is blatant and she seemingly is unaware of inappropriate remarks which she inserts within the context of her activities. Fathers are described on projective tests by her as being shy, ineffectual and always losing to mothers, while mothers are seen as powerful and rejecting. The psychiatric diagnosis given this child was schizophrenia, childhood type.

During the speech and hearing examination, this child for an entire hour refused to speak to the examiner. Instead, she held her hands over her ears and made biting movements with her mouth. When she began to make noises like a horse, the examiner made some whinnying noises like a horse which allowed some communication to ensue. This was followed by some sound similar to a violin which in turn changed into a sound like a child crying. At that point, she demonstrated essentially adequate articulatory patterns for consonants. Formal tests of this child's auditory capacities could not be totally completed. She was unable to cooperate. However, it was possible to demonstrate her sensitivity for pure tones in the critical speech frequencies was within normal limits.

This child represents an individual with gross disturbances in communication which are reflective of her gross psychological disorganization. It is of importance to notice her dependence on vowel sounds as a means of communicating with her environment. Such a finding is not inconsistent with the notion which has been advanced by the writer of the present chapter regarding the basic significance of vowels as indicators and expressions of drives. Thus, one should expect in a child of this chronological age who depends so much on vowel sounds for establishing contact during the course of a speech examination that this child should be seen by the psychiatric examining team as schizophrenic. The heavy dependence on vowels at this time is understood as reflecting the predominance of the primary process in this child's thought patterns and as not being related to mental retardation. Although this child behaviorally would be seen as quite disturbed regardless of the outcome of the speech examination, she is a good illustration of the basic meanings which sounds come to express. When or if one discusses emotional problems as found in individuals with speech and hearing difficulties, one is accustomed to thinking of them as secondary to the speech problem. That is, the assumption is made that if only the speech problem is cured then the emotional reactions which are present will go away. It seems to us that the aforementioned explanatory formulation misses the essential richness which is present when one understands speech behavior is indicative of psychic states. Understanding of emotional disturbances in individuals with speech problems as usually secondary reactions also leads to, in our opinion, mismanagement of the case clinically and perpetuation of a disturbed emotional state. Elsewhere P. Kernberg and Rousey (1969) and Fleming and Rousey (1969) have described how speech behavior changes coincident with recovery in the course of psychiatric treatment. The implications of such an assertion are revolutionary in the sense that new dimensions of training for students and practitioners become mandatory. Similarly, our professional interrelationships with the disciplines of psychology need to be explored and expanded in much the same way as we have done with otologists, laryngologists and special educators.

EXAMPLE NO. 3

This patient is a twenty-year-old girl who left college after only one year because of increasing withdrawal, depression and persistent weight loss. Following the patient's birth, the mother had little to do with her for several days because a boy had been desired. Finally when the attending physician insisted that the child be taken or given up for adoption, the mother was then able to take the child and try to accept her. The early relationships with the mother were unusual in that the child was on a strict four-hour feeding schedule and developmental tasks, such as toilet training, were completed early (around thirteen months). There was a great deal of unpleasantness in the home situation. There were open fights going on between the parents and the mother engaged in extramarital affairs. Even though her grades in her early school years were above average, as she entered junior high school following an episode of infectious mononucleosis she began to do poorly in school and her interests turned more to dating and being out with her girlfriends. An affair with a boy in her high school years resulted in an abortion. Following her failure in the first year of college, she for a time worked in a secretarial job but finally became increasingly depressed and was referred for psychotherapy. The neurological examination performed on her was within normal limits.

The attending psychiatrist described her as "a small child who is helpless and frightened by demands of the big, confusing, demanding world." Although her thinking at times bordered on suspiciousness, she was described as an extremely sensitive, self-conscious, narcissistically oriented, helpless young lady. Her intelligence on the Wechsler scale was within normal limits for all the various scales. The psychiatrist's diagnosis was of a depressive reaction and that the patient sustained anorexia nervosa.

During psychological testing, the patient had first complained that she was too upset to do well on the tests but was with some support able to complete them. The patient's style of thinking was described as reflecting a passive stance. The psychologist felt there was a certain flaccidity of ego functioning which limited the patient's development and use of her intellectual resources. Her interests were described as being egocentrically determined and confined to elemental things, such as her body, clothes and her own experiences. The patient's psychosexual development was considered to have been arrested at the oral aggressive stage with a good deal of resulting anger and consequent depression ensuing. The patient continues to struggle with unsolved problems of sexual identity and heterosexual adjustment. Indeed, the patient's personality organization is considered to be poorly differentiated and at a primitive level. There were glimpses on phychological testing of behaviors typical of what is labeled a borderline state of personality organization.

The patient's speech examination revealed the substitution of *f* for the voiceless *th* sound as well as a pronounced whistle on sibilant sounds. The pitch range to her voice was within normal limits. Her voice quality was felt to be normal. No tongue thrust was present in her swallowing pattern. Her sensitivity for pure tones was within normal limits. During the test of intracranial sound localization, she perceived a simultaneously and binaurally presented pure tone as emanating variously from both ears, one ear, and approximately one foot off her head.

Again, we see that this patient would not primarily have been referred for speech services or hearing diagnosis but again we find speech and hearing pathology coexisting in the presence of known psychopathology. Of significance diagnostically in this patient's

case is the substitution of *f* for the voiceless *th* sound. Elsewhere
(Rousey, 1970) it has been noted that the *f* sound is believed
associated primarily with the phallic stage of psychosexual development. Hence, the sound substitution pattern in this particular
instance reflects early and continuing difficulties with phallic
aspects of her personality and inferentially of her sexual identity.
In another paper, LaFon and Rousey (1969) have demonstrated
that there is an unusually high incidence of substitution of *f* for
the voiceless *th* in individuals who sustained a deprivation experience in terms of interaction with their father during their early
years. In this particular patient's case, this inference is completely
substantiated as her father was out of the home during her first
five years developing a successful business. It is also known that
one of the functions of fathering in a child's early life is to help
develop a positive and appropriate sexual identity. Such a problem area was substantiated by both the examining psychologist
and psychiatrist. Indeed one would expect a twenty-year-old girl
with confusions over such issues to have major relationship problems as well as major struggles around sexual issues. This patient's
abortion and difficulties in establishing any lasting relationships
attests to such problems. Of further importance are the deviant
responses seen during the test of intracranial sound localization.
These test patterns are indicative of a borderline personality state
and hence would, when taken together in interaction with her
articulation difficulties, emphasize an incapacity on her part to
think logically. Diagnostically, this possibility is portrayed by the
diagnosis of infantile personality on the part of the psychiatrist
and by the borderline personality inferred on the basis of psychological testing (cf. O. Kernberg, 1967 and 1968). It is also of
importance to note that none of the indicators on the audiological
examination of neurological dysfunction were present and similarly none were noted during the course of the patient's neurological
examination. The client was concerned at the time of the speech
examination about her pitch being too soft and low causing her to
strain in talking. Dynamically, it was understood that this symptom probably reflects her shift via her voice toward a masculine
identity over which she had major feelings of conflict. This client

had some psychotherapy but she interrupted this treatment early in a manner which the psychotherapist understood as resulting from the patient becoming frightened over establishing a deep relationship. It was felt at the end of her treatment that she was not as depressed as she was when she entered the hospital. It will be recalled that the pitch range data on the speech examination did not support the diagnosis of her being depressed at the beginning. Whether or not this represented a more accurate indication of the client's genuine state (that is, as some sort of pseudo-depression) or whether it reflected an accurate prognosis or whether it was totally wrong cannot be stated with certainty at this time. However, a divergence in the speech findings in this particular instance points up an interesting possibility in the sense that diagnosis cannot only be corroborated for psychiatric patients but in many cases perhaps can be extended and modified if the speech data is taken into consideration. Again, such a concept of the meaning of speech problems implies a wider role for the speech pathologist than is customarily believed and requires additional training experiences for both the clinician and the instructors. Obviously, such diagnostic work cannot be done by people trained on an elementary level. What is required seemingly instead of the substantial number of subprofessionals advocated nowadays is rather a more thorough training of the doctoral level personnel. Put another way, what is probable is that the so-called shortage of personnel serving the speech and hearing impaired in this country may be more a reflection of inadequate training and conceptualization of the problem rather than inadequate numbers of people. For diagnostically, if one conceives of speech difficulties as reflecting psychological states, it is obvious that retraining of speech patterns is not the treatment of choice in most of the cases. Rather, what is the treatment of choice is a dynamic understanding of the symptomatology and resulting psychological intervention. This also means that providing speech therapy for everyone in the schools may be a totally erroneous goal. For under the present conception, this would represent an invasion of privacy in terms of the client's illness which would be unwarranted unless requested. What should become obvious in this stage of our examination of the diagnostic assessment of patients is that the differing theoretical orientation of the present writer opens up diagnostic and professional issues which are a good deal broader than the conventional diagnostic stance allows.

EXAMPLE NO. 4

The patient involved is a seventeen-year-old girl whose psychiatric problems included impulsive behavior, drinking, running away and deteriorating relationships at school and at home. This is an adopted child. The parents were reported to be on the verge of being divorced. During the first year of the patient's life, she was hospitalized repeatedly for allergic reactions. The patient experienced a good deal of fear when she went to the hospital to have a tonsillectomy. With the exception of continuing allergic reactions, the physical examination was negative. The neurological examination was within normal limits. The patient reported she has an aversion to her father touching her. Yet frequently she is involved in planning various family activities or having dinner together with him. At the same time, she feels her mother is rather weak. Her relationship with her peers is described as superficial and lacking in depth. Her plans for the future appear extremely naive and poorly founded in reality. The patient's diagnosis was of an adjustment reaction of adolescence; group delinquent reaction manifested by truancy, sexual misbehavior, refusal to abide by any limitations of the parents and episodic alcoholism.

Intellectual capacities as measured during psychological testing revealed the patient to be of superior intelligence. At times, however, she was rather naive in her knowledge and demonstrated a marked vulnerability to powerful affect. Thought style was characterized as being rather fluid and uncrystalized. One of the ways she tries to cope with her emotions is through impulsive action which leads to ill-conceived and ill-considered behavior. She also uses her angry rebellion as a way of concealing her fears. There was marked confusion over her sexual identity. Psychological testing also revealed the indications of suicidal tendencies.

The results of the speech examination disclosed an inconsistent substitution of *f* for the voiceless *th* and inconsistent omission of *L* in dobule consonant combinations. Further, her voice quality at times was slightly hoarse. The pitch range to her voice was only one octave in spread. There was a tongue thrust present in her swallowing pattern. Her hearing sensitivity for pure tone stimuli was within normal limits as were her speech reception thresholds and speech discrimination ability. During the test of intracranial sound localization, she perceived a simultaneously and binaurally presented pure tone variously as emanating from both ears, both sides of her mandible, and from two to three inches to one foot outside of her head.

Once again, it is possible to infer from the speech and hearing data on the basis of the substitution of *f* for the voiceless *th* and the omission of *l* that this child's early relationships with both of her parents have been poor although for the most part they have been generally sealed over. The stabilizing effect of normal paternal relationships in a child's growth is well known and the absence of such a stabilizing relationship is often clearly associated with later emotional disturbances. In this instance, speech data provides us with inferences which are independently confirmed by the psychological examination and family history. Of further interest is the inference already alluded to in Example No. 3 where the association was made between the confusion over sexual identity and the persisting substitution of *f* for the voiceless *th* sound. As in the previous case, we see abundant confirmation of this diagnostic inference based not only on psychological testing but on psychiatric interviews. In a similar fashion, we see the disregard for reality which this patient is able to manifest at times in her interactions with others. There is further confirmation of this client's disturbance in thinking based on the test of intracranial sound localization. The responses are more typical of a client with a borderline personality disorder. This conclusion does not appear in the psychiatric diagnosis of this client. Again, follow-up of this client's hospital course reveals that she was discharged at her parents' request after only four months and considered unimproved in terms of social adjustment, character structure, and her psychiatric syndrome. She continued numerous instances of antisocial behavior, making treatment difficult within the present setting. Of further interest in this particular client is the persisting tongue thrust. When this is viewed dynamically, one conceives of this as occurring in patients who have a capacity for inappropriate display of competitiveness and aggression. This inference is also abundantly confirmed by the social history as well as what went on in the hospital and precipitated her premature termination of treatment. Such an interpretation is obviously a far cry from viewing this as a "tongue habit" which can be effected by swallowing exercises. In our view, this approach to treatment, i.e. swallowing exercises, again demonstrates the simplistic notions about speech and hearing behavior which are perpetuated because of the field's restrictive orientation via organic and/or learning theories. Certainly, if the diagnostic impression regarding the tongue thrust as proposed in this paper is correct, then one would consider the treatment of such a disturbance in an entirely different light than is usually done. This is not to say that there are not orthodontic conditions which necessitate appliances but it does argue that the often made association of tongue thrust solely with dental conditions may indeed be in error. In the view held by the present writer, the persistent pressure of the tongue against the teeth is a displacement of the competitiveness in such a manner as it is directed against the self, resulting in structural dental abnormalities. In such a case, while some dental intervention is needed to stabilize dentition what may be needed is psychiatric treatment.

With respect to the client's voice quality being slightly hoarse, it is our inference that this often occurs in clients who attempt to be overly mature and masculine. It is not surprising then that in a client who is severely concerned over her own sexual identity that we find such a disturbance occurring. The pitch range to the client's voice is constricted, being only eight steps in spread (cf. Fairbanks, 1960) and clearly suggests the possibility of some depression. The depression as inferred through the restricted pitch range was abundantly confirmed in the psychological and psychiatric examinations.

The speech and hearing behavior in this client undoubtedly has been present for some time. Probably she was not picked up for speech therapy because of the "relative mildness" of the speech symptom. In this particular case, it is possible to see that our usual conception of what is a "mild speech symptom" may have little if any reality with what is really serious in the client's life. This client could have been treated earlier if the speech and hearing had been used as a diagnostic instrument for early detection of mental illness. Another issue which arises out of the examination of this patient is that our usual indices of severity of speech problems may be inadequate and merit significant revision. Such a revision cannot be done as long as we are theoretically calcified in our present manner of viewing speech and hearing disorders.

EXAMPLE NO. 5

This 3½-year-old child was brought for an initial consultation on referral of her pediatrician because of lack of intelligible speech patterns. At that time, she talked little, with the mother estimating that she had only approximately one hundred words in her vocabulary. She had never attended nursery school nor had been seen anywhere else for treatment for her speech and language difficulties. At the time of this consultation, it was possible to demonstrate that her hearing sensitivity was within normal limits. Her attempts to communicate were primarily by use of vowel sounds. On the Ammons Full Range Picture Vocabulary Test, Form A and Form B, it was possible to demonstrate an average awareness of receptive language in terms of her chronological age. There was no specific neurological involvement of the child's speech mechanism. Often with children of this age having a lag in speech and language acquisition, the recommendation is made to place them in a nursery school in hopes that this will somehow or other help them grow out of their difficulties. As the author of this chapter and a colleague have written elsewhere (Fillippi and Rousey, 1968), the hope in many of these cases is that somehow or other there will be some significant maturation occurring in their communication abilities over a period of time. However, in this particular child's case, after approximately six months it became clear that this child, while making some progress, was decidedly still underachieving in terms of her communication efforts. In addition, the child continued to have difficulty with episodes of bed wetting and being reticent in terms of separating from her parents. Accordingly, a brief period of conventional speech stimulation procedures was entered into. When the child's receptive vocabulary level began to decrease, she was referred for psychological testing. The subsequent report emphasized separation difficulties appearing in the course of psychological testing. As a result, one parent had to stay with the child during testing. During the course of testing, the child would often look to her mother for support and for permission to proceed. There was no intrinsic difference in her style of relating to the test procedures whether the examiner was male or female. It was possible, however, in spite of her disturbance in speech and language, to demonstrate that she was capable of at least average intellectual achievement. The examining psychologist felt that there was unusual inability to separate from her mother together with some recurrent apparent negativism expressed towards the mother.

The developmental history reported for this child is one which could lead a person to suspect some organic reasons for her delay in use of langauge and correct speech. That is, both the mother and father were carriers of galactosemia. Although pregnancy and labor were considered as normal, shortly after the child was born she steadily lost weight and as a result she was taken to a university medical center where the diagnosis of galactosemia was made. Because of the special diet which was required for this disorder, both parents were exteremly watchful of the child in her early life. Although her language development early in life was described as normal in terms of age on onset of the first word and apparent attempts at using language in terms of length, the child could never be very clearly understood at any time by anyone. There are no reported examples of motor dysfunction. A complete neurological examination revealed no significant disturbances of the nervous system.

Conceptualizing this child's disturbance of unintelligibility in speech as indicative of marked fearfulness and anxiety necessitated placing an emphasis on psychotherapeutic aspects of her speech and language performance rather than on the speech and language patterns. The psychological inferences made on the basis of the diagnostic examination of this child in comparison to the previous cases are somewhat limited in view of the failure of any intelligible articulation patterns which could allow us to discuss or predict problem areas. Diagnostically, one would certainly be concerned that there may be some other hidden problems which would become apparent as soon as this child's speech becomes more intelligible.

It is therefore instructive to summarize some of the significant points in this child's psychotherapy to determine the psychological meanings which inferentially were thought to be embodied in her unintelligible patterns of speech. At the beginning of psychotherapy, this child expressed a good deal of anxiety that her mother would leave her, running to the door whenever she heard a noise outside of the office or insisting that the therapist's office door remain open so that she could keep track of her mother. Therapy took the course of the child playing out through water play and other "messing" activities her concern about her toilet training problems which it will be recalled were continuing at the time of her referral to psychotherapy. In addition to the play with water and other messing activities, a good deal of flatus occurred during the course of the therapy with her. Along with this play around toilet training, the child began to indicate an interest in the differences between sexes. In her play, she examined the genital areas of the dolls. As the child was able to express her anger more towards the therapist without being penalized, her speech became clearer. What also became clearer was the impact of father's repeated absences from the home on business trips, with the mother thus assuming a dominant role in the upbringing of this child. Thus, the psychological conditions considered to be necessary for the delay in onset of intelligible speech became more and more apparent in this child (cf. Filippi and Rousey, 1968).

It will be recalled that at the beginning of the treatment there was not enough evidence to consider this child as completely meeting the conditions of the syndrome described by the above mentioned writers. With the increasing involvement of the parents in casework, the child in turn became increasingly more concerned about the differences between boys and girls and her speech patterns became even more intelligible. As it became increasingly intelligible, the child was able to verbalize her wish to be a boy rather than a girl. At this point during the course of treatment when she injured a finger slightly, she requested a bandaid. The injury was not sufficient enough to really put a bandaid on and so it was not done. However, in subsequent sessions the child continued to ask for a bandaid and did so for some time. The child at a later stage in treatment was able to share her fantasy that a bandaid placed over her buttocks if removed would result in the appearance of a penis for her. At this time with almost totally intelligible speech, it became clear that her only sound substitution error was the substitution of *f* for the voiceless *th*. If it is recalled that the sound substitution of *f* for the voiceless *th* sound is believed to occur in children who have sustained a significant disturbance with their father and who have significant confusion over their sexual identity, one can see that in this case treatment seems to bear out the diagnostic implication of the meaning ascribed to this sound in the other cases which we have so far talked about. Working through this disturbance in her relationship with her father and inferentially between the father and the mother took some considerable time. During the course of working through of this problem the child sustained numerous times when she would mistakingly label an older brother as a girl or look very carefully at dolls to see if a penis were present. During a time when her mother underwent an operation on her legs, the child clearly expressed the fantasy that her mother's penis had been cut out and that this was the reason for the lack of the mother's genitals. Towards the end of the treatment when she had largely worked through these problems, she at one stage drew a picture of a female dog with a long tail which she redrew so that the dog's tail was short. With an appropriate interpretive remark concerning the symbolism expressed through such a drawing, she was then able to easily and consistently change her sound substitution pattern of *f* for the voiceless *th* to the correct phonemic patterning.

This is an appropriate case to show that one's diagnostic inferences can be validated successfully through therapy if they are explored in the proper fashion. The argument with such an assertion, of course, is that one finds what one is looking for and that this does not confirm or negate the diagnosis. This argument in and of itself has its own weaknesses inasmuch as the diagnosis of a physical disease, such as a tumor or other malignancy, is confirmed by the finding of such a malignancy during an operation and one does not have to go through any academic gyrations to demonstrate its presence. While admittedly the psychopathology noted here in some respects hardly merits comparison with a malignant tumor on the one hand, yet in another way it does. That is, the psychological significance attributed to speech and communication problems by the present author suggests a serious psychological malignancy present in people which if not diagnosed and treated correctly may lead to significant handicaps for the patient in a later stage of life. One cannot claim to investigate a theory unless one understands the theory perfectly and unless one has a rigorous understanding of the system itself. Hence, opponents of a diagnostic schema, such as suggested in this chapter, can hardly hope to demonstrate either its validity or incorrectness unless they are totally cognizant of the procedures which are involved. Additionally, it should also be noted that one cannot hope to use the diagnostic position expounded in this chapter in a clinical sense with any degree of success unless one has thorough training in the appropriate subject matter. For if one were to do so it is unlikely that one would be successful in adequately using it for its intended purpose.

POSTSCRIPT

In this chapter, we have summarized a diagnostic approach to communication disorders which emphasizes dynamic rather than educational, learning, neurological or linguistic approaches. Specific illustrations of this diagnostic process as well as issues which arise during its application are discussed. The position which is taken is that basically nearly all speech disorders save the most obvious instances of cerebral palsy, cleft palate or known insults to the central nervous system have diagnostic significance in terms of psychopathology. Put another way, the development of articulatory patterns without errors is assumed to be one indicator of normal development and any deviation from this pattern is assumed to reflect an ongoing developmental crisis and/or fixed psychopathology in the individual. Such a diagnostic view offers immense possibilities for early detection and treatment of emotional disturbances as well as secondarily raising controversial issues for the field of speech pathology and audiology.

ACKNOWLEDGMENTS

A deep sense of gratitude must be recorded to Mrs. Carol Rousey, Dr. Larry Bradford, and Mrs. Bernice Flaherty for their critical reading and editorial assistance in the preparation of this chapter.

REFERENCES

Fairbanks, G.: *Voice and Articulation Drillbook,* 2nd ed. New York, Harper and Brothers, 1960, pp. 122-126.
Filippi, R., and Rousey, C.L.: Delay in onset of talking: A symptom of in-

terpersonal disturbance. *J Amer Acad Child Psychiat, 7* (2) :316-329, 1968.

Filippi, R., and Rousey, C.L.: Positive carriers of violence: An exploratory study of detection by speech deviations. Accepted for publication. *Ment Hyg,* 1970.

Fleming, P.D., and Rousey, C.L.: Quantification of psychotherapy change by study of speech and hearing patterns. Unpublished manuscript, 1969.

Kernberg, O.: Borderline personality organization. *J Amer Psychoanal Ass, 15* (3) :641-685, 1967.

Kernberg, O.: The treatment of patients with borderline personality organization. *Int J Psychoanal, 49:* (4) :600-619, 1968.

Kernberg, P., and Rousey, C.L.: Variations in speech sounds during psychotherapy—An independent indicator of change. Presented at annual meeting, American Association of Psychiatric Clinics for Children, Boston, Massachusetts, 1969.

LaFon, D.N., and Rousey, C.L.: Residues of early father-child conflict. Accepted for publication. *J Nerv Ment Dis,* 1969.

McReynolds, L.V.: Contingencies and consequences in speech therapy. *J Speech Hearing Dis, 35:*12-24, 1970.

Mehrhof, E.G., and Rousey, C.F.: Speech difficulties symptomatic of destructive behavior toward self or others. Accepted for publication. *J Nerv Ment Dis,* 1970.

Menninger Clinic, Children's Division: *Disturbed Children.* San Francisco, Jossey-Bass, 1969.

Menninger, K.; Mayman, M., and Pruyser, P.: *The Vital Balance.* New York, Viking, 1963.

Milisen, R.F.: A rationale for articulation disorders. *J Speech Hear Res, (suppl No. 4):*5-17, 1954.

Norris, V.L.: Speech disturbances and the assessment of mental retardation in children. Presented at annual meeting, American Association of Psychiatric Clinics for Children, Boston, Massachusetts, 1969.

Rousey, C.L.: A Theory of Speech. Presented at annual meeting, American Association of Psychiatric Clinics for Children, Boston, Massachusetts, 1969.

Rousey, C.L.: The psychopathology of articulation and voice deviations. To be published in Travis, L.E. (Ed.) : *Handbook of Speech Pathology.* New York, Appleton-Century-Crofts, 1970.

Rousey, C.L., and Moriarty, A.: *Diagnostic Implications of Speech Sounds: The Reflections of Developmental Conflict and Trauma.* Springfield, Thomas, 1965.

Van Riper, C.: *Speech Correction: Principles and Methods,* 4th ed. Englewood Cliffs, N.J., Prentice Hall, 1963.

Weston, A., and Irwin, J.: The Use of Paired Stimuli in the Modification of Articulation. *J Percept Motor Skills, 32:*947-957, 1971.

CHAPTER TWELVE

THE PROCESS OF THERAPY FOR COMMUNICATIVE DISORDERS

LOUISE M. WARD

Speech pathology and audiology's broad base in human communication is reflected in the verbal construct, "process of therapy for communicative disorders." When one considers how incomplete is our understanding of the nature and function of man's ability to communicate, it is not surprising that the activities of a profession based in this phenomenon are also incomplete. Nevertheless, knowledge evolves by a process of creating new conceptions of the unknown from expanding knowns. This process implies the continual back and forth movement of inquiry from the whole to the part, the general to the specific, the abstract to the concrete. Over time, such inquiry results in new syntheses of both levels, although particular investigations may focus more on one or the other. For example, the investigations of psycholinguistics have been largely focused toward the nature of language, while the investigations of behavior modification have been largely focused toward the shaping of specific behaviors. Eventually the contribution of each will give rise to new syntheses of what is valid in both. The broad base of speech pathology and audiology in human communication implies that any conceptual model of the process of therapy must be considered at best a temporarily useful walking stick along the path of evolving knowledge.

The phrase, *process of therapy*, suggests the dynamic, changing nature of therapy. Therapy is, indeed, a process, not a static entity. Any attempt to conceptualize its critical elements in the present stage of knowledge must be cautious and flexible. This field has had a proliferation of theories and forms of therapy. Such a proliferation is characteristic of an evolving body of knowledge and

351

simply means that the phenomena under consideration are not yet sufficiently understood to allow an encompassing theory and precise forms. It has been the history of other disciplines that as a science evolves, conflicting theories by responsible workers tend to be subsumed under new, more comprehensive theories. In spite of their fragmentary and incomplete nature, the articulation of varied conceptions of the process of therapy for communicative disorders should stir new questions and evolving models. It is in this spirit that this chapter is advanced.

Human development appears to be characterized by movement toward increasing expressiveness of the organism in general and also by increasing sophistication and differentiation of symbolic expressiveness. The increasing expressiveness of the organism in general is seen in such examples as progressive accomplishment of more complex motor tasks or progressive differentiation and development of sexual organs and functions. The increasing sophistication and differentiation of symbolic expressiveness underlies the whole of cognitive development.

It is acknowledged that man's capacity for creating and manipulating symbols is the source both of his highest capabilities and some of his most complex problems. Hayakawa (1949) stated:

> The symbolic process, which makes possible the absurdities of human conduct, also makes possible language and therefore all human achievements dependent upon language (p. 26).

So central to humanness is symbolic expressiveness that no discipline within the science of man can ignore it. Increasing recognition of its centrality to human functioning is evidenced by the place given communication in the scholarship of the behavioral sciences. As Barnlund (1968) points out:

> During the last two decades a number of academic disciplines have been stimulated by viewing some of their persistent problems from the vantage point of communication. Sociologists, social psychologists, speech pathologists and linguists might be expected to find the concepts and terminology of communication congenial to their work. But it is no longer unusual for anthropologists, neurologists, mathematicians and psychotherapists to use similar rationale and vocabulary. No longer can the serious student of communication consider himself adequately informed if he is not familiar with the work of investigators outside his particular specialty (p. 2).

There is reason to believe that the potential for symbolic expression is an innate ability that is part of the given equipment of a human being. Lenneberg (1966) has hypothesized that there may be biological endowments in man that make the human form of communication uniquely possible for our species. He cites evidence supporting his contention as follows: (a) evolution has produced a number of sensory and cognitive specializations in man; (b) the onset and development of speech follow extremely regular developmental schedules in all children, the order of developmental milestones remaining invariable from culture to culture; (c) it is difficult to suppress children's development of language, rudimentary forms appearing even in children who experience physiological trauma or psychological deprivation; (d) language appears and can be nurtured but is extremely difficult to teach; (e) all languages are based on the same universal principles of semantics, syntax, and phonology. In light of this evidence Lenneberg states, ". . . it becomes plausible to hypothesize that language is a species-specific trait, based on a variety of biologically given mechanisms" (p. 69).

While the capacity for symbolic expression appears to be innate, in any specific case the individual's development of it into human communication is subject to a texture of promoting and impeding forces. Thus, in any individual we see a relativistic development of an innate capacity. In certain individuals, however, the impeding forces have attacked the physiological, psychological, and/or neurological integrity of the organism's movement toward symbolic expression in such ways that the acoustic and/or cognitive adequacy of verbal communication is markedly limited. The expression of these impeding forces in the conventional categories of inadequate verbal communication (e.g. stuttering, voice disorders, etc.) are delineated in other chapters of this book. This discussion of the process of therapy for communicative disorders addresses itself to critical elements of the situation in which persons with disordered communication are confronted and helped.

With the initiation of the therapeutic process a new dynamic equation is formed. This equation consists of the clinician and client interacting in a creative directedness toward enhancement and development of the client's potential for adequate speech and language.

Both client and clinician bring to this human equation the uniqueness of their own personhoods. Each brings his own particular configuration of personality, knowledge and experience, his developed and underdeveloped potentialities. Thus, in each new client-clinician interaction there is the quality of a new creation with its decisions and risks. There are, nevertheless, certain general principles and bodies of accumulated knowledge which have bearing on the decisions and risks. Therapy as a process moves between this polarity of the general, as principles and knowledge, and the particular, as the uniqueness of each client-clinician interaction.

The process of therapy appears to consist of three broad types of activity which overlap and interact in circular rather than linear fashion. They do, however, have distinctions which can be recognized for purposes of discussion. These three types of activity are the following: (a) those designed to enhance the forces promoting adequate verbal communication, (b) those designed to reduce the effects of forces which have impeded the development and/or functioning of verbal communication, and (c) those activities designed to integrate the effects of the previous two in developing more effective modes of perceiving, evaluating, and behaving. Identification and evaluational procedures are implied in each of these types of activity, however, these are detailed in another chapter of this book and will not be the focus of this discussion.

These types of activity will be discussed in terms of general principles and criteria which can serve as a framework for application of knowledge specific to the traditional categories of disorders and implementation of forms of therapy specific to each clinician's particular configuration of personality, knowledge and experience.

Activities Designed to Enhance the Forces Promoting Adequate Verbal Communication

As stated earlier, increasing sophistication and differentiation of symbolic expressiveness appears to be a tendency characteristic of human growth and development. The most pervasive form of such symbolic expressiveness is verbal communication in human interactions. A profession committed to alleviate communicative disorders exists by virture of man's stringent need to symbolize his experience to himself and to communicate it meaningfully to others. While modification of the acoustic effect of verbal communication has been the historical focus of this profession and continues to be its major goal, activities designed to enhance verbal communication in human interaction have a significant place in attainment of this goal.

The communicative process between clinician and client is the matrix in which all the activities of therapy take place. This process is the vehicle for interaction, influence, change.

This first type activity is concerned with providing communicative experience which would nurture the client's basic tendency toward verbal communication in human interaction. The clinician's task is to utilize the clinician-client communicative process in ways which respect the client's individuality and also promote his ability to interact with others with greater relative satisfaction, security and productivity. Whether such communication is referred to as "establishing rapport," "getting the client's involvement," "social motivation," "indirect therapy," or in other terminology, it is recognized implicity, if not explicitly, as a dimension of the process of therapy.

It seems important to consider what characteristics of the communicative process allow people to use their potentialities more constructively and cooperatively. At the present time most of the studies of such characteristics of the communicative process between clinician and client have been done outside the field of speech pathology and audiology. Barnlund (1968) attempts to describe in summary form the attributes of a communicative relationship that are likely to contribute to social and psychological health. He considers that a constructive communicative relationship is likely when:

1. there is a willingness to become involved with the other person, i.e. a willingness to concentrate on this situation, this person and this message.
2. one or both persons communicate positive regard for the other in

that the other is valued as a human being and there is respect for his integrity; this attribute is conveyed more by presence and attitude than by explicit statement.

3. there is a permissive climate which allows the communicants to express and explore their experience openly and honestly.

4. there is a desire and capacity to listen without anticipating, interfering, competing, or forcing meanings into preconceived channels of interpretation.

5. emphatic understanding is communicated, i.e. when one participates as fully as he can in the meaning the speaker's experience has for him.

6. there is accurate reflection and clarification of feeling, which of all verbal techniques seems most appropriate to apply widely to the ordinary interactions of men.

7. the communicators are genuine and congruent, the opposite of presenting a facade in the interest of maintaining a particular image in the eyes of the other (p. 638 and following).

While Barnlund acknowledges that these verbal behaviors and attitudes were first enunciated for psychotherapy, he believes good communication, free communication, within or between man, is always therapeutic. As Lennard and Bernstein (1960) state:

Our position is that the social sciences and the depth psychological fields have developed concepts useful for description and analysis of human interactions of all kinds, whether they occur in a therapeutic setting, a family setting, a political decision—making group or social work supervisory conference. In our view, many of the basic questions regarding the nature of interaction, communication, influence and change are the same for all the relationships listed (p. 1).

Certainly persons with communicative disorders have experienced some degree of lack in the fullness of human communicative experience. Thus providing some amount of the most constructive communication possible is considered to have an important effect on the perceiving, evaluating, and behaving of such persons.

In attempting to provide therapeutic communicative experience, it has seemed important to simplify the communicative environment of the client to the level of his ability to assume responsibility and to provide for successive approximations in the direction of increased responsibility. Special type situations and interactions have been created which have allowed for maximum simplification of the communicative process for the client and maximum attention on the part of the clinician to behaving consistently with the attributes of a therapeutic communicative relationship. Such situations have been designated as play therapy, communicative play, counseling, role playing, etc. It is important, however, to point out that therapeutic communication is not limited to such situations. Ruesch (1961) says:

> Communication is a universal function of man that is not tied to any particular place, time, or context; and basically communication which produces a therapeutic effect in no way differs from what happens in ordinary interchanges. Therapeutic communication, therefore, is not confined to an appointed hour in the doctor's office. On the contrary, it occurs almost anywhere—on the play field, in battle, on the ward, at home, or at work. Neither is it bound to the use of certain props such as couch or chair, nor does it run off according to a special formula. . . . . Therapy is done all day long by many people who do not know they act as therapists, and many people benefit from such experiences without knowing it. Therapeutic communication is not a method invented by physicians to combat illness; it is simply something that occurs spontaneously everywhere in daily life, and the physician is challenged to make these naturally occurring events happen more frequently (p. 30-31).

Communicative play, counseling and role-playing situations, used in a variety of ways by different clinicians, have the advantage of focusing the communicative interactions more intensively toward therapeutic communication and for many clients are a valid and significant part of the process of therapy.

This dimension of activity within the process of therapy for communicative disorders may occur in situations designed especially for this purpose or it may be more of a quality running through a variety of situations. It is properly called an activity because it requires active attention and careful participation on the part of the clinician, but can occur as an integral thread of the fabric of the clinician-client communication whether it be in a two minute walk down the hall or in a communicative play or counseling situation.

Van Riper (1957) seemed to be making a similar point when

he took the position that stuttering always involves a disturbance in interpersonal relationships and speech clinicians should be sophisticated enough in the knowledge of psychotherapy that whatever is done in symptom modification would not interfere with psychotherapeutic change (p. 879). Attention to this type activity has been more prevalent in the literature on stuttering than most other communicative disorders. It seems likely that this may be more a historical accident than necessarily reflecting only the uniqueness of stuttering. The contribution of persons who stutter to the development of the literature in this area would have given a "playing field" orientation in this area rather than the "grand-stand" orientation of the literature in other areas. In no other area have the major contributors to theories and therapies been participants in the day by day living with the effects of the disorder rather than experiencing these effects only by looking on from the outside. It seems reasonable that the uniqueness of the client's particular configuration of personality, rather than the type disorder, would determine the kind and amount of therapeutic communicative experience. It also seems that any person who has lived whatever number of years with a communicative disorder has experienced some lacks and thus has legitimate needs in this area.

In an age where there is such broad concern for better qualities of communication which would allow people to communicate more constructively and cooperatively, professional personnel dealing with communicative disorders should be increasingly aware of these qualities. There is a rich microcosm for such continuing study in each client-clinician relationship.

Activities Designed to Reduce the Effects of Forces Which Have Impeded Development and/or Functioning of Verbal Communication

The goal of this type activity is to increase the intrinsic power of the client's capabilities for development of verbal communication. Such activities may be corrective or may be compensatory. They may be done inside this profession or through referral to other professional specialties or through some joint endeavor of several professional specialties.

Here again the communicative process between clinician and client is the matrix in which the clinician uses his knowledge, experience and constructive concern to identify and evaluate the effects of impeding forces and institute procedures which would appear to restore in so far as possible the physiological, neurological and/or psychological integrity of the client's basic capacity to communicate.

In time sequence the majority of the activity designed to reduce impeding forces may precede the majority of the activity designed to enhance forces promoting verbal communication. This latter type was discussed first because of its application to broadly human communicative needs which nevertheless may have particular urgency in persons with disordered communication. It becomes obvious that in actual practice there is no clear-cut point at which the three types of activity are separated.

Just as this profession has borrowed heavily from bodies of knowledge developed in other disciplines, so too it stands in an interdependent relationship with other professional specialties in the accomplishment of its goals. Especially for restoring the structural and functional integrity of the client's capacity to communicate, medical treatment, surgical correction or prosthetic compensation often indicate referral to the medical and dental professions. Psychological specialties may be indicated for evaluation, treatment and/or consultation in determining compensatory procedures and/or corrective treatment. Various other professionals such as regular classroom teachers, special education teachers, social workers, rehabilitation counselors, physical therapists, etc., often participate in achieving the goal of this dimension of the process of therapy.

Efforts to reduce the effects of forces which have impeded development and/or functioning of verbal communication may indicate the extension of the clinician's abilities through referral to other professions. However, modification of a variety of intrapersonal, interpersonal and extrapersonal variables which contribute to increasing the client's intrinsic capacity for adequate communication also fall within the province of this profession.

Some activities may be directed toward the client himself and others may be directed toward modification of his environment.

Familiar activities designed for reducing impeding forces in the client himself include provision of hearing aids, auditory training, perceptual-motor training, concept-symbol training, relaxation training, and muscle control. While therapeutic communicative experience was discussed as enhancing the basic drive toward communication with application to the broad base of communication, it also has functions applicable here.

As stated earlier, referral to psychological specialties may be indicated for severely impeding forces in this area, however, many activities within this profession provide corrective emotional experience and thus increase the client's psychological integrity. Individual clinicians have different degrees of competency in this area but each should have intelligent awareness of his strengths and limitations. Backus (1952) stressed "regions of shared activity" with the field of psychotherapy stating that: (a) each field should share with the other at the level of theory, i.e. the subject matter of each should stem from a common scientific base; (b) each should have a knowledge of the working principles of the other; (c) each should share with the other an area at the level of clinical practice.

Modification of the client's environment may be done through work with important persons in the environment. For example, counseling of a child's parents will be discussed by Webster (Chap. 13) . Environmental modification may include providing of appropriate social experiences, development of vocational skills or providing for other experiential lacks. It may also include specific environmental controls such as absence of distracting stimuli, inhibition of movement, etc.

This dimension of activity occupies an important place in alleviating communicative disorders; however, as McDonald (1964) has pointed out, the human being has amazing ability to compensate for deficiencies of structure and/or function except where a deficiency is too gross or when several deficiencies coexist, any one of which, by itself, might be compensated for by the individual.

Activities Designed to Develop Effective Modes of Perceiving, Evaluating, and Behaving

The two previous types of activity are applied to the dynamics of communication while this type activity applies to the form. That is to say, the first two are directed toward the forces under-lying man's communication while this type is directed toward the modes of its manifestation. At any given time acceptance and/or development of one or the other pole of this relation may have temporary precedence. Ultimately, however, the uniqueness of this client's own selfhood must find expression while adapting to his need to establish an appropriate relation to the outside world. Actual communication unites dynamics and form, for what is real must have form and the form must be adequate to the dynam-ics it represents.

In attempting to develop more adequate modes of perceiving, evaluating and behaving in verbal communication we see the bipolar, yet interactive, self-world relation characteristic of human communication and indeed, all of human life. A major criterion for all the activities of therapy is that they express an adequate self-world relation. The two-fold dynamism of man's tendency toward symbolic expressiveness and the organism's capacity for expressiveness are realized only in the forms of its manifestation as human communication.

In activities designed to develop more adequate modes of per-ceiving, the clinician is concerned with helping the client develop more differentiated perception. A major direction of this activity is toward the acoustic effect of voice, articulation rate and rhythm in speech production. Perception of similarities and differences may be directed toward any of the range and variety of character-istics of the clients own speech and that of others in various situa-tions at various points in time. The clinician is concerned with maximum utilization of all the channels of perception in pro-moting such differentiated modes of perceiving.

More differentiated perception of language forms for many clients will be an important direction of activities. The forms of such activity through semantics, syntax and morphology will include perception of the uniqueness of the client's own language forms and perception of the language forms of others.

More accurate and differentiated perception of the total communicative situation is also a needed development for many clients. Perceiving the character of the communicative situation before one at a given time, its demands and risks, like all the activity of perception, ties in closely with evaluation.

Effective modes of evaluating are rooted in the client's differentiated perception of the communicative situation, his own speech and language forms and those of others. The clinician is concerned with promoting the client's appropriate use of his evaluative abilities. Common target areas for evaluation are the client's immediate and long-term goals for communication, paths he has taken in meeting these goals and consequences of his ways of coping with communicative situations. The client often needs more adequate evaluative procedures in differentiating his own responsibility and that of others, assessing others' reactions to his communication and appraising his own abilities and level of functioning.

The clinician promotes modes of evaluation which are differentiated. He encourages the client to use modes of evaluation which are based on perceptual data rather than broad generalizations, open to change with the availability of new data and formed in thought patterns of "in what ways" and "to what extent" rather than "either—or" concepts such as success or failure, good or bad, etc.

The development of more effective modes of perceiving and evaluating is the foundation of more effective modes of behaving. A multiplicity of specific behaviors may be targets for modification through the activities of the clinician-client interaction. Such activities attempt to build on the client's present abilities. Goals, though sequential, continue closely enough related to present abilities to provide reinforcement for experimentation with and successive approximations at desired behaviors. The specific modes of behaving are developed within the context of appropriate self-world relation in order that the giving and receiving nature of communication is expressed.

Finally, it should be noted that the three types of activity which comprise the process of therapy for communicative disorders are present in each client-clinician relationship. The kind and amount of each type is determined by the particular conditions in each concrete situation.

It was stated earlier that inquiry moves back and forth from the whole to the part, the general to the specific, the abstract to the concrete. This discussion has considered the process of therapy for communicative disorders from a holistic viewpoint. In deciding to take this viewpoint, one takes on the risk of any decision—the inescapable threat of excluded possibilities. Cherry (1966), in discussing the study of human communication pointed out that there are both values and dangers in "intense cultivation of small gardens of specialized interest" and to the values and dangers of broad attempts at unification. It is only in acknowledging the dangers and trusting there will be values that one overcomes the threat of excluded possibilities enough to discuss, at all, so complex an endeavor as the process of therapy for communicative disorders.

REFERENCES

Backus, O.: Collaboration among psychiatrists, pediatricians, clinical psychologists and speech therapists. *Nervous Child, 9:* 1952.

Barnlund, C.: *Interpersonal Communication: Survey and Studies.* New York, Houghton-Mifflin, 1968.

Cherry, C.: *On Human Communication.* Cambridge, M.I.T. Press, 1966.

Hayakawa, S.I.: *Language in Thought and Action.* New York, Harcourt, 1949.

Lennard, H., and Bernstein, A.: *The Anatomy of Psychotherapy: Systems of Communication and Expectation.* New York, Columbia U Press, 1960.

Lenneberg, E.H.: A biological perspective of language. In Lenneberg, E. H. (Ed.): *New Directions in the Study of Language.* Cambridge, M.I.T. Press, 1966.

McDonald, E.T.: *Articulation Testing and Treatment: A Sensory-Motor Approach.* Pittsburgh, Stanwix House, 1964.

Ruesch, J.: *Therapeutic Communication.* New York, Norton, 1961.

Van Riper, C.: Symptomatic therapy for stuttering. In Travis, L. (Ed.): *Handbook of Speech Pathology.* New York, Appleton-Century, 1957.

Webster, E.J.: Parents of children with communication disorders. In Weston, A. (Ed.): *Communicative Disorders: An Appraisal.* Springfield, Thomas, 1971.

CHAPTER THIRTEEN

PARENTS OF CHILDREN WITH COMMUNICATION DISORDERS

ELIZABETH J. WEBSTER

At this stage of knowledge about parents of children with speech, hearing, and language disorders, it is necessary to keep our generalizations tentative. Although a number of studies have been done with these parents, we still know little about ways in which parents of communicatively handicapped children differ from parents of children who develop communication within normal range.

Another caution against overgeneralization arises from the fact that many of the studies have involved mothers rather than both parents. There are two reasons for this fact. First, in our society, mothers bear chief responsibility for child rearing. The second reason for the paucity of studies of fathers is that their working hours often make them unavailable for research. Therefore, we must understand that we infer about parents from information largely obtained from groups of mothers.

It is obvious that grouped data about variables found in mothers do not reveal problems faced by an individual mother. Nor do these data reveal how a mother's problems may be compounded when she interacts with her family. Thus, it is necessary to avoid global judgments about the nature of individual mothers, about fathers, and about the family's interactions; indeed it is prudent to try to delay judgment until we have information about those individuals and their interactions.

Because of these limitations on our knowledge about parents of children with disorders, we are not yet certain about how best to help them. However, where professional personnel deal with children with disorders, they also deal with those children's parents. And the needs of parents and their children are impelling;

they cannot wait for further studies. Professionals must work from available knowledge. They must also work from a value system in which they attempt to assist children, to assist their parents, and to damage neither in the process.

In order to provide a frame of reference in which to think about work with parents of children with communication disorders, this chapter will (a) discuss various viewpoints about such parents; (b) suggest implications of these conceptions; and (c) suggest several directions for further study.

VIEWPOINTS ABOUT PARENTS OF CHILDREN WITH COMMUNICATION DISORDERS

In the field of speech pathology there has been a tendency to consider parental attitudes and parent-child interactions as significant factors in the development and maintenance of certain language and speech disorders. For example, Johnson (1946, 1957) and Bloodstein (1952) linked stuttering to parental functions of labeling and reacting to a child's nonfluencies; Moncur (1951, 1952) linked stuttering with parental domination. Clinicians who follow these lines of reasoning advocate counseling for parents of stuttering children either as an integral part of the child's therapy program, or in preference to direct work with the child if he is just beginning to stutter. In the same vein, it has been thought that parents of children with cerebral palsy play a vital role in their children's development of language and speech; these parents have been included in various ways in their children's treatment programs (e.g. Bice, 1952; Denhoff and Robinault, 1960).

Thus, parents of children with certain types of communication problems have received considerable attention from clinicians and researchers. Parents of children with other types of disorders have received less attention. However, studies such as those by Beckey (1942) and Wood (1946) raised questions regarding possible relationships between parental attitudes and/or behaviors and such other communication disorders as defective articulation, delayed language, etc.

Currently the trend in speech pathology seems to be toward a broader view which considers parent-child interactions as possibly influencing all types of communication disorders (Beasley, 1956; Wyatt, 1962; McDonald, 1962). Many professional persons think that parent-child interactions are so central as to effect every aspect of the child's development, including his language and speech development. Therefore, speech pathologists now assess parent-child relationships as a basic part of the diagnostic workup. Many clinicians also advocate some form of parent counseling for numbers of parents; their judgment of which parents need counseling now seems based more on their assessment of parent-child relationships and less on the category of disorder the child presents. Some clinicians (Rittenour, 1964; Webster, 1966) consider parents as the central members of their child's treatment team, viewing professional personnel as serving an adjunctive role to that of the parent.

Parents as Reinforcers of Communication Disorders

Parents' roles in the causation of communication disorders still are unclear. Professional personnel agree that the child's communicative environment plays a major role in shaping his language and speech behavior (Kanner, 1950; Lewis, 1951; McCarthy, 1952, 1953, 1954; Peckarsky, 1953; Murphy and Fitzsimons, 1960; Wyatt, 1962; Deutsch, 1967; Filippi and Rousey, 1968). It is axiomatic that the child's parents play the earliest and most important roles in his environment.

Perhaps, as Beasley (1956) postulated, stressful environmental variables are crucial in the acquisition and maintenance of inadequate communication. Beasley stated:

> Since a child develops speech in an interpersonal setting, speech or language difficulties inevitably mean that he has encountered emotional stress within his family deeper or different than that of a child who has developed adequate speaking skill. Disorders such as mutism, faulty articulation, or stuttering may have occurred as a child's way of coping with unfavorable attitudes and treatment from family members. Disorders of other kinds, as those associated with cleft palate, hearing loss, or brain injury, may have been aggravated in the child as much by the expectations, disappointments and anxieties of the family members as by the original organic involvement (p. 317).

Mowrer (1950) believed that warm and loving communicative relationships were essential if the child was to acquire normal language and speech. Mowrer saw the child's earliest speech sounds as reflecting his attempts to call back or recapture objects and relationships, including the warm feelings associated with the attentions of his mother.

McCarthy (1952; 1953) also cited evidence to support the centention that psychic strain imposed by the environment may prevent rapid or adequate speech development. McCarthy (1954) concluded from her studies of parents and children that the atmosphere in the home, as determined by the parents' personalities, seems to be the most important single factor influencing the child's acquisition of language.

Particularly noteworthy on the subject of environmental influences on speech development is such work as that of Goldfarb (1945), in which he cited evidence of children developing severely disordered speech as an aftermath of severe psychological deprivation. Brodbeck and Irwin (1946) also reported serious language and speech deficits in children placed in an orphanage at an early age.

Although environmental factors are crucial to the child's language and speech, we cannot overlook the fact that each child also acts on his environment. The child's own unique physiology and personality help to shape the environment in which he will develop language and speech. When we view the communicative equation as including the uniquenesses of the child, his parents, and their interactions with each other, it is inaccurate to say that parents or parental functions are the cause of a communication disorder. Rather, it is more accurate to say that parents and parental functions play a part in the development of the disorder, while the child and his functions also play a part in its development. Wolpe (1957) summed up this thinking when she said, "It is neither the parents nor the child who are responsible for the emergence of a problem . . . It is a two-way channel, and the parent is neither entitled to total credit nor to total blame for the child's behavior" (p. 1016).

It is quite likely that parents and/or parental functions serve to reinforce and maintain a child's communication disorder. However, we still are unclear about the mechanism by which parents reinforce disordered communication. Perhaps parents' personalities play an important part; perhaps their attitudinal responses to the child are important variables. Professional persons no longer rely on the simplistic explanation that children's communication disorders arise from the absence of "good speech models" (McCarthy, 1954). Lack of speech models cannot be the whole story because so many children speak more adequately than do their parents (Deutsch, 1967). Further, we no longer think children learn their communication skills simply through imitation (Lenneberg, 1966; McNeill, 1966; Dees, 1970). However, parents do provide attitudinal and behavioral models with which the child identifies and which contribute to the child's subsequent adequacy in communication.

The next section will discuss various attitudinal and behavioral variables found in parents whose children have communication disorders.

Information about Parents of Children with Communication Disorders

Findings on the subject of differences between parents of communicatively handicapped children and parents of normally speaking children are somewhat equivocal, but they may indicate some attitudinal and behavioral differences.

Wood's (1946) study sought to describe emotional adjustment of both mothers and fathers of children with articulatory defects. Fifty sets of parents were studied. Emotional adjustment was rated by means of the California Test of Personality, the Bernreuter Personality Inventory, and the Thematic Apperception Test. Wood found that at least one parent in each of the fifty sets was rated as emotionally maladjusted. From these data Wood concluded that parental emotional factors may be important in the etiology of articulation defects. He also believed these emotional factors must be dealt with in any corrective treatment for the child.

Despert (1945) reported that many of the mothers of stuttering children she studied had personality profiles tending toward obsessive-compulsiveness. Goodstein and Dahlstrom (1956) also reported maladaptive personality characteristics in parents of stuttering children. Other observers (see, for example, Murphy and Fitzsimons, 1960) concur that children's maladaptive behavior reflects maladaptive parental attitudes and behaviors; nevertheless, these observers caution that many parental problems are not classifiable as serious psychological disturbances.

Moll and Darley (1960) studied attitudes of a group of mothers of children with articulation disorders and a group of mothers of children diagnosed as having delayed speech. Each of the two groups was compared with a group of mothers of normally speaking children. The investigators administered the Parental Attitude Research Instrument (PARI) and Wiley's Attitudes Toward the Behavior of Children (ATBC). Although these scales as a whole did not isolate differences among the three groups of parents, differences were observed on three of the PARI subscales. These indicated that mothers of speech-retarded children were reluctant to permit their children to express their feelings and problems verbally. Mothers of the speech-retarded also indicated a reluctance to permit their children to take part in family discussions. Mothers of children with articulation disorders differed from those in the control group on two scales within the factor of "Excessive Demand for Striving"; this finding was interpreted to mean that mothers of articulatory-impaired children tend to have high standards for their children and tend to be dissatisfied with their children's present activities and accomplishments. Moll and Darley also stated that such high maternal standards and general disapproval of the child's functioning may be related causally to the speech defect, or may be partially an effect of the child's speech problem.

Other researchers have reported that parents of children with communication disorders set high standards for their children. For example, Goldman and Shames (1964a; 1946b) described two studies of goal-setting behavior by parents of children who stutter. The investigators hypothesized that parents of stuttering children set higher goals for themselves than do parents of nonstuttering children. In their first study (1964a), goal-setting behavior was

measured by obtaining a parent's pretest estimate of his performance on a Rotter Board motor coordination task; the parent's estimate of his performance was then compared with his actual task
performance. The authors found that "Parents of stutterers and
parents of non-stutterers did not differ significantly in goal-setting
behavior for themselves . . . " In their second study (1964b), the
authors investigated whether differences exist in the goals set for
their children by parents of stutterers and parents of nonstutterers. Goal-setting behavior was measured by having the parents
predict their children's performances on two tasks: (a) the Rotter
Board motor coordination task and (b) telling a story. Parents of
stuttering children were found to set higher goals for their children generally, as measured by their Rotter Board prediction, and
higher speech goals, as measured by their prediction of their children's story-telling performance, than did parents of nonstutterers.

Johnson (1946) also observed that parents of stuttering children set perfectionistic standards for their children. He particularly noted high parental standards with respect to cleanliness,
toilet training, eating habits, and speech.

In another study of attitudes of parents of children who stutter, Kinstler (1961), attempted to measure the variable of maternal rejection. Kinstler defined two types of rejection: overt, i.e.
open and direct, and covert, i.e. more subtle and hidden. He then
developed a "self inventory projective questionnaire" designed to
measure overt and covert rejection. The questionnaire was administered to thirty mothers of young stuttering boys and thirty
control mothers. Kinstler found significant differences between
the two groups of mothers in their patterns of responses, which he
summarized as follows:

> (a) Mothers of young male stutterers reject their children cov-
> ertly far more but overtly far less than do mothers of normal speakers.
> (b) Mothers of stutterers accept their children covertly less and
> overtly only slightly more than do the mothers of normal speakers.
> (c) Mothers of stutterers reject their children more than they
> accept them while mothers of normal speakers accept their children
> more than they reject them.

Filippi and Rousey (1968) have been interested in observing

communication patterns in parents of young nonverbal children whose lack of communication cannot be accounted for by physiological problems. The first pattern they reported is a marked lack of pleasant verbal communication between the child's parents; often these parents engage in discourse with each other only in anger or annoyance. The second pattern which emerges is lack of verbal communication between parents and child.

> They (the parents) are at a loss to an unusual degree to know what to say to their child. They are actually uncomfortable just to talk with him. When left to their own devices to relate to him they are either attempting to 'teach him something' or engage in some nonverbal activity (p. 320).

Filippi and Rousey suggested that the child's lack of verbal communication is associated both with his attempts to emulate the models provided by the parents and with his extreme ambivalence about the purposes of speech in communication.

Eaton (1967) found some indication that parents of children with organically based communication disorders may be less responsive to their environment, and thus less responsive with their children, than are parents of normally speaking children. She compared parents of children with organically based disorders with parents of children with normal communication. She assessed personality attributes through the Draw-A-Person procedure, Travis Projective Pictures, Jourard Self-disclosure Scale, and Jersild Self-concept Scale. From the analysis of these tests, Eaton concluded, "Statistically significant differences were found only in contact dimensions measured by an objective scale for scoring the Draw-A-Person test and the Travis Picture responses" (p. 54). Parents of children with organically based handicaps did more poorly with contact dimensions than did control parents. On the other hand, findings of a study by Gerth (1969) suggested that parents of children with communication disorders may be very sensitive to the details of their environment, and thus sensitive to their children. Gerth administered the Myers-Briggs Type Indicator, designed to measure normal dimensions of personality, to a group of mothers of children with various types of speech and hearing disorders and to a group of control mothers whose children communicated normally. More mothers of the communicatively handicapped preferred the personality category labelled "Sensing" than did control mothers, indicating a preference in the former for direct perception by way of sensory modalities and indicating attention to details of the environment.

It has been postulated that perhaps parents of children with communication disorders are more sensitive to variations in speech than they are to other aspects of their children's behavior. To test this hypothesis, Berlin (1960) assessed parents with respect to their sensitivity to stuttering. Berlin presented contrived and controlled samples of nonfluent speech under two conditions to a group of parents of children who stuttered, a group of parents of children with misarticulations, and a group of parents of normally speaking children. In Condition 1 each parent was asked if the child's speech caused concern, and if so, what caused the concern; in Condition 2 the parent was asked if the child stuttered. Mothers of normally speaking children did not change their diagnoses significantly from Condition 1 to Condition 2, but parents in the other two groups diagnosed significantly more stuttering in Condition 2 than they did in Condition 1. Berlin concluded in part that the wording of the instructions seemed to be a factor in parental diagnoses; when the word *stuttering* was introduced in the directions, parents diagnosed more stuttering. Berlin also concluded that "parents of stuttering children were not unusually intolerant of nonfluency compared to the other parents, since members of all parent groups misdiagnosed some normal nonfluency as stuttering."

Laubenthal (1970) also reported findings on mothers' sensitivity to their children's communication disorder. She used Flanagan's Critical Incident Technique (1954) in individual interviews with mothers of children with communication disorders. Laubenthal asked mothers to describe specifically (a) aspects of their children's behaviors that they liked, and (b) aspects of their children's behaviors that they disliked. She found that in her population, mothers were able to describe their children's behavior in great detail. Laubenthal reported:

. . .mothers seemed very aware of and able to describe children's behaviors. This ability was evidenced not only by the numbers of Critical Incidents offered, but also by the specificity of details of description. Many times these descriptions were not prompted by specific questions asked by the interviewer, but initiated by the mother as she discussed what her child was doing in school, how he got along with siblings, etc.

Mothers in this population were as able to describe their children's general behavior as they were to describe their children's speech behavior; i.e. in this situation, these mothers did not overemphasize their children's communicative behavior and difficulty with communication (p. 37).

Laubenthal reported further that these mothers offered more incidents describing behavioral characteristics of their children that they liked than that they disliked, although she thought it possible that in an initial interview situation mothers might be reluctant to describe their children's undesirable behaviors.

Parents' Experience of Stress

Even as parents produce stressful situations for their children, they also experience stress. Certainly parenthood *per se* imposes its unanswerable questions, quandaries, and anxieties. Perhaps these are different or more constant for some parents; perhaps the important variables are those related to ways in which parents express their troubled feelings. Various authors have attempted to conceptualize the distress parents experience in relation to their communicatively handicapped children, but again we do not yet know whether parents of children who develop communication disorders experience greater or different stress than do other parents.

Several authors (e.g. Beasley, 1956; Matis, 1961; McDonald, 1962; Rittenour, 1964; Webster, 1966) have stated that parents of communicatively handicapped children experience guilt in relation to these children. Parents question what they have done to cause or compound the disorder. They wonder if they might have taken steps which would have prevented or alleviated the child's condition. Experience indicates that many parents harbor such feelings of guilt, whether or not there is physiological causation in the child's condition.

Parents of the communicatively handicapped are also thought to experience anxiety in relation to their children (Wolpe, 1957; Murphy and Fitzsimons, 1960; Rittenour, 1964). Parents' anxiety may take the form of worrying about the future of their children (McDonald, 1962). This anxiety may be reflected in a variety of ways: questions about the child's mental abilities, his educational possibilities, his social and emotional future. Parents often ask, "Will my child be able to go to a regular classroom?" or "What will happen to him when other children tease him about his speech?" Such questions reflect concern for the child's future. These parents recognize that communication is central to human life and so they worry about the child's future well-being if he cannot communicate adequately.

Many parents also experience embarrassing situations because of their child's communication problem (McDonald, 1962). Often other family members, neighbors, and friends may volunteer quantities of advice about what to do for the child, sometimes embarrassing if not confusing the parent (McDonald, 1962; Laubenthal, 1970). Other parents feel so sensitive to their child's disorder as to feel other people stare at the child as if in ridicule of them and their child (Webster, 1968).

McDonald (1962) also has reminded professional personnel that no parent really likes to hear that there is something wrong with his child, and may resist the person who tells him so. This seems important to keep in mind. Very often clinicians confirm a parent's fears about his child by delineating and describing the child's problem. It seems inevitable that we will meet parents' expressions of disappointment, distress, or resentment.

IMPLICATIONS OF THESE CONCEPTIONS FOR WORK WITH PARENTS

The question is not *whether* professional persons should involve parents in their child's treatment; parents are always involved in some way in what happens to their children. A more constructive question seems to be, "In what ways should we involve parents?" It is likely that many parents of children with communication disorders need to be actively included in their child's treatment program.

Clinicians sometimes also wonder who should do the direct work with parents. It is this writer's assertion that even as speech pathologists, audiologists, special educators and other professionals, *do in fact* have direct contact with parents, they also *should* do this, i.e. it is right and proper that we should and do deal directly with parents. In this view, constructive questions center around the kind of approach we will take in encounters with parents. We must question how we shall ask parents to involve themselves in their child's treatment, how we shall treat the parents themselves, whether we shall seek out parent contacts or wait till parents come to us, and how we can make parent-clinician contacts therapeutic.

Again, our knowledge is incomplete in relation to these questions, but at this date there seem to be two major avenues utilized by professional persons in dealing with parents. These avenues are (a) parent counseling, and (b) training of parents for direct work with their children.

PARENT COUNSELING

Let us first consider what the term counseling means. It is often used as a synonym for *therapy* or *a therapeutic approach*. It is widely recognized that therapy can take place in a variety of interpersonal encounters, whatever the initial reason for the contact (Mowrer, 1964; MacLennan and Felsenfeld, 1968; Brodey, 1968). Rogers (1951) illustrated the point when he stated that a variety of professionals utilize a therapeutic approach:

> . . .we find educators who are eager to keep pace with the development (in counseling and psychotherapy) in order that they may adapt and use these findings through the work of school and college counselors and adjustment teachers. Ministers and religious workers are seeking training in counseling and psychotherapy in order to improve their skill in dealing with personal problems of their parishioners. Sociologists and social psychologists have a keen interest in this field because of its possible adaptations to work with groups, and because it helps to shed light on the dynamics of groups as well as individuals. And last, but far from least, the average citizen is supporting the rapid extension of psychotherapeutic work. . . (p. 3).

Thus, any professional person who attempts to use interpersonal encounters therapeutically can be said to be utilizing a counseling approach. The counseling approach is thought of as the process which underlies one person's attempts to implement therapeutic attitudes and perspectives toward another in an interpersonal encounter. The crucial feature of a counseling approach seems to be centered in attitudes rather than in techniques or situations; counseling techniques stem from the counselor's attitudes, values and experience.

Clinicians perform counseling functions when they give information, assist clients to cope with issues which face them in light of this information, and help clients explore and clarify their roles. Thus, it does not seem to be a leap from logic that clinicians also should consider themselves as counselors. Therefore, in this section on Parent Counseling the terms *clinician* and *counselor* will be used interchangeably.

Counseling requires continuous decision-making. The counselor's primary decision seems to be made at low levels: First, there is the stratum at which he decides the basic values, attitudes and goals to which he will commit himself and from which he will attempt to respond. At the second level the counselor makes on-the-spot decisions about his responses as each counseling session unfolds. Notice the use of the word "attempt." No counselor can implement his basic values, attitudes and goals 100 per cent of the time. As Rogers (1951; 1961; 1967) pointed out, the important factors are the counselor's willingness to see where he strays from his basic values and his attempt to return once again to their implementation.

This author (Webster, 1966) has maintained that the many varieties of clinician-parent contacts can be thought of as opportunities for parent counseling, whether they are short-term contacts, as for example, in a one-session diagnostic interview, or whether they are long-term contacts, as in a series of counseling sessions. However, it should be noted that, as Russell and Halfond (1965) pointed out, clinicians cannot hope to adequately counsel parents if they do it in brief, hurried contacts.

The next section will discuss some attitudinal variables thought to be important when clinicians approach parent counseling.

An Approach to Parents and Parent Counseling

The clinician must decide his rationale for parent counseling. Traditionally, many clinicians have seemed to verbalize a rationale which makes the child the central concern and work with parents an additional channel for helping the child (Wolpe, 1957; Denhoff and Robinault, 1960; Matis, 1961; Rittenour, 1964; Webster, 1966). The view that the child is the central concern, and that parent counseling is adjunctive to the chief work of clinicians, seems to lead to a narrow, if not dangerous, rationale for counseling. It is this writer's opinion that clinicians should try to operate in a frame of reference which is more parent-centered than child-centered.

Indeed, in the view presented here, we should enlarge our notions to embrace parents as an additional clinical population. Traditionally, clinicians have thought of attempting to meet needs of children and/or adults with such classified communication disorders as stuttering, articulation disorder, hearing impairment, etc. Granted that parents of children with communication disorders come to us by the route of concern for their children, it is erroneous to consider the route by which they arrive for help as descriptive of their total human needs. These parents have their own difficulties, including their own difficulties with communication. They may not visualize a need for counseling—or they may. But it seems most productive for clinicians to think of parents as people with human needs, people who may be in trouble and who need help. The clinician can then go on to teach each parent for his own sake, a procedure which is consistent with the clinical approach of treating each client as a unique individual.

As the clinician interacts with the parent as the client who is his immediate concern, he has many opportunities to develop positive regard for that person.

Murphy and Fitzsimons (1960) reflected a basically positive view of parents when they stated,

> Most parents want to do right by their child. They want to be the good parent and to have a good parent-child relationship—no matter how far removed their day-to-day course of interaction appears to take them from this aspiration (p. 423).

Beasley (1956) urged the professional worker to reach out to parents "as people who are operating in the best way they know at the moment, who probably have a lowered sense of self-worth because of the difficulties the child is having, and who have need to express their doubts and uncertainties" (p. 317).

Other authors (Wolpe, 1957; Wyatt, 1962, Rittenour, 1964; Webster, 1966; Satir, 1967) concurred that parents may seek help for their child because they experience a breakdown in communication with that child and seek to alleviate the communication difficulty. These authors viewed the parent's desire for better communication with his child as a growth-promoting factor.

These essentially positive approaches presume the counselor's respect for parents as individuals, his acceptance of their wish to do what they see as right for their children, and his understanding that parents have needs of their own.

The clinician's development of a more parent-oriented approach and his positive view of parents as clients will govern the manner in which he will counsel them. Murphy and Fitzsimons (1960) discussed options open to clinicians:

> It (parent counseling) may embrace many approaches and many levels of intensity from supportive to reconstructive therapy. Treatment may be authoritarian or directive, concerning itself with the intellectual imparting of information concerning the child, his speech symptom, and the best methods of coping with the . . problem. Or counseling may be client-centered, focusing upon feelings, attitudes, insights, and the parent's inner capability to find emotional growth (p. 426).

The parent-oriented clinician can develop his compassion for parents. He will learn more often to avoid what Murphy and Fitzsimons (1960) called "directive advice-giving therapy," some dangers of which they listed as the following: (a) the parent may experience emotionally debilitating effects, such as intensified guilt or inadequacy feelings; (b) the clinician-parent exchange is definitely an intellectual one; and (c) parents may develop feelings of ambivalence concerning the clinician's advice, and have no chance to explore these feelings. In preference to advice giving, Murphy and Fitzsimons suggested that clinicians' attitudes should provide for "the discharge and realignment of parental feelings and attitudes rather than the parceling out of advice," and for the possibility that, "The deeper the parent's psychic prejudices are, the more permissive counseling therapy is needed" (p. 427).

If we are not aware of the parent as a client in his own right, we run the risk of manipulating and using that parent for our own short-range purposes to the possible detriment of his long-range needs. We may give the parent advice, instruct him in the care and keeping of speech notebooks, teach him sound games, or show him films; and we may entirely miss his human needs. If we are aware of a given parent as our client-of-concern we may ultimately have him keep a speech notebook, learn a sound game, or see films, but we would do these things because they seem appropriate as the clinician came to know and understand the parent's needs. We would not rely on these procedures because they are our standard way to operate.

A more parent-oriented approach to counseling may avoid several other counselor hang-ups. First, in this approach the counselor need not make judgments about the relative appropriateness of the content parents bring to counseling. The child-oriented clinician may think he has to judge whether or not parent verbalizations relate to the chief concern, i.e. to the child in therapy. If the child-oriented clinician can see that a given parental verbalization relates to the child, the parent may continue; if not, that clinician may feel compelled to divert the parent to clinician-chosen topics. Consider the problems the child-oriented clinician has in responding to a parent who says, "I am so worried about my older boy (who is not in therapy) who is sixteen years old and has started to borrow my car without permission." That clinician is faced with such poor options as trying to stretch the parent's concern to relate to the child in therapy, ignoring the parent's expressed concern so as to "get down to business," or viewing subsequent conversation about the older boy as irrelevant.

The parent-oriented frame of reference also seems likely to avoid some dangerous clinician biases. The logic of biases seems to be that one must be *for* something or someone and *against* something or someone else. In the case of the clinician using a child-oriented rationale it seems quite easy to be biased on the side of the child and against the parents. Clinicians sometimes verbalize their biases very unsubtly, e.g. "Johnny won't talk because he doesn't get a chance;" "He (the child)) would be all right if you (the parents) wouldn't put pressure on him;" etc. Clinicians' biases are a deterrent to adequate parent counseling; several dangers inherent in such biases were elaborated well by Russell and Halfond (1965).

The clinician can develop attitudes of open-mindedness toward parents to the extent that he is willing to become a more open-minded person. To this extent the clinician will be willing to clarify his impressions about parents as he interacts with them. Many authors (Bice, 1952; Rogers, 1951, 1961; Murphy and Fitzsimons, 1960) have stressed the importance of the counselor's ability to listen to the client. Beasley (1956) stated the cogent advice to professionals to "listen to what people are saying— really listen— and *attempt to understand the emotional import* (italics mine) of the topics parents choose to raise, the problems they describe, the observations they make about their child, and the relationships among family members on which they comment (p. 318)." It also seems crucial that the clinician listen to parents with regard to the topics they do not introduce, what they cannot seem to say, and the subjects they discuss with difficulty.

A more parent-centered approach to counseling requires that the counselor attempt to keep in touch with his own emotions so as to be more aware of that with which he approaches parents. This approach also requires a good deal of flexibility and spontaneity on the part of the clinician. Self-awareness, flexibility, and spontaneity, although difficult to develop, are thought to be essential characteristics of clinicians in any successful clinical practice (Ward and Webster, 1965; for an excellent discussion of this point, see Murphy, 1969).

Goals For Parent Counseling

The clinician's goals for parent counseling follow from his decisions regarding his rationale for counseling, his view of parents, and his conceptions of his clinical role. In the view presented here, the parent counselor is encouraged to establish and maintain goals for himself as counselor rather than to set narrow, discreet goals for parents as clients. Said in another way, goals for parent counseling are set with reference to the clinician's functions rather than with reference to describable changes in parents. The clinician bears sole responsibility for making the proper decisions consistent with his values. The clinician does not bear responsibility for the parent's immediate or eventual use of the counseling experience; that responsibility is reserved for the parent.

Goals for clinicians were advanced and elaborated by Backus (1957) in discussing aspects of the therapist's role. They will be restated here only as they relate to the clinician-counselor. For further discussion of crucial elements of the therapeutic process, see Chapter 12 of this text.

First, the clinician attempts to create and maintain an atmosphere in which the parent has a chance to feel free to discuss and clarify issues which confont him (Webster, 1966, 1968). As Murphy and Fitzsimons summarized this goal: "The aim of parent counseling is to provide parents with conditions in which they may find for themselves greater confidence, comfort, and competency" (p. 422).

Within this atmosphere of respect, understanding, and freedom for the parent, the clinician attempts to help the parent reduce some of the barriers which prevent his adequate functioning and productive communication. He attempts to provide parents with successful experiences in discovering, verbalizing, and clarifying attitudes, concerns, and behaviors (Webster, 1966, 1968).

Another of the counselor's goals is to provide the parent with tools for clarifying his attitudes and behaviors. The term *tools* is used here to cover the variety of items the counselor thinks important to include in his own unique counseling situation. Certainly information about the child's disorder is a vital tool for the use of parents; it is the counselor's responsibility to draw on his training and experience to give parents accurate information (McDonald, 1962; Rittenour, 1964; Webster, 1966; Giolas *et al.,*

1968). Other more general tools also may be deemed important by a given clinician in his own counseling program. Matis (1961) introduced parents to the concepts of general semantics as a means of attempting to help them clarify their attitudes toward their children. Sander (1958) described normal speech development for parents so that they could understand this process in their children. This author (1966) elaborated several general tools she thought important to introduce to groups of parents.

Bice (1952) made the point that parents receive much education during the process of counseling, but that such education is meaningful to parents only when they actively seek it and after they have clarified some issues which block their learning.

The clinician's final goal is to provide parents with opportunities to experiment with new modes of dealing with their attitudes and/or behaviors (Webster, 1966, 1968). Other authors have described a similar point of view. For example, Wyatt (1962) stated that the counseling situation can be a "sort of experimental laboratory" where parents can experiment with new ways of looking at problems and can plan more constructive ways of dealing with them.

These goals are probably achieved more readily in long-term counseling where parents have a chance to discuss over time the issues which concern them. Long-term counseling situations also provide opportunities for contrived situations, such as role playing, to supplement discussion (Webster, 1968). However, one cannot overlook the fact that there are always time limitations on clinician-parent contacts; these same goals can be set for himself by the clinician who interacts with parents in a single short period of time as well as by the one who sees parents more frequently.

Forms of Parent Counseling

What has been said previously about parent counseling can be applied to parents seen individually or in groups, in short-term or long-term contacts.

Although clinicians often see both fathers and mothers during the child's diagnostic interview (Rittenour, 1964), when clinicians conduct long-term counseling, their population is largely made up of mothers (Bice, 1952; McDonald, 1962; Russell and Halfond, 1965). The typical pattern of involving mothers in counseling has the advantage of reaching those persons with primary responsibility for implementing child rearing practices; it has such disadvantages in that the two parents may not grow in parallel fashion (Satir, 1967), certain fathers may resent their lack of involvement in the treatment of their wives and children, and certain fathers may use their lack of involvement to reinforce their passivity (Sander, 1959). Fathers also experience deep concern for their communicatively handicapped children (McDonald, 1962; Webster, 1968) and may have little chance to explore and clarify their concern. Another important disadvantage of having only the mother in counseling is that the counselor gets a one-sided view of the family's interactions.

Long-term counseling may be done either in two-person or multiperson situations. Further, Wilson, Ginott and Berger (1959) noted that grouping parents can be an effective way for clinicians to see them for an initial interview. The clinician can explain his program, obtain parents' initial responses to plans for their children, hear about some ways they perceive their child's problems, etc. While counseling principles are the same regardless of the number of individuals participating, group counseling has the advantage of providing parents with opportunities to learn from each other (Webster, 1968; Laubenthal, 1970).

Family Counseling

A special instance of group parent counseling is family counseling (Satir, 1967; Brodey, 1969). In this procedure mother and father are seen together. Depending on the age and status of the children in the family, they, too, may be included in the counseling group. Family counseling recognizes the premise stated by McDonald (1962):

> In a very real sense we are never faced with just a handicapped child but rather a handicapped family. To be maximally effective, a treatment program should regard the family as the patient and provide not just treatment for the child but also a program designed to help parents understand their feelings (p. 5).

Family counseling also is based on the premise that if a family is to gain or maintain its equilibrium, the parents must grow and develop together (Satir, 1967). For example, the family of a child with a communication disorder may identify its problem as having arisen from the child's disorder. It is often the case, however, that the child presents additional difficulties, rather than being the original cause of family problems (McDonald, 1962; Satir, 1967). Satir (1967) observed the frequently seen paradox that as the child improves, other family members seem to get worse; this indicates that the child is not the whole of the family problem. Family counseling seeks to help families develop together by means of each individual's recognition and clarification of issues which confront them.

A major advantage of this approach is that each family member involved is apprised of what the other verbalizes during the counseling sessions. Family members, past and present problems in communicating with each other can be aired openly and honestly with the counselor serving as catalyst, referee, and understanding listener. Procedures for family counseling have been detailed most readably by Satir (1967).

It is to be noted that multiperson counseling, and particularly family counseling, requires a great deal of openness, flexibility, and security on the part of the counselor. These requisites are necessary if the counselor is to respond to and support more than one client at a time, and if he is to cope with potentially threatening conflicts which may arise between group members (Satir, 1967; Webster, 1968).

Results of Parent Counseling

At this date clinicians must be humble about the changes they help to effect in any client through counseling. We do not yet have conclusive evidence about the outcomes of counseling in terms of clients' behavior changes (Rogers, 1951, 1961; Webster, 1966; Carkhuff, 1970). However, it is thought that understanding and support of clients in their clarification of attitudes, if not the whole of what they need, at least cannot be harmful to them (Rogers, 1951, 1961, 1967; Mowrer, 1964; Murphy and Fitzsimons, 1960; Webster, 1966).

Laubenthal's study (1970) supported clinical impressions that the experience of counseling had various positive meanings to mothers of children with communication disorders. In Laubenthal's group, mothers described counseling as helping them to (a) feel understood by other persons; (b) cope more confidently with their children's behavior; (c) communicate more effectively with their children; and (d) communicate more effectively with other adults. Although there is yet little description of ways parents implement these perceived changes in their parent-child interactions (Laubenthal, 1970; Carkhuff, 1970), it seems possible that parents' perceptions of greater confidence and comfort are worthwhile results of counseling.

Parent Training

Professional persons who attempt to assist parents use a variety of terms to describe their work; the term "training" is used by many to include various approaches to teaching parents to improve their children's communicative behavior.

Wyatt and her associates (1962) described a program in which, in addition to counseling, mothers of children with communication disorders were instructed to emulate clinical procedures for improving their children's communication. Each mother ultimately worked with her own child under the supervision of a trained clinician. Wyatt advocated that counseling should accompany the use of such procedures if they were to benefit both mothers and children. Her studies showed that both mothers and children changed their communicative behavior constructively under this program.

Other workers who have been concerned with training have focused on parent training rather than on more global benefits to parents and children. For example, Sommers and associates (1964) used personality tests to divide mothers of children with articulation disorders into a well adjusted and poorly adjusted group. They trained both groups of mothers to imitate clinicians' procedures for correcting articulation errors. These authors found these mothers could learn such drills quite easily; there was no significant difference in the effective use of such procedures by well-adjusted and poorly adjusted groups.

More recently, Cazden (1966) reviewed studies of mothers' verbal behavior with their children. In the populations studied mothers tended to converse with their children by means of two classifiable processes: expansions, i.e. repeating the child's verbalization, lengthening it, supplying missing elements, but keeping the meaning of the utterance intact; and expatiation, i.e. elaborating on both the utterance and its meaning. Expatiations were thought to be the most productive of those two language intervention techniques. The extension of these ideas is that mothers who do not use these techniques easily can be taught to do so in order to improve the child's communicative behavior.

Carkhuff and associates (1970) use the term "training" to describe their preferred treatment for parents of emotionally disturbed children. In one of a series of procedural studies (Carkhuff and Bierman, 1970), both parents of twenty-one emotionally disturbed children were divided into the following treatment groups: Group one: ten parents (five couples) met in a group for twenty-five hours of systematic training in the developing of interpersonal skills, with emphasis on improving their communication; Groups Two, Three, Four: twenty-four parents (12 couples) were equally divided into three groups for twenty-five hours of more traditional parent counseling from counselors assessed as high, moderate, and low in their therapeutic functioning; Group 5: eight parents (four couples) served as a time-control group. Each parent responded to several measures prior to and following the treatment period. Included in testing were stimuli designed to measure parental functioning in several affect areas, assessment of functioning in the role of helper to the spouse, and a personality change index which was constructed by using those items on the Minnesota Multiphasic Personality Inventory on which the examinee could change constructively. In addition, both parents conducted a play session with their child.

Results of this study showed that ". . . in a relatively brief period systematic group training can effect changes in interpersonal skills that traditional counseling groups cannot" (p. 161). It was noted that parents in the therapy group led by the counselor at the highest level of functioning also functioned at the highest level of all the therapy groups studied; however, the level of functioning of the most improved therapy group was not as high as that of the training group.

Parents in Group One (training) showed statistically significant constructive change or gain in level of communication and discrimination in general; there was also a significant constructive gain in communication between parents. However, while parents perceived themselves as communicating at a higher level with their children, there was little evidence that they did in fact communicate at a higher level in the experimental play situation. In discussing this finding, Carkhuff and Bierman made the point that people learn best what they practice most, and "if we wish to effect changes in play situations, methodologies ought to be advised where parents are trained specifically and progressively to understand and work with their children in these situations" (p. 161).

Following similar thinking Risley and his associates (Risley and Wolf, 1967; Risley and Hart, 1968; Reynolds and Risley, 1968; Risley, Reynolds, and Hart, 1970) have not only used a number of behavior modification procedures to alleviate various language and speech deficits in children, but have also taught mothers to be teachers (Reynolds and Risley, 1968).

In one series of studies, Risley, Reynolds, and Hart (1970) introduced and assessed various behavior modification procedures to train mothers of disadvantaged preschool children to use social reinforcement (praise) to shape their children's behavior. The object was to provide mothers with positive reinforcement for successful performance in the use of praise to reinforce their children's appropriate behaviors. Before training, the investigators found mothers in this population to be poor teachers, particularly with their own children; they tended to nag and threaten rather than to use positive reinforcement.

Among the interesting findings of these studies, the following seem particularly noteworthy. Positive reinforcement for the mother effected higher praise rates with her child. When mothers began the training program by working with their own children in a lesson situation, their rates of praise increased under several conditions of reinforcement; however such praise rates were still thought inadequate at the end of a year. Mothers' nagging of their children persisted in other less structured situations, such as play. When the training condition was changed so that each mother worked with children other than her own until she attained an adequate praise rate prior to beginning work with her own child, mothers were found to achieve higher praise rates. Under the latter condition mothers also generalized their behavior to less structured situations, e.g. they praised their children more and nagged them less during play. Another increment of training seemed to be that many mothers expanded their interests, e.g. devoting time to the preschool, doing other volunteer work, taking jobs, etc. It is also interesting to note that a parent cooperative preschool was thought to be a more efficient training site than the mother's own home.

The implications of the studies cited in this section should stir the thinking of clinicians who train parents of the communicatively handicapped.

IMPLICATIONS FOR FURTHER RESEARCH

Those who work with parents hold various, and sometimes conflicting, theories about parental roles in child rearing and about clinicians' functions with them. For example, Axline (1947, 1964) asserted that it is not necessary to involve parents in their child's treatment, while Russell and Halfond (1965) noted the prevalence among speech clinicians of the notion that all parents of the communicatively handicapped need counseling or training. Such assertions, formulations outlined previously in this chapter, and studies cited herein raise crucial questions for further study.

We need to know more about the personalities, attitudes, and behaviors of parents of children with communication disorders. There are many problems inherent in such studies (Schaefer, 1962).

Future studies need to be carefully controlled so that meaningful comparisons can be made between parents of children with communication disorders and parents whose children develop adequate communication (Bayley and Schaefer, 1960 a). We have learned that socioeconomic variables are important in determining child rearing practices (Bayley and Schaefer, 1960 b; Risley,

Reynolds, and Hart, 1970) ; early studies in speech pathology did not adequately control for socioeconomic status.

As noted previously, mothers rather than both parents typically have served as research subjects; this pattern appears too in work done in fields other than speech pathology (Schaefer and Bell, 1958). It is thought that meaningful descriptions of the child's milieu will emerge as both parents are studied with respect to their personalities, attitudes, behaviors, and interactions. There is need for longitudinal as well as cross-sectional descriptive data from which to assess variables common to parents whose children develop communication disorders.

There seems to be a paramount source of difficulty in assessing speech pathologists' findings about parents. Part of the work of this field is to diagnose pathology, and many of the studies seem to have evolved from the concept of diagnosis of parental pathologies. That is, many studies seem to have been based on a model of parental illness, or at least deviance from normalcy, rather than on a model of normalcy. For example, the tendency toward covert rejection was found in mothers of stuttering children (Kinstler, 1961). This may be a very reliable finding. The point is that findings were determined by a scale designed to measure only the variable of rejection. Such parental traits do not occur in isolation from other traits; we do not know what other variables might have vitiated the variable of rejection in parent-child relationships.

We need to recognize that most of the parents we see are functioning adequately in many areas; their adequate functioning can also be measured and taken into account (Roth 1961; Gerth, 1969). The larger context of a texture of strength and weakness in every parent should serve as a more valid background against which to judge specific problem areas.

Again, some studies (Berlin, 1960) have used parents of children with one type of disorder as a control group in comparing groups of parents of children with other types of disorders. These findings also may be quite reliable. The continued use of such controls seems risky, however, if we are to compare parents of the communicatively disordered with parents of normally speaking children.

Besides the need for further description of our population, we need much more research regarding clinicians' functions with parents. We have been concerned about the procedures for parent counseling or training (Weinstein, 1968). We have also been concerned about the results of work with parents in terms of behavior change (Carkhuff, 1970). We also must raise and study questions about the meanings to these people of our work with them. We seem to have only begun to do this. Laubenthal's study (1970) described mothers' verbalized expressions of positive and negative perceptions of their counseling experience. Marshall and her associates (1970) are developing a questionnaire to help them assess the types of assistance parents of mentally retarded children say they need and benefit from. Such a questionnaire also seems beneficial in that it reveals parents' understanding of suggestions made by clinicians. Risley *et al.* (1970) thought mothers in their population developed into more productive people living fuller lives following their experience of positive reinforcement training; it would be of interest to describe further such changes in these people.

Just as clinicians' work settings vary, so also may their parent populations vary. Gerth (1969) questioned possible relationships between the personalities and attitudes of parents who seek help for their children and the type of help they seek.

We also don't yet know a great deal about how children with communication disorders view their mothers, their fathers, and their family constellation. We might well question children's responses to parents, including the extent to which they perceive their parents as changing through treatment, and the direction of this change.

We are faced with the situation of having a Pandora's Box of questions for research. We have made only a beginning in our understanding of parents, particularly those whose children have disordered communication. It follows that we have made only a beginning in being able to work creatively and productively with these people. We must respect these beginnings. At the same time we must actively seek to expand our conceptual models and to behave in keeping with our bits of enlightenment.

REFERENCES

Axline, V.: *Play Therapy*. Boston, Houghton-Mifflin, 1947, Chap. 6.

Axline, V., and Dibs: *In Speech of Self*. Boston, Houghton-Mifflin, 1964.

Backus, O.: Group structure in speech therapy. In Travis, L. (Ed.) : *Handbook of Speech Pathology*. New York, Appleton, 1957, Chap. 33.

Bayley, N., and Schaefer, E.S.: Maternal behavior and personality development data from the berkeley growth study. *Psychiatr Res Rep, 13:* 1960 (a).

Bayley, N., and Schaefer, E.S.: Relationships between socioeconomic variables and the behavior of mothers toward young children. *J Genet Psychol, 96:*61-77, 1960(b).

Beasley, J.: Relationship of parental attitudes to development of speech problems. *J Speech Hearing Dis, 21:*317-321, 1956.

Becky, R.E.: A study of certain factors related to retardation of speech. *J Speech Dis, 7:*223-249, 1942.

Berlin, C.I.: Parents diagnoses of stuttering. *J Speech Hearing Res, 3* (4) : 372-379, 1960.

Bice, H.V.: *Group Counseling with Mothers of the Cerebral Palsied*. Chicago, Nat Soc Crippled Children and Adults, 1952.

Bloodstein, O.; Jaeger, W., and Tureen, J.: A study of the diagnosis of stuttering by parents of stutterers and parents of nonstutterers. *J Speech Dis, 3:*308-315, 1952.

Brodbeck, A.J., and Irwin, O.C.: The speech behavior of infants without families. *Child Develop, 17* (3) :145-156, 1946.

Brodey, Warren M.: *Changing the Family*. New York, Clarkson N. Potter, 1968.

Carkhuff, R.F., and Bierman, R.: Training as a preferred mode of treatment of parents of emotionally disturbed children. *J Counsel Psychol, 17* (2) :157-161, 1970.

Cazden, C.: Some implications of research on language development for preschool education. Report to Social Science Research Council Conference on Preschool Education, 1966.

Dees, J.: *Psycholinguistics*. Boston, Allyn and Bacon, 1970, Chap. 1.

Denhoff, E., and Robinault, I.P.: *Cerebral Palsy and Related Disorders*. New York, McGraw-Hill, 1960, Chap. 7, 10.

Despert, J.L.: A psychosomatic study of fifty stuttering children. *Amer J Orthopsychiat, 16:*100-116, 1945.

Deutsch, M. *et al.: The Disadvantaged Child*. New York, Basic Books, 1967, Chap. 1, 2, 9, 16.

Eaton, M.J.: An investigation of selected personality dimensions of mothers whose children have severe communication problems. Unpublished doctoral dissertation, University of Alabama, 1967.

Filippi, R., and Rousey, C.L.: Delay in onset of talking. *J Amer Acad Child Psychiat, 7* (2) :1968.

Flanagan, J.C.: The critical incident technique. *Psychol Bull, 51*:327-358, 1954.

Gerth, Marilyn N.: Two indices of personality variables in parents of children with communication disorders. Unpublished master's thesis, University of Alabama, 1969.

Giolas, T.C.; Webster, E.J., and Ward, L.M.: A diagnostic-therapy setting for handicapped children. *J Speech Hearing Dis, 33* (4) :345-350, 1968.

Goldfarb, W.: Effects of psychological deprivation in infancy and subsequent stimulation. *Amer J Psychiat, 102*:18-33, 1945.

Goldman, R.: A study of goal-setting behavior of aprents of stutterers and parents of non-stutterers. *J Speech Hearing Dis, 29*:192-194, 1964(a) .

Goldman, R., and Shames, G.H.: Comparisons of the goals that parents of stutterers and parents of non-stutterers set for their children. *J Speech Hearing Dis, 29*:381-389, 1964(b) .

Goldstein, L., and Dahlstrom, W.: MMPI differences between parents of stuttering and nonstuttering children. *J Consult Psychol, 20*:365-370, 1956.

Johnson, W.: *People in Quandaries.* New York, Harper Bros., 1946.

Johnson, W.: Perceptual factors in stuttering. In Travis, L. (Ed.) : *Handbook of Speech Pathology.* New York, Appleton-Century-Crofts, 897-915, 1957.

Kanner, L.: *Child Psychiatry,* (2nd ed.) Springfield, Thomas, 1950, p. 181.

Kinstler, D.B.: Covert and overt maternal rejection in stuttering. *J Speech Hearing Dis, 26* (2) :145-155, 1961.

Laubenthal, S.: A descriptive study of mothers' attitudes toward their communicatively handicapped children and toward their parent counseling experience. Unpublished masters' thesis, University of Alabama, 1970.

Lenneberg, E.H.: The natural history of language. In Smith, F., and Miller, G. A. (Eds.) : *The Genesis of Language.* Cambridge, M.I.T. Press, 1966.

Lewis, M.M.: *Infant Speech: A Study of the Beginnings of Language.* New York, The Humanities Press, 1951.

McCarthy, D.: Organismic Interpretation of infant vocalizations. *Child Develop, 23*:273-280, 1952.

McCarthy, D.: Some possible explanations of sex differences in language development and disorders. *J Psychol, 35*:155-160, 1953.

McCarthy, D.: Language development in children. In Carmichael, L. (Ed.) : *Manual of Child Psychology.* New York, Wiley, 1954.

McCarthy, D.: Language disorders and parent-child relationships. *J Speech Hearing Dis, 19*:514-543, 1954.

McDonald, E.T.: *Understand Those Feelings.* Pittsburgh, Stanwix House, 1962.

McNeill, D.: Developmental psycholinguistics. In Smith, F. and Miller, G. A. (Eds.) : *The Genesis of Language.* Cambridge, M.I.T. Press, 1966.

MacLennan, B.W., and Felsenfeld, N.: *Group Counseling and Psychotherapy with Adolescents.* New York, Columbia U Press, 1968.

Marshall, N.R.: Unpublished questionnaire for parents of retarded children. University of Oregon Medical School, Portland, 1970.

Matis, E.: Psychotherapeutic tools for parents. *J Speech Hearing Dis, 26:* 164-170, 1961.

Moll, K.L., and Darley, F.L.: Attitudes of mothers of articulatory-impaired and speech retarded children. *J Speech Hearing Dis, 25* (4) :377-384, 1960.

Moncur, J.P.: Environmental factors differentiating stuttering children from non-stuttering children. *Speech Monogr, 18:*312-325, 1951.

Moncur, J.P.: Parental domination in stuttering. *J Speech Hearing Dis, 17:*155-165, 1952.

Mowrer, O.H.: *Learning Theory and Personality Dynamics.* New York, Ronald, 1950.

Mowrer, O.H.: *The New Group Therapy.* Princeton, N.J., D. Van Nostrand, 1964.

Murphy, A.T., and Fitzsimons, R.M.: *Stuttering and Personality Dynamics.* New York, Ronald, 1960, Chap. 12.

Murphy, A.T., and Fitzsimons, R.M.: Love may be enough: The passionate investments of clinicians. *Seminars Psychiat, 1* (3) :262-269, 1969.

Myers, B.: *The Myers-Briggs Type Indicator.* Princeton, Educational Testing Service, 1962.

Peckarsky, A.K.: Maternal attitudes toward children with psychogenically delayed speech. Unpublished doctoral dissertation, New York University, 1953.

Reynolds, N. J., and Risley, T.R.: The role of social and material reinforcers in increasing talking of a disadvantaged preschool child. *J Appl Behav Anal, 1* (3) :253-262, 1968.

Risley, T.R., and Wolf, M.M.: Establishing functional speech in echolalic children. *Behav Res Ther, 5:*73-88, 1967.

Risley, T.R., and Hart, B.M.: Developing correspondence between the non-verbal and verbal behavior of preschool children. *J Appl Behav Anal, 1:* 267-281, 1968.

Risley, T.R.; Reynolds, N., and Hart, B.: Behavior modification with disadvantaged preschool children. In Bradfield, R. (Ed.) : *Behavior Modification: The Human Effort.* San Rafael, California, Dimensions Press, in process, 1970.

Rittenour, M.: Counseling with parents of children with abnormal speech and language development. *J Med Ass Alabama, 34:*62-65, 1964.

Rogers, C.R.: *Client-Centered Therapy.* Boston, Houghton-Mifflin, 1951.

Rogers, C.R.: *On Becoming a Person.* Boston, Houghton-Mifflin, 1961.

Rogers, C.R., and Stevens, B.: *Person to Person: the Problem of Being Human*. Layfette, Calif., Real People Press, 1967.

Roth, R.M.: *The Mother-Child Relationship Evaluation*. Beverly Hills, Western Psychological Services, 1961.

Russell, L.H., and Halfond, M.M.: Crucial issues in parent counseling. Adapted from a paper presented at ASHA Convention, 1965.

Sander, E.K.: Counseling parents of stuttering children. *J Speech Hearing Dis, 24* (3) :262-271, 1959.

Satir, V.: *Conjoint Family Therapy*. Palo Alto, Science and Behavior Books, 1967.

Schaefer, E.S.: Social science contributions to the measurement of parent behavior. In *Quantitative Approaches to Parent Selection*. New York, Child Welfare League of America, 1962.

Schaefer, E.S., and Bell, R.Q.: Development of a parental attitude research instrument. *Child Develop, 29* (3) :339-361, 1958.

Sommers, R.K.; Furlong, A.K.; Rhodes, R.E.; Fichter, G.R.; Bowser, D.C.; Copetas, F.G.; Saunders, Z.G., *et al.:* Effects of maternal attitudes upon improvement in articulation when mothers are trained to assist in speech correction. *J Speech Hearing Dis, 29* (2) :126-132, 1964.

Ward, L.M., and Webster, E.J.: The training of clinical personnel: II. A concept of clinical preparation. *ASHA 7* (4) :103-106, 1965.

Ward, L.M.: Process of therapy for Communicative Disorders. In Weston, A. (Ed.) : *Communicative Disorders: An Introduction*. Springfield, Thomas, 1971.

Webster, E.J.: Parent counseling by speech pathologists and audiologists. *J Speech Hearing Dis, 31:*331-340, 1966.

Webster, E.J.: Procedures for group parent counseling in speech pathology and audiology. *J Speech Hearing Dis, 33:*127-131, 1968.

Weinstein, B.: The parent counseling conference: A programmed learning experience. *Rehab Lit, 29* (8) , 1968.

Wilson, D.K.; Ginott, H.G., and Berger, S.L.: Group Interview: Initial parental clinic contact. *J Speech Hearing Dis, 24* (3) :282-284, 1959.

Wood, K.S.: Parental maladjustment and functional articulatory defects in children. *J Speech Dis, 11:*255-275, 1946.

Wolpe, Zelda: Play therapy, psychodrama, and parent counseling. In Travis, L. (Ed.) : *Handbook of Speech Pathology*. New York, Appleton, 1957, Chap. 32.

Wyatt, Gertrud L.: Treatment of stuttering children and their parents; report of the Wellesley research project. Presented at the ASHA convention, 1962.

CHAPTER FOURTEEN

SPEECH PATHOLOGY AND SPECIAL EDUCATION

WILSON L. DIETRICH

IN RECENT years, greater attention has been given to those children in our society who, for some reason, differ from the average. Historically, some attention was paid to that type of child but usually out of curiosity, fear or superstition. The word "exceptional" has managed to be attached to the child who is different. This word has caused confusion in many people's minds as they tended to correlate it only with superior achievement. Kirk (1962) defines the exceptional child as "that child who deviates from the average or normal child in mental, physical, or social characteristics to such an extent that he requires a modification of school practices, or special educational services, in order to develop to his maximum capacity." While many professionals continue to struggle with new definitions, Kirk's continues to stand alone in both its simplicity and comprehensiveness.

Exceptional children have been known from earliest recorded time. The earliest reported efforts to educate the exceptional children involved those who were deaf or blind. In 1760, the first public school for deaf children was founded in Paris by Charles Michel, Abee de l'Epee (Obermann, 1965). In the United States, residential settings were the beginnings for special education for exceptional children. Special classes were begun in the early 1900's. This correlated closely with the mental testing movement begun at approximately the same time. While the notion of individual differences was not begun at this time, the interest of psychologists in developing instruments to measure differences gained wide attention. Most significant was the development of the Binet-Simon Scale to measure intelligence in 1905 (Anastasia, 1964). This test was revised and most famous was the revision by

L. M. Terman at Stanford University, now known as the Stanford-Binet (Anastasia, 1964). This test originated the use of the Intelligence Quotient (IQ) or the ratio between mental age and chronological age for the first time (Anastasia, 1964). When an instrument was available to more closely determine the extent of a child's problem, attention was then given to classifying or categorizing the child.

EXCEPTIONALITIES

The Mentally Retarded

The definition of mental retardation has been the subject of more controversy and change than any other area of special education. Various terms have been used through the years to describe this problem such as mental deficiency, idiot, imbecile, moron, amentia (used in England), mental subnormals, and feebleminded, to include just a few. Typically, those individuals were placed in "asylums." The most widely accepted definition of mental retardation at this time is that of the American Association on Mental Deficiency which states "mental retardation refers to subaverage general intellectual functioning which originates during the developmental period and is associated with impairment in adaptive behavior" (Heber, 1961). Educators have classified the mentally retarded into three categories. They are:

Educable Mentally Retarded

This child will usually be in the IQ range of 50 to 80 depending on individual state laws. They generally are recognized as children who may become independent citizens able to carry on a vocational task. A significant number of these children will be found in lower socioeconomic groups which may indicate that early intervention and specific training techniques could help to alleviate the problem. The majority of the mentally retarded are in this category.

Trainable Mentally Retarded

The trainable child will usually be functioning in the IQ range of 25 to 50. This child will eventually function in sheltered workshops under supervision and rarely becomes an independent citizen. The trainable child usually shows some visible stigmata with a high incidence of brain damage. Educational techniques center around developing self-help skills, language development and social adjustment. Emphasis is placed on practical skills. No societal boundaries are placed on this problem.

Custodial Mentally Retarded

The custodial child will be in the IQ range of 0 to 25. They are typically found in institutions or in their homes. They are totally dependent and some never gain the ability to speak. Many rare syndromes are found in this category.

The Auditorally Handicapped

Special classes are available for children who suffer from a hearing loss. Estimates on the numbers of children who suffer such a loss vary but it is safe to estimate about 5 per cent of the school population could benefit from special education (Kirk, 1962). The auditorally handicapped are divided into two categories:

The Deaf

These children essentially suffer such a loss that their hearing is nonfunctional for life purposes. They may either have been born deaf or hearing may have been lost through an illness or accident. Sensory training is utilized in an effort to enable the child to communicate and be educated.

The Hard of Hearing

Hearing itself may be functional with or without amplification. The loss may vary from a mild to severe loss and educational techniques are modified to accommodate the child. Many of these children can be accommodated in regular class with the services of a trained resource special education teacher assisting the regular education teacher. Early identification is critical for planning of the educational future of the child.

The Visually Impaired

The visually impaired are divided into two areas based on the extent of the loss of vision.

The Blind

The blind are defined as those individuals with less than 20/200 usable vision in the best eye after correction. Few school children are in this category and the majority attend institutions for the blind.

The Partially Sighted

The partially sighted have tested vision within the range of 20/70-20/200 in the best eye after correction. There are many children in this category and with proper training and instruction they can adapt to the seeing world. The resource room is utilized with the child attending regular class part of the day and receiving special attention the remainder of the day.

The Physically Handicapped

The area of the physically handicapped covers a wide spectrum of disabilities. Cerebral palsy represents the largest group served by the public schools. Some other common disabilities found in special classes for the physically handicapped are heart defects, spina bifida, congenital deformities, accident victims, muscular dystrophy, health conditions, such as tuberculosis, and the multiply handicapped who are identified as having two or more handicaps. Because of the Salk and Sabin vaccines, poliomyelitis has practically been eliminated but there are still post-polio individuals who require special educational techniques for proper training.

The Emotionally Disturbed

Children experiencing emotional problems vary from behavior problems in the classroom or at home to the seriously involved child in need of intensive therapeutic intervention in an institution or clinic. Special education primarily deals with those children with mild problems as compared with schizophrenic forms of behavior. Classification of emotional problems is a difficult one and should involve a highly trained team of professionals.

Learning Disabilities

A "new" category of exceptionality has attracted great attention in recent years. There has been controversy over defining this problem. Basically, the child experiencing a learning disability has the potential to learn but, because of some intervention such as a neurological defect, is restrained from acceptable progress. This indicates the need to alter the process of teaching and requires special techniques by a trained special educator. These children generally have average to high intelligence. Further research is indicated in order to best meet the needs of the learning disabled (Johnson and Myklebust, 1967).

The above represent a rather brief overview of the field of special education. Speech problems as related to special education will receive attention later in this chapter.

PUBLIC SCHOOLS

In recent years, the public schools have become the focal point for serving the needs of the handicapped. The school officials of this country have begun to live out the philosophy of "education for all," partly out of a recognition of the need and partly from concerted efforts of organized parent and professional groups. Special laws have been passed in most states to provide for exceptional children. Local districts have voted bond issues to implement the need. Training institutions of higher education have begun or increased programs preparing teachers of the handicapped. Major impetus in training of special education teachers came about through the passage by the Federal Government of Public Law 85-926 as amended by Section 301 of Public Law 88-164. This action created funds for the training of prospective teachers of the handicapped. Probably no other single action of the Federal Government has meant as much to the field of Special Education as PL 85-926 as amended.

One important issue that is raised in the involvement of public schools in the education of the handicapped is that those children should be maintained in close proximity to the general mainstream of public education. In the past, isolation for the handicapped was the rule and the chances for an exceptional child of either entering the mainstream or approaching his full capacity were virtually nil. It has become apparent to the public and general educators that the majority of the handicapped are more like normal children than they are unlike normal children.

INSTITUTIONS

The placing of handicapped children in institutions has historical roots. Recorded history shows that institutions for the blind and deaf were begun in the 1700's. Care of individuals was the primary objective of early institutions and it is only in modern times that we have witnessed the emphasis shifting to the training of individuals in the hope that they may leave the institution and return to their communities. While there are institutions today that retain some of the older characteristics, there does appear to be an effort to update living quarters, training programs and the quality of personnel. The lack of funds appropriated for public institutions is a serious problem. Antiquated institutions will remain as long as the citizens of communities and states continue to ignore this need.

VOCATIONAL PLACEMENT

The major goal of Special Education is for vocational placement of students who have been classified as handicapped. This should be recognized from the time of identification throughout the curriculum. Emphasis should be placed on practical training. A close working relationship should be maintained between special education, vocational education and vocational rehabilitation. With such a team approach, realistic goals can be established for individual children. Challenging, but not frustrating, opportunities should be made available.

THE ROLE OF SPEECH PATHOLOGY

Probably no other two disciplines share as much in common as do speech pathology and special education. Much of their training overlaps. The pattern of organization of training varies with some universities combining the two areas into one program, others operate separately within the same college, while still others are physically located in separate colleges within the same university. As long as communication remains open and opportunities to exchange students exists, this is not a serious problem. Speech pathology programs should enable prospective special education teachers to participate in coursework that encompasses not only deviant speech behavior but normal patterns of language acquisition. This should also include psychological and social factors that influence communication disorders.

A major concern for speech clinicians should be in developing techniques for the implementation of therapy programs that can be carried out by the special education teacher. This cooperative venture should enable the child to receive optimal training as opposed to a once or twice a week exposure to the therapist. Careful planning by the two professionals involved should be the initial step. It should be the responsibility of the speech clinician to not only indicate sounds that should be emphasized but the rationale of identification, diagnosis and treatment of the disorder. As much information regarding individual children as possible should be collected. Medical histories, past school performances, home visitations, and the sharing of each other's impressions of the child should be included. Such an approach for a mutual endeavor in assisting the speech impaired child will only be successful if appreciation for each other's professional training is recognized.

The goal of the special educator for the individual child should closely involve the work of the speech clinician. If the two work in isolation from each other maximum efficiency of their talents will not be achieved. Utilizing the prescriptive teaching approach can unite the two disciplines. After the speech clinician has arrived at a differential diagnosis of the speech impairment, the teacher and the speech clinician should meet together and decide on how best to meet the needs of the child. A developmental program should be constructed incorporating the curriculum goals of the teacher and the remediation of speech problems by the speech clinician. It is important that the child remain as the focal point of attention and not just the problem that the child may be manifesting at a point in time. Occasionally professional people become so concerned with a child's problem that involves their training specialty that they overlook the fact of a child being a complex individual with many sides and interest areas.

Repeated conferences by the special educator and speech clinician are essential through the school year. For one or the other not to be willing to share their experiences or a successful technique with the child is a mistake. Each must consider themselves as a resource person to the other. Obviously, all of the above indicates the need for desire to work together. It has been proven that merely placing professional people from different disciplines together will not guarantee the "team approach." A mutual respect for the competencies that each brings to a situation is the most expedient way to develop a team approach to a child's problem. To act in competition defeats the purpose of combining disciplines. Because of the one to one situation in much of speech therapy, the speech clinician may develop a closer relationship with the child than the special education teacher can attain. Rather than reacting out of jealousy, the teacher can utilize this relationship to gain insight about the child as he functions in the general classroom environment. Likewise, the speech clinician may gain greater understanding of the child and his problems through discussion with the teacher about the child's general attitude and progress through the typical school week.

Responsibility for the success of such a mutual program rests heavily on both professionals. It is the author's opinion that it is the only way to assist children with problems. No longer should one discipline operate in isolation with the naive impression that they can meet all of a child's needs. We must work together and continue to explore new avenues to help insure the best possible life for all children.

It has fallen the lot of the special education teacher and the speech clinician to be considered "different" from the regular school faculty. Physical education instructors, music and art specialists, remedial reading teachers and school counselors are more easily accepted into the school community. Perhaps this is because of the functioning level of exceptional students. Regardless of the reason, special educators and speech clinicians must make a concerted effort to become an integral part of the school.

Various means are available to accomplish this and some suggestions are the following: (a) to attend all faculty meetings; (b) to involve regular classes in programs performed by special classes; (c) to offer to discuss in faculty meetings the exceptional child and the curriculum and educational goals for the special students; (d) to offer to "trade off" with other teachers so that they will have an opportunity to experience teaching or speech therapy with exceptional children; and (e) to be tolerant of criticism because of the limited number of students in special classes as opposed to the large pupil-teacher ratio often found in regular classes.

Special education and speech pathology represent two of the many professional disciplines working together to assist exceptional children in leading a worthwhile life to the maximum of their abilities. Speech pathology will always have an important contribution to make in the lives of children because the ability to communicate is a necessity for individuals to exist happily in an ever-changing world.

REFERENCES

Anastasia, Anne: *Psychological Testing.* New York, Macmillan, 1964.

Heber, R.F.: A manual on terminology and classification in mental retardation. *AJMD,* 1959, 64, Monogr. Suppl. (Rev. ed.), 1961.

Johnson, Doris J., and Myklebust, Helmer R.: *Learning Disabilities.* New York, Grune & Stratton, 1967.

Kirk, Samuel A.: *Educating Exceptional Children.* Boston, Houghton Mifflin, 1962.

Obermann, C. Esco: *A History of Vocational Rehabilitation in America.* Minneapolis, Denison, 1965.

NAME INDEX

Adler, S., 303, 304, *328*
Agranowitz, A., 251, *259*
Anastasia, A., 395, 396, *403*
Andrews, G., 211, *217*
Ansberry, M., 182, 191, *198*
Arnold, G. E., 101, 109, 110, 114, 116, 117, *124*
Aronson, A. E., 117, *124*
Aronson, M., 253, *259*
Ash, J., 110, *124*
Auer, J. J., 12, *13*, 78, *98*
Axline, V., 388, *391*

Bach, E., 96, *98*
Backus, O., 192, *196*, 360, *363*, 381, *391*
Bankson, N., 176, *196*
Barbara, D. A., 105, *124*, 192, *196*
Barnlund, C., 352, 355, 356, *363*
Bay, E., 252, *259*
Bayley, N., 388, *391*
Baynes, R. A., 106, *124*
Beasley, J., 192, *196*, 366, 373, 378, *391*
Beavin, J., 75, *100*
Beckey, R. E., 365, *391*
Bekesy, G. von, 65, 70, 72
Bell, A. G., 60
Bell, R. Q., 389, *394*
Bellugi, V., 80, 83, 88, 91, 95, *98*
Benton, A., 233, *259*
Berger, S. L., 383, *394*
Berlin, C. I., 372, 389, *391*
Bernstein, A., 356, *363*
Berry, M., 102, *104*, 251, *259*
Berry, M. F., 211, *217*, 304, 324, *328*
Bice, H. V., 365, 382, 383, *391*
Bierman, R., 386, 387, *391*
Birdwhistell, R. L., 8, *13*
Bloch, P., 117, *124*
Bloodstein, O., 200, 203, 210, 211, 213, 217, 365, *391*

Bloom, I., 253, *259*
Bloomer, H., 176, *196*
Bluemel, C. S., 200, 217
Bock, D., 225, 226, *261*
Boone, E., 245, *259*
Bordeaux, J., 251, *260*
Bosma, J. F., 175, *196*
Bouillaud, 233, 234
Bragg, V. C., 102, *125*
Brain, R., 227, 232, *259*
Braine, M., 82, 91, *98, 99*
Broca, P., 234
Brodbeck, A. J., 367, *391*
Brodnitz, F. S., 101, 107, 111, 113, 114, *124*
Brody, W. M., 375, 383, *391*
Brooks, K., 3, *13*
Brown, R., 80, 83, 88, 91, 95, *98*
Brutton, E. J., 215, *217*
Bryngelson, B., 203, *217*
Buck, McK., 221, 245, 250, *259*
Butler, K. G., 214, *219*
Butler, R., 221, *261*
Byrne, M. C., 176, *196*

Campbell, E. J. M., *72*
Carhart, R., 277, *296*, 323, *328*
Carkhuff, R. F., 384, 385, 386, 387, 390, *391*
Carney, P. J., 134, 157, *159*
Carr, A., 182, 191, *198*
Cazden, C., 81, *98*, 386, *391*
Chalfant, J. C., *328*
Chall, J., 316, *328*
Chapman, M., 199, *218*
Charlton, M. H., 254, *260*
Chase, 157
Cherry, C., *363*
Chew, W., 106, *124*
Chomsky, N., 95, *98*, 165, 171, *196*

Note: Numbers appearing in italics apply to reference entries.

405

SUBJECT INDEX

A

Adenoids, 146, 147
Adolescents, male and pitch, 108
Aerodynamic-myoelastic theory, 40
Agnosia, 225, 226
American Association on Mental Deficiency, 396
Analphabetia partialis and therapy, 324-328
Animals, speech, 30, 31
Apasia, adult, 220-261
Aphonia, hysterical, 116, 117, 118
Apraxia, 227
Articulation, 31, 32, 49-58, 161-198
    acquisition and behavior, 161
    deficits, 180, 181
    errors
        classification, 181, 182
        cleft palate, 131-135
    evaluation, 182, 183
    intervention and behavioral model, 194, 195
    mechanism and paralysis, 49, 50
    patterns and cleft palate, 134-138
    structures, 50, 51
    testing and cleft palate, 138-140
Arytenoids, 40, 41
Asai operation, 123
Attention and auditory perceptual disturbances, 300, 301
Audiograms, 277-281
Audiometry
    puretone, 276-282
    speech, 282-284
Auditory disorders, 262-296
Auditory perceptual disturbances, 297-330

B

Base and generative grammar, 96
Behavioral and personality alterations and brain damage, 239, 240
Behavioral theory and articulation, 194, 195
Bernoulli effect, 44, 45
Bernreuter Personality Inventory, 368
Binet-Simon Scale, 395
Binits, 7
Biological bases for language development, 353
Birth defects and cleft palate, 128-130
Bone conduction of sound, 69
Brain damage and aphasia, 237-240
Brain dysfunctions, minimal
    characteristics and auditory perceptual disturbances, 305-308
Breathiness, 106, 107
Breathing
    speech, 37
    ventilation, 35-37
Broca's area, 234, 235
Broca's aphasia, 234, 235

C

California Test of Personality, 368
Carcinoma
    hoarseness, 106
    laryngeal, 115, 116
Castration, and falsetto register 109
Central nervous system dysfunction and aphasia, 225, 226
    auditory perception, 302-304
Cerebral hemispheric dominance and aphasia, 255-258
Cerebral lesions and aphasia, 223, 233, 234
Cerebral vascular accidents and aphasia, 237
Channel of transmission, 4
Children
    auditorally handicapped, 397

411